T0257742

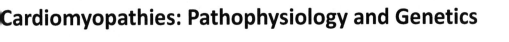

Cardiomyopathies: Pathophysiology and Genetics

Cardiomyopathies: Pathophysiology and Genetics

Edited by **Bernard Tyler**

New Jersey

Published by Foster Academics,
61 Van Reypen Street,
Jersey City, NJ 07306, USA
www.fosteracademics.com

Cardiomyopathies: Pathophysiology and Genetics
Edited by Bernard Tyler

International Standard Book Number: 978-1-63242-070-1 (Hardback)

Contents

Preface

In my initial years as a student, I used to run to the library at every possible instance to grab a book and learn something new. Books were my primary source of knowledge and I would not have come such a long way without all that I learnt from them. Thus, when I was approached to edit this book; I became understandably nostalgic. It was an absolute honor to be considered worthy of guiding the current generation as well as those to come. I put all my knowledge and hard work into making this book most beneficial for its readers.

Cardiomyopathies are related to the destructed heart muscle, impacting the functionality of the heart. This book is a compilation of an up to date analysis of the current information regarding cardiomyopathies. It presents the complete cardiovascular system as a functional unit, and the various contributors to this book analyze pathophysiological mechanisms from diverse viewpoints, including genetics, metabolic and drug-induced cardiomyopathies, imaging techniques and surgical procedure. This book will be helpful for readers interested in this field.

I wish to thank my publisher for supporting me at every step. I would also like to thank all the authors who have contributed their researches in this book. I hope this book will be a valuable contribution to the progress of the field.

Editor

Pathophysiology and Genetics of Cardiomyopathies

Heart Muscle and Apoptosis

Angelos Tsipis

1st Department of Pathology, Medical School, University of Athens
Greece

1. Introduction

Significant progress has been made in demonstrating the role of apoptosis in various heart diseases, and in elucidating the molecular mechanisms of cardiac apoptosis. Apoptosis has been attributed an essential role in cardiomyopathy. The progressive loss of cardiac myocytes is one of the most important pathogenic components of the heart failure. While initial studies reported unrealistically high levels of cell death, probably due to methodological problems, later work has consistently shown that approximately 80–250 heart muscle cells per 10^5 cardiac nuclei commit suicide at any given time in patients with late-stage dilated cardiomyopathy. In contrast, the base-line rate of apoptosis in healthy human hearts is only one to ten cardiac myocytes per 10^5 nuclei (Anversa & Kajstura, 1998; Yue et al., 1998). Even though the rate of apoptosis in heart failure is relatively low in absolute numbers, it is significantly higher than that in the normal heart, which has essentially negligible baseline apoptosis. Recently, animal models of heart failure incorporating transgenic technology have confirmed that myocyte apoptosis itself is sufficient to induce heart failure. Apoptosis has been implicated in a wide variety of physiological and pathological processes. The importance of apoptosis in cardiovascular system is also becoming increasingly clear, and the inhibition of apoptosis is emerging as a potential therapeutic tool for various forms of cardiovascular disease. In this chapter, we examine the evidence for apoptosis in cardiovascular disease and the molecular mechanisms of cardiac apoptosis.

2. Apoptosis

2.1 Concept and morphologic characteristics of apoptosis

There are two primary pathways by which cells die. The path for accidental cell death is called necrosis. Accidental cell death occurs when cells receive a structural or chemical insult from which they cannot recover. Examples of such insults include ischemia, extremes of temperature, and physical trauma. The hallmark of necrosis is that cells die because they are damaged. In contrast, cells that die by programmed cell death commit suicide actively as the results of activation of a dedicated intracellular program. For programmed cell death, the most commonly described pathway is apoptosis. Apoptosis begins with a signal that can come from within the cell (e.g., detection of radiation-induced DNA breaks) or from without (e.g., a decrease in the level of an essential growth factor or hormone). This pro-apoptotic signal induces the cell to make a decision to commit suicide. Initially, cells that are committed to undergo programmed cell death are in a latent phase of apoptosis. The latent phase can be subdivided into two stages: a condemned stage, during which the cell is proceeding on a pathway toward death but can still be rescued if it is exposed to anti-apoptotic activities, and a committed stage, beyond which rescue is impossible. Ultimately, the cells enter the execution phase of apoptosis, in which they undergo the dramatic morphologic and physiological changes (Pollard & Earnshaw, 2004). Apoptosis is characterized by a reproducible pattern of structural alterations of both the nucleus and cytoplasm. In order of appearance, these include: (1) Loss of microvilli and intercellular junctions. (2) Shrinkage of the cytoplasm. The cell is smaller in size. The cytoplasm is dense. The organelles, although relatively normal, are more tightly packed. (3) Dramatic changes in cytoplasmic motility with activation of a violent program of blebbing. (4) Loss of plasma membrane asymmetry, with the distribution of phosphatidyl serine being randomized so that it appears in the outer membrane leaflet. (5) Changes in the organization of the cell nucleus, typically involving the hypercondensation of the chromatin. This is the most characteristic feature of apoptosis. The chromatin aggregates peripherally, under the nuclear membrane, into dense masses of various shapes and sizes. The nucleus itself may break up, producing two or more fragments. (6) Formation of cytoplasmic blebs and apoptotic bodies. The apoptotic cell first shows extensive surface blebbing, then undergoes fragmentation into membrane-bound apoptotic bodies composed of cytoplasm and tightly packed organelles, with or without nuclear fragments. (7) Phagocytosis of apoptotic cells or cell bodies, usually by macrophages. The apoptotic bodies are rapidly degraded within lysosomes, and the adjacent healthy cells migrate or proliferate to replace the space occupied by the now deleted apoptotic cell. Because the vesicles remain membrane bound, the cellular contents are never released into the environment. As a result, apoptotic death does not lead to an inflammatory response. (Kumar et al., 2005; Pollard & Earnshaw, 2004).

2.2 Molecular mechanism and pathway description
The process of apoptosis may divided into an initiation phase, during which caspases become catalytically active, and an execution phase, during which these enzymes act to cause cell death. Initiation of apoptosis occurs principally by signals from two distinct but convergent pathways: the extrinsic, or receptor-initiated, pathway and the intrinsic or mitochondrial pathway. Both pathways converge to activate caspases and they may be interconnected at numerous steps.

2.2.1 The extrinsic (death receptors) pathway
This pathway is initiated by engagement of cell surface death receptors on a variety of cells. Death receptors are members of the tumor necrosis factor receptor family (Fas, TNFαR, DR3, DR4, DR5) that contain a cytoplasmic domain involved in protein-protein interactions that is called death domain because it is essential for delivering apoptotic signals.. Death receptor ligands characteristically initiate signaling via receptor oligomerization, which in turn results in the recruitment of specialized adaptor proteins and activation of caspase cascades. Binding of FasL induces Fas trimerization, which recruits initiator caspase-8 via the adaptor protein FADD. Caspase-8 then oligomerizes and is activated via autocatalysis. Activated caspase-8 stimulates apoptosis via two parallel cascades: it can directly cleave and activate caspase-3, or alternatively, it can cleave Bid, a pro-apoptotic Bcl-2 family protein. Truncated

Bid (tBid) translocates to mitochondria, inducing cytochrome c release, which sequentially activates caspase-9 and -3. TNF-α and DR-3L can deliver pro- or anti-apoptotic signals. TNFαR and DR3 promote apoptosis via the adaptor proteins TRADD/FADD and the activation of caspase-8. Interaction of TNF-α with TNFαR may activate the NF-κB pathway via NIK/IKK. The activation of NF-κB induces the expression of pro-survival genes including Bcl-2 and FLIP, the latter can directly inhibit the activation of caspase-8. Some viruses and normal cells produce FLIP, which binds to pro-caspase-8 but cannot cleave and activate the enzyme because it lacks enzymatic activity, and use this inhibitor to protect infected and normal cells from Fas-mediated apoptosis (Kumar et al., 2005). FasL and TNF-α may also activate JNK via ASK1/MKK7. Activation of JNK may lead to the inhibition of Bcl-2 by phosphorylation. In the absence of caspase activation, stimulation of death receptors can lead to the activation of an alternative programmed cell death pathway termed necroptosis by forming complex IIb. (Humphreys & Halpern, 2008; Logue & Martin, 2008; Yuan, 2010)

2.2.2 The intrinsic (mitochondrial) pathway

This pathway of apoptosis is the result of increased mitochondrial permeability and release of pro-apoptotic molecules into the cytoplasm, without a role for death receptors. Growth factors and other survival signals stimulate the production of anti-apoptotic members of the Bcl-2 family of proteins. The Bcl-2 family of proteins regulates apoptosis by controlling mitochondrial permeability. The anti-apoptotic proteins Bcl-2 and Bcl-xL reside in the outer mitochondrial wall and inhibit cytochrome c release. The proapoptotic Bcl-2 proteins Bad, Bid, Bax, and Bim may reside in the cytosol but translocate to mitochondria following death signaling, where they promote the release of cytochrome c. Bad translocates to mitochondria and forms a pro-apoptotic complex with Bcl-xL. This translocation is inhibited by survival factors that induce the phosphorylation of Bad, leading to its cytosolic sequestration. Cytosolic Bid is cleaved by caspase-8 following signaling through Fas; its active fragment (tBid) translocates to mitochondria. Bax and Bim translocate to mitochondria in response to death stimuli, including survival factor withdrawal. Activated following DNA damage, p53 induces the transcription of Bax, Noxa, and PUMA. Upon release from mitochondria, cytochrome c binds to Apaf-1 and forms an activation complex with caspase-9. Although the mechanism(s) regulating mitochondrial permeability and the release of cytochrome c during apoptosis are not fully understood, Bcl-xL, Bcl-2, and Bax may influence the voltage-dependent anion channel (VDAC), which may play a role in regulating cytochrome c release. Mule/ARF-BP1 is a DNA damage activated E3 ubiquitin ligase for p53, and Mcl-1, an anti-apoptotic member of Bcl-2 (Brenner & Mak, 2009; Chalah & Khosravi-Far, 2008; Yuan 2010). The essence of this intrinsic pathway is a balance between pro-apoptotic and protective molecules that regulate mitochondrial permeability and the release of death inducers that are normally sequestered within the mitochondria (Kumar et al., 2005).

2.2.3 The execution phase

The final phase of apoptosis is mediated by a proteolytic cascade, toward which the various initiating mechanisms converge. Caspases, a family of cysteine proteases, are the central regulators of apoptosis. They are mammalian homologues of the ced-3 in the nematode Caenorhabditis elegans. The caspase family, now including more than 10 members, can be divided functionally into two basic groups – initiator and executioner – depending on the order in which they are activated during apoptosis. Caspases exist as inactive pro-enzymes, or zymogens, and must undergo an activating cleavage for apoptosis to be initiated. Caspases have their own cleavage sites that can be hydrolyzed not only by other caspases but also autocatalytically. After an initiator caspase is cleaved to generate its active form, the enzymatic death program is set in motion by rapid and sequential activation of other caspases. Executioner caspases act on many cellular components. They cleave cytoskeletal and nuclear matrix proteins and thus disrupt the cytoskeleton and lead to breakdown of the nucleus. In the nucleus, the targets of caspase activation include proteins involved in transcription, DNA replication, and DNA repair (Haunstetter & Izumo, 1998; Kumar et al., 2005) (Table 1). Initiator caspases (including caspase-2, -8, -9, -10, -11, and -12) are closely coupled to pro-apoptotic signals. Once activated, these caspases cleave and activate downstream effector caspases (including caspase-3, -6, and -7), which in turn execute apoptosis by cleaving cellular proteins following specific Asp residues. Activation of Fas and TNFR by FasL and TNF, respectively, leads to the activation of caspase-8 and -10. DNA damage induces the expression of PIDD which binds to RAIDD and caspase-2 and leads to the activation of caspase-2. Cytochrome c released from damaged mitochondria is coupled to the activation of caspase-9. XIAP inhibits caspase-3, -7, and -9. Mitochondria release multiple pro-apoptotic molecules, such as Smac/ Diablo, AIF, HtrA2 and EndoG, in addition to cytochrome c. Smac/Diablo binds to XIAP which prevents it from inhibiting caspases. Caspase-11 is induced and activated by pathological proinflammatory and pro-apoptotic stimuli and leads to the activation of caspase-1 to promote inflammatory response and apoptosis by directly processing caspase-3. Caspase-12 and caspase-7 are activated under ER stress conditions. Anti-apoptotic ligands including growth factors and cytokines activate Akt and p90RSK. Akt inhibits Bad by direct phosphorylation and prevents the expression of Bim by phosphorylating and inhibiting the Forkhead family of transcription factors (Fox0). Fox0 promotes apoptosis by upregulating pro-apoptotic molecules such as FasL and Bim (Degterev & Yuan, 2008; Kurokawa & Kornbluth, 2009; Yuan 2010).

Nuclear proteins
Lamin, Rb protein, DNA-dependent protein kinase, 70-kDa subunit of U1 small nuclear ribonucleoprotein, Poly (ADP)-ribosylating protein (PARP), Mdm2
Regulatory proteins
MAPK/ERK kinase kinase 1 (MEKK1), Protein Kinase Cδ, G4-GDI GDP dissociation inhibitor, Sterol regulatory element binding protein, DNA fragmentation factor/inhibitor of caspase-activated DNAse
Cytoskeletal proteins
Fodrin, Gelsolin, Actin, Gas2

Table 1. Downstream targets of Caspases. (Haunstetter & Izumo, 1998)

2.3 Study of apoptosis

Light and electron microscopy are two of the classical techniques for the study of this process. Because of the lack of cellular synchronization in apoptosis and of the fact that the apoptotic cell is rapidly disposed of through phagocytosis, study methods based on morphologic criteria are adequate for the demonstration of the process, but are not useful for quantifying it. Further to these procedures, the study of DNA fragmentation in agarose gels has been considered to be identificative for apoptosis. A number of techniques take advantage of this DNA fragmentation for labelling the fragments and thus for quantifying the proportion of apoptotic cells. Each DNA fragment has a 3'OH terminal portion. This terminal fragment can be labelled in various ways (for instance, with the help of a modified terminal deoxynucleotidyl transferase), so that the labelling rate is proportional to the degree of DNA fragmentation. In TUNEL assay (terminal deoxyribonucleotidyl transferase [TdT]-mediated dUTP-digoxigeninnick end labeling), TdT transfers a fluorescent nucleotide to exposed breakpoints of DNA. Apoptotic cells that have incorporated the labeled nucleotide are then visualized by fluorescence microscopy or flow cytometry. Apoptotic cells that have extruded some of the DNA have less than their normal diploid content. Automated measurement of the amount of DNA in individual cells by flow cytometry thus produces a population distribution according to DNA content (cytofluorograph) (Rubin et al., 2005). At present, the most widely accepted and standardized technique takes advantage of the changes in the membrane phospholipids that occur early in apoptotic cells (Vermes et al., 1995). The negatively charged membrane phospholipids exposed to the external environment by the apoptotic cell are labeled with fluorochrome-conjugated molecules, and the percentage of fluorescent cells can be easily quantified (Chamond et al., 1999).

2.4 Apoptosis in developmental and physiological processes

Cell death is extremely important in embryonic development, maintenance of tissue homeostasis, establishment of immune self-tolerance, killing by immune effector cells, and regulation of cell viability by hormones and growth factors. Apoptosis is a normal phenomenon that serves to eliminate cells that are not longer needed and to maintain a steady number of various cell populations in tissues. It is important in the following physiologic situations. During molecular maturation of T-cell antigen receptors, immature T cells in the thymus rearrange the genes encoding the receptor α and β chains. Cells with receptors recognizing self-antigens are potentially harmful and are eliminated through programmed cell death. Cells with damaged DNA tend to accumulate mutations, and they are potentially harmful to the organism. DNA damage induces programmed cell death in many cell types. Furthermore one of the mechanisms to eliminate infected cells is through the action of cytotoxic T lymphocytes, which kill cells, by inducing them to undergo programmed cell death. T lymphocytes whose T-cell receptors cannot interact with the spectrum of MHC glycoproteins expressed in a given individual are ineffective in the immune response. Up to 95% of immature T cells die by apoptosis without leaving the thymus. Fetal development involves the sequential appearance and regression of many anatomical structures: some aortic arches do not persist, the mesonephros regresses in favor of the metanephros, interdigital tissues disappear to allow discrete fingers and toes, and excess neurons are pruned from the developing brain. Cells in these conditions serve no purpose in humans and are eliminated by programmed cell death. Excess neurons that do not make appropriate connections have no function and so are eliminated by apoptosis. Up to 80%of neurons in certain developing ganglia die this way (Rubin et al., 2005). Apoptosis also eliminates the constituent cells of mullerian ducts in males. Epithelial cells must die to allow fusion of palate and mammary and prostate cells die when deprived of hormones (Pollard & Earnshaw, 2004).

2.5 Apoptosis and disease

Death by apoptosis is also responsible for loss of cells in a variety of pathologic states. The diseases in which apoptosis has been involved can be divided into two groups: those in which there is an increase in cell survival (or diseases associated to inhibition of apoptosis), and those in which there is an increase in cell death (and hence hyperactive apoptosis) (Chamond et al., 1999). The group of diseases associated to apoptosis inhibition includes those diseases in which an excessive accumulation of cells occurs (neoplastic diseases, autoimmune diseases) (Table 2). It was classically believed that the excessive accumulation of cells in these diseases occurred because of an increased cell proliferation. In recent years, the study of apoptosis in these patients has led to a new and different approach, according to which this accumulation of cells would be due to defective apoptosis. Increased cell apoptosis has also been implicated in the aetiopathogenesis of a number of diseases.

A large group of neurodegenerative diseases, among them Alzheimer's disease, Parkinson's disease, amyotrophic lateral sclerosis and retinitis pigmentosa, are associated to selective apoptosis of the neurones. This neuronal death appears to be associated to increases susceptibility to apoptosis in these cells. Oxidative stress, mitochondrial defects and neurotoxic agents have been postulated as the inductors of neuronal death. The disease associated to infection by the Human Immunodeficiency Virus (HIV) has been defined as an imbalance between the number of CD4+ lymphocytes and the ability of the bone marrow to generate new mature cells. The CD4+ cells of the HIV(+) patients die through apoptosis when stimulated in vitro. Also, HIV infection of cells from healthy subjects induces apoptosis of CD4+ cells. However, further to this, not only the infected cells but also non-infected cells undergo apoptosis. Replicative exhaustion of the responding cell clones has been demonstrated in a number of diseases (among them AIDS, in which the responding clone is the CD4+ one); in these diseases the responding clone, after an initial phase of intense response to the stimulus, become exhausted and undergo apoptosis (Ameisen, 1995).

Through inhibition of apoptosis	Through excess apoptosis
Cancer	**AIDS**
Colorectal	T lymphocytes
Glioma	**Neurodegenerative diseases**
Hepatic	Alzheimer's disease
Neuroblastoma	Amyotrophic lateral sclerosis
Leukaemias and lymphomas	Parkinson's disease
Prostate	Retinitis pigmentosa
Autoimmune diseases	Epilepsy
Myastenia gravis	**Haematologic diseases**
Systemic lupus erythematosus	Aplastic anaemia
Inflammatory diseases	Myelodysplastic syndrome
Bronchial asthma	T CD4+ lymphocytopenia
Inflammatory intestinal disease	G6PD deficiency
Pulmonary inflammation	**Tissue damage**
Viral infections	Myocardial infarction
Adenovirus	Cerebrovascular accident
Baculovirus	Ischaemic renal damage
	Polycystic kidney

Table 2. Diseases associated to apoptosis

2.6 Apoptosis and cardiovascular disease

The myocardial cells allocate a limited faculty of proliferation and correspondingly, apoptosis is observed infrequently in adult hearts. On the contrary at the duration of organogenesis and in the formation of heart the apoptosis plays an important role, as an example in the formation of septa between the cardiac chambers and the valves. As consequence the defects in apoptosis can constitute basic causative factor of relatives of congenital heart disease. Apoptosis of myocardial cells is also observed afterwards the birth and concretely in the interventricular septum and right ventricular wall, at the duration of passage from the fetal circulation in the adult circulation. Moreover the phenomenon of apoptosis is also distinguished in the conducting system and can lead to congenital heart block, syndrome of long QT, and the existence of accessory pathways (Table 3) (Bennett, 2002). Until recently, the loss of myocytes was attributed to necrosis; however, it is now clear that apoptosis may play an important role in the pathogenesis of a variety of cardiovascular diseases. For instance, apoptosis has been detected in myocardial samples obtained from patients with end-stage congestive heart failure, arrhythmogenic right ventricular dysplasia and myocardial infraction. In addition, apoptosis has been detected in cardiac myocytes under hypoxia/reoxygenetion, mechanical stretch and in animal models of cardiac ischemia/reperfusion injury (Table 4) (Gustafsson & Gottlieb, 2003).

Myocyte
Idiopathic dilated cardiomyopathy
Ischaemic cardiomyopathy
Acute myocardial infarction
Arrhythmogenic right ventricular dysplasia
Myocarditis
Conducting tissues
Pre-excitations syndromes
Congenital complete atrioventricular heart
Long QT syndromes
Vascular
Atherosclerosis
Restenosis after angioplasty / stenting
Vascular graft rejection
Arterial aneurysm formation

Table 3. Apoptosis and cardiovascular disease (Bennett, 2002; Haunstetter & Izumo, 1998)

Stimulus	Signaling pathway	Potential inhibitor
Ischaemia/reperfusion Pressure overload Neurohormonal factors Ischaemia Death receptor ligands	ERK/SARK ERK/SARK G protein coupling Lack of growth factor signaling Adapter molecules / caspases	Activation of ERK, inhibition of SARK signaling Activation of ERK, inhibition of SARK signaling β blockers Activation of Akt/ERK pathways Decoy receptors / receptor antagonists IAPs / caspase inhibitors
ERK, extracellular signal related kinase; IAP, inhibitor of apoptosis protein; SAPK, stress activated protein kinase		

Table 4. Potential inhibitors and signaling pathways of cardiomyocyte apoptosis (Bennett, 2002).

2.6.1 Apoptosis and atherosclerosis

Apoptosis constitutes basic characteristic of vessels remodeling that takes place in organogenesis and in pathological situations like injury and atherosclerosis. The significance of apoptosis in atherosclerosis depends on the stage of the plaque, localization and the cell types involved. Apoptosis of vascular smooth muscle cells (SMC), endothelial cells and macrophages may promote plaque growth and pro-coagulation and may induce rupture, the major consequence of atherosclerosis in humans. Apoptosis of macrophages is mainly present in regions showing signs of DNA synthesis/repair. SMC apoptosis is mainly present in less cellular regions and is not associated with DNA synthesis/repair. Even in the early stages of atherosclerosis SMC become susceptible to apoptosis since they increase different pro-apoptotic factors. Moreover, recent data indicate that SMC may be killed by activated macrophages. The loss of the SMC can be detrimental for plaque stability since most of the interstitial collagen fibres, which are important for the tensile strength of the fibrous cap, are produced by SMC. Rupture of atherosclerotic plaques is associated with a thinning of the SMC-rich fibrous cap overlying the core. Rupture occurs particularly at the plaque shoulders, which exhibit lack of SMCs and the presence of inflammatory cells. Apoptotic SMCs are evident in advanced human plaques including the shoulders regions, prompting the suggestion that SMC apoptosis may hasten plaque rupture. Indeed, increased SMC apoptosis occurs in unstable versus stable angina lesions. Apoptosis of macrophages could be beneficial for plaque stability if apoptotic bodies were removed. Apoptotic cells that are not scavenged in the plaque activate thrombin, which could further induce intraplaque thrombosis (Kockx & Knaapen, 2000). Most apoptotic cells in advanced lesions are macrophages next to the lipid core. Loss of macrophages from atherosclerotic lesions would be predicted to promote plaque stability rather than rupture, since macrophages can promote SMC apoptosis by both direct interactions and by release of cytokines (Bennett, 2002). It can be concluded that apoptosis in primary atherosclerosis is detrimental since it could lead to plaque rupture and thrombosis.

2.6.2 Apoptosis and ischaemia/infarction

Cardiac myocyte death during ischemic injury has been thought to occur exclusively by necrosis, but recently several studies have demonstrated that large numbers of myocytes undergo apoptosis in response to ischemic disorders (Saraste et al., 1997). In humans, apoptosis seems to occur primarily in the border zone of the ischemic region and, according to some studies, in the remote from ischemia regions. However, in vivo animal studies have demonstrated apoptosis both in the ischemic region and the ischemic border zone. Apoptosis of cardiomyocytes occurs in a temporally and spatially specific manner. The central, unperfused region also manifests apoptosis, particularly within the first six hours, although between 6-24 hours necrosis is more common (Bennett, 2002). In contrast, in some studies ischemia caused apoptosis in the ischemic region alone, whereas reperfusion caused a decrease in apoptotic cells in the ischemic region and an increase in apoptotic cells in the ischemic border zone and the remote from ischemia regions. These differences theoretically could be explained by the different methods of measuring apoptosis that were used (Krijnen et al., 2002). Apoptosis in the remote non-infarcted myocardium may be partly responsible for myocardial remodelling and dilatation after myocardial infarction, and may be amenable to treatment. Apoptosis is a highly regulated process in which several regulatory proteins play a significant part. P53 limits cellular proliferation by inducing cell cycle arrest and apoptosis in response to cellular stresses such as DNA damage, hypoxia, and oncogene activation. P53 mediates apoptosis through a linear pathway involving bax activation, cytochrome c release from mitochondria, and caspase activation (Shen & White, 2001). The Bcl-2 family of proteins constitutes a critical checkpoint in cell death. These proteins contain agonists and antagonists of apoptosis and alterations of their ratio determine the life or death of a cell (Anversa & Kajstura, 1998). Proapoptotic proteins include Bax, Bak, Bad, and Bcl-xs whereas Bcl-2 and Bcl-xL are antiapoptotic. Several studies have demonstrated that Bcl-2 protein is induced in salvaged myocytes surrounding infracted areas in the regions at risk in acute stage of infraction. Bcl-2 positive myocytes were not seen in the infracted myocytes in the heart with acute infraction. Bcl-2 positive immunoreactivity was not evident in salvaged myocytes of hearts with old infraction, in chronic ischemic disease or in normal hearts. P53 and Bax protein expression was rare in salvaged myocytes within the risk area at the acute stage of infraction. P53 and Bax positive immunoractivity was evident in the infracted myocytes. P53 protein is induced in salvaged myocytes at the old stage of infraction and in chronic ischemic disease. P53 positive immunoreactivity of normal control heart tissue was slight in most of myocytes. Myocytes exposed to various stress, such as chronic ischemia (salvaged myocytes at the old stage of infraction, myocytes at chronic ischemic disease) induced the overexpression of p53 protein (Tsipis et al., 2007). Consequently, the expression of bcl-2 or P53 protein in myocytes of human hearts with infarction may play an important role in the protection or the acceleration of cellular damage after infarction (Figure 1, Figure 2).

2.6.3 Apoptosis and heart failure

Congestive heart failure occurs as a late manifestation in diverse cardiovascular diseases characterized by volume or pressure overload and significant loss of contractile muscle mass. Cardiac output is initially maintained in these disorders by the development of compensatory myocardial hypertrophy and dilatation. However, the early mechanical adaptations to growth stimulus soon fall short of adequate compensation. The mechanism by which compensatory

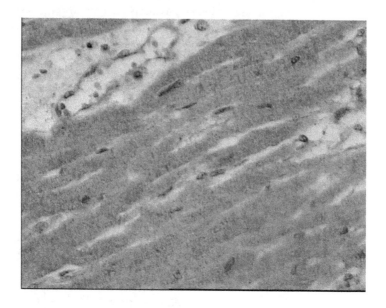

Fig. 1. Immunohistochemical staining for Bcl-2 in myocardial infarction (X400).

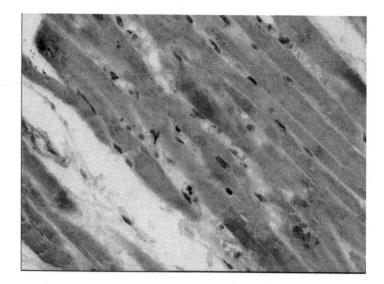

Fig. 2. Immunohistochemical staining for P53 in myocardial infarction (X400).

response triggered by myocardial failure culminates in myocardial dysfunction is not clear. In the past few years, several scientists have proposed apoptosis as the basis of the inexorable decline in ventricular systolic function (Narula et al., 2000). Although the initial studies reported unrealistically high levels of apoptosis in failed heart (as much as 35%), recent studies show an apoptosis rates of <1% (TUNEL-positive cells) during heart failure (Kang & Izumo, 2000). Because of the limitations with TUNEL staining and the difficulties in interpreting these findings, the use of TUNEL alone to detect the presence of apoptosis is not sufficient to define the role of apoptosis in heart failure. Later studies have consistently shown that approximately 80–250 heart muscle cells per 10^5 cardiac nuclei commit suicide at any given time in patients with late-stage dilated cardiomyopathy. In contrast, the base-line rate of apoptosis in healthy human hearts is only one to ten cardiac myocytes per 10^5 nuclei (Anversa & Kajstura, 1998; Yue et al., 1998). Even though the rate of apoptosis in heart failure is relatively low in absolute numbers, it is significantly higher than that in the normal heart, which has essentially negligible baseline apoptosis. Recently, animal models of heart failure incorporating transgenic technology have confirmed that very low levels of myocyte apoptosis, levels that are four- to tenfold lower than those seen in human heart failure, are sufficient to cause a lethal, dilated cardiomyopathy (Wencker et al., 2003).

It has been long believed that apoptosis does not occur in terminally differentiated cells such as adult cardiomyocytes. However, all mechanisms responsible for induction of apoptosis are operative in myocytes and are particularly activated during heart failure. Actually, the onset of myocardial failure leads to systemic and myocardial neurohumoral alterations and cytokine expression to maintain cardiac output. Upregulation of these adaptive responses also induces growth response and leads to compensatory myocardial hypertrophy and dilatation. Cardiac myocytes differentiate and withdraw from the cell cycle during the neonatal period, and persistent growth stimulus in the adult myocardium (such as that in heart failure) is perceived as a contradictory genetic demand, and programmed cell death occurs (Narula et al., 2000). P53 (tumor suppressor protein) is involved in the regulation of cell cycle progression in response to DNA damage. This p53 typically causes the cell to delay its entry into S phase until the damage has been repaired. P53 also is involved in triggering an apoptotic response in instances in which the damage is too severe to repair. P53 is a transcriptional regulator of the bcl-2 and bax genes. P53 mediates apoptosis through a linear pathway involving bax transactivation, Bax translocation from the cytosol to membranes, cytochrome c release from mitochondria, and caspase-9 activation, followed by the activation of caspase-3, -6, and -7 (Kim et al., 1994; Shen & White, 2001). P53 down-regulates the antiapoptotic gene product Bcl-2 and up-regulates the proapoptotic gene product Bax. Immunohistochemistry of p53 and antiapoptotic Bcl-2 protein demonstrated higher levels of both of these proteins in heart failure as compared with normal hearts (Figure 3, Figure 4). Tsipis et al. have observed that the percentage of p53- and bcl-2 positive samples in the end-stage dilated cardiomyopathy was 100% (20/20 diseased group samples). A 2- and 2.5-fold increase in p53 and bcl-2 positive samples was observed in the diseased group as compared with the control group. The diseased group had a larger number of samples with strong p53 staining as compared with the control group, which demonstrated weak p53 staining. Bcl-2 staining in the positive samples of the diseased group was generally weak as in the control group (Tsipis et al., 2010). Latif and colleagues, in a quantitation of the bcl-2 family of proteins after Western Immunoprobing, demonstrated a 2.9- and 5.35-fold increase in the levels of Bax and of Bcl-2, respectively,

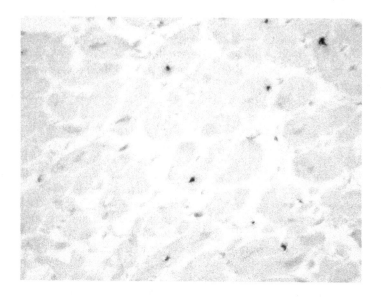

Fig. 3. Immunohistochemical staining for p53 protein in dilated cardiomyopathy (X400).

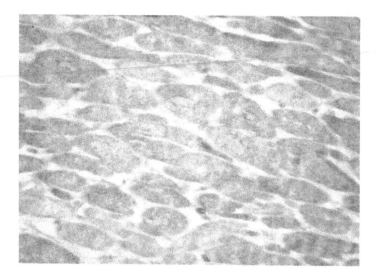

Fig. 4. Immunohistochemical staining for bcl-2 in dilated cardiomyopathy (X400).

in patients with dilated cardiomyopathy (Latif et al., 2000). Narula and colleagues demonstrated a release of cytochrome c from mitochondria in patients with heart failure (Narula et al., 2000). In the study of Tsipis et .al, increased expression of P53 protein was seen, but p53 up-regulates the proapoptotic gene product Bax (Tsipis et al., 2010). Elevated levels of Bax and Bak may mediate the release of cytochrome c, as it has been demonstrated that Bax and Bak accelerate the opening of the voltage-dependent anion channel (Latif et al., 2000; Shimizu et al., 1999). These results suggest that increased expression of p53 may be associated with apoptosis in heart failure of end-stage dilated cardiomyopathy. Moreover, various factors present in the failing myocardium have been shown to stimulate apoptosis in cardiac myocytes. Such factors include inflammatory cytokines, reactive oxygen species, nitric oxide, hypoxia, reperfusion, growth factors, and mechanical stretch (Foo et al., 2005). Ventricular decompensation and failure impose an elevated diastolic load on myocytes, resulting in stretching of sarcomeres and the stimulation of multiple second messenger systems which have been linked to the initiation of myocyte reactive hypertrophy in the pathologic heart. Abnormal levels of resting tension may lead to the local release of angiotensin II (Ang II) and the induction of programmed cell death in the myocardium. Sarcomere elongation in vitro results in Ang II release and activation of p53 and p53-dependent genes (Leri et al., 1998). Moreover, overstretching appears to be coupled with oxidant stress, expression of Fas, programmed cell death, architectural rearrangement of myocytes, and impairment in force development of the myocardium (Cheng et al., 1995). Using Western blotting, Olivetti et al. demonstrated a 2.4-fold increase in bcl-2 in patients with heart failure (Olivetti et al., 1997). However, the expression of Bax protein was not altered in the diseased group. This low expression of Bax protein may represent the prevalence of bcl-2 compensatory mechanism. The elevated presence of p53-positive cells, as demonstrated by immunohistochemistry, suggest that apoptosis may be significantly higher in dilated cardiomyopathy than that in the normal heart. On the other hand, increased expression of the antiapoptotic protein bcl-2 in human myocardium with dilated cardiomyopathy may be a compensation for the loss of myocytes and a possible compensatory antiapoptotic mechanism in the diseased group (Tsipis et al., 2010). In conclusion the etiology of heart failure in dilated cardiomyopathy involves multiple agents. The heart failure involves not only the contractile dysfunction, but also the progressive loss of myocytes by apoptosis. The elevated expression of proapoptotic is associated with progressive loss of myocytes in heart failure, and the increased expression of antiapoptotic proteins represent a possible compensatory mechanism. The prevalence of the apoptotic mechanism or this of compensatory antiapoptotic may influence the evolution of heart failure in cardiomyopathy.

3. Conclusions

Cells are poised between survival and apoptosis, and their fate rests on a balance of powerful intracellular and extracellular forces, whose signals constantly act upon and counteract each other. In many circumstances, apoptosis is a self-protective programmed mechanism that leads to the suicide of a cell when its survival is deemed detrimental to the organism. In other instances, apoptosis is a pathological process that contributes to many disorders. Thus, the pharmacological manipulation of apoptosis represents an active frontier of drug development. Recognition of the inducing mechanisms of apoptosis could open up ways to inhibit cell death in cardiovascular tissues and possibly help to define targets for future drug design. Furthermore, end-stage events of apoptosis, such as the activation of downstream caspases are essentially uniform in all cell types; although some regulatory mechanisms may be unique to cells in cardiovascular tissues. Elucidation of proapoptotic and antiapoptotic mechanisms in cardiomyocytes and vascular smooth muscle cells could delineate potential targets for intervention. In conclusion, various factors present in the diseased myocardium have been shown to stimulate apoptosis in cardiac myocytes. Changes in the induction of genes promoting or opposing apoptosis may modulate the total amount of myocyte damage. There is still a need to clarify the role played by different genetic and environmental factors implicated in cell death or survival.

4. References

Ameisen JC. From cell activation to cell depletion. The programmed cell death hypothesis of AIDS pathogenesis. Adv Exp Med Biol 1995; 374:139-163.

Anversa P & Kajstura J. Myocyte Cell Death in the Diseased Heart. Circulation Research. 1998;82:1231-1233.

Bennett Martin R. Apoptosis in the cardiovascular system, Heart 2002; 87: 480-487

Brenner D. & Mak TW. Mitochondrial cell death effectors. Curr. Opin. Cell Biol 2009; 21(6):871-7

Chalah & Khosravi-Far R. The mitochondrial death pathway. Adv. Exp. Med. Biol. 2008;615:25-45.

Chamond R.R, Añón J.C, Aguilary C.M. & Pasadas F.G. Apoptosis and disease. Alergol Inmunol Clin 1999; 14(6): 367-374

Cheng W, Li B, Kajstura J, Li P, Wolin MS, Sonnenblick EH, Hintze TH, Olivetti G & Anversa P. Stretch-induced programmed myocyte cell death. J Clin Invest. 1995;96:2247–2259.

Degterev A & Yuan J. Expansion and evolution of cell death programmes. Nat. Rev. Mol. Cell Biol. 2008;9(5), 378–90.

Foo RSY, Mani K. & Kitsis RN. Death begets failure in the heart. J Clin Invest. 2005;115: 565–571.

Gustafsson A.B. & Gottlieb R.A. Mechanisms of apoptosis in the heart. J Clin Immunol. 2003;23(6):447-59

Haunstetter A & Izumo S. Apoptosis: Basic mechanisms and implications for cardiovascular disease. Circulation Research. 1998;82:1111-1129.

Humphreys R.C. & Halpern W. Trail receptors: targets for cancer therapy. Adv. Exp. Med. Biol. 2008;615:127-58.

Kang P & Izumo S. Apoptosis and heart failure: A critical review of the literature. Circ Res. 2000;86 (11): 1107-13.

Kim KK, Soonpaa MH, Daud AI, Koh GY, Kim JS & Field LJ. Tumor suppressor gene expression during normal and pathologic myocardial growth. J Biol Chem. 1994; 269 (36): 22607-13.

Krijnen PA, Nijmeijer R, Meijer CJ, Visser CA, Hack CE & Niessen HW. Apoptosis in myocardial ischemia and infarction. J Clin Pathol. 2002;55(11):801-811.

Kockx M M & Knaapen MW. The role of apoptosis in vascular disease. J Pathol. 2000;190(3):267-80

Kumar V, Abbas Ak, Fausto N. Robbins and Cotran: Pathologic Basis Of Disease. 7th ed. Philadelphia: Elsevier Saunders;2005:26-32

Kurokawa M & Kornbluth S. Caspases and kinases in a death grip. Cell. 2009;138(5), 838-54.

Latif N, Khan MA, Birks E, O'Farrell A, Westbrook J, Dunn MJ & Yacoub MH. Upregulation of the Bcl-2 family of proteins in end stage heart failure. J Am Coll Cardiol. 2000;35 (7):1769-1777.

Leri A, Claudio PP, Li Q, Wang X, Reiss K, Wang S, Malhotra A, Kajstura J & Anversa P. Stretch-mediated release of Angiotensin II induces myocyte apoptosis by activating p53 that enhances the local renin-angiotensin system and decreases the bcl-2-to-bax Protein ratio in the cell. J Clin Invest. 1998;101(7): 1326-42.

Logue SE & Martin SJ. Caspase activation cascades in apoptosis. Biochem. Soc. Trans. 2008;36(1) :1-9

Narula J, kolodgie FD & Virmani R. Apoptosis And cardiomyopathy. Curr Opin in Cardiol 2000;15:183-88

Olivetti G, Abbi R, Quaini F, Kajstura J, Cheng W, Nitahara JA, Quaini E, Di Loreto C, Beltrami CA, Krajewski S, Reed JC & Anversa P. Apoptosis in the failing human heart. N Engl J Med. 1997;336(16): 1131-41.

Pollard T & Earnshaw W. Cell biology. Updated Edition 2004. Philadelphia: Saunders. An imprint of Elsevier, 2004; 772-776.

Rubin E, Gorstein F, Rubin R, Schwarting R, Strayer D. Rubin's Pathology: Clinicopathologic Foundations of Medicine. 4th ed. Philadelphia: Lippincott Williams & Wilkins; 2005:566-70

Saraste A, Pulkki K, Kallajoki M, Hennksen K, Parvinen M & Voipio-Pulkki LM. Apoptosis in human acute myocardial infarction. Circulation 1997; 95(2):320-3.

Shen Y & White E. P53-dependent apoptosis pathways. Adv Cancer Res. 2001; 82:55-84.

Shimizu S, Narita M & Tsujimoto Y. Bcl-2 family proteins regulate the release of apo-ptogenic cytochrome c by the mitochondrial channel VDAC. Nature 1999;399:483-87

Tsipis A, Athanassiadou AM, Athanassiadou P, Kavantzas N, Agrogiannis G & Patsouris E. Apoptosis-related factors p53, Bcl-2 in acute and chronic ischemic cardiac disorders. Virchows Arch 2007;451(2):483-84

Tsipis A, Athanassiadou AM, Athanassiadou P, Kavantzas N, Agrogiannis G & Patsouris E. Apoptosis-related factors p53, Bcl-2 and the defects of force transmission in dilated cardiomyopathy. Pathol Res Pract 2010;206(9):625-30

Vermes I, Haanen C, Steffens-Nakken H & Reutelingsperger C. A novel assay for apoptosis. Flow cytometric detection of phosphatidilserine expression on early apoptotic cell using fluorescein labelled Annexin V. J Immunol Methods 1995; 184(1):39-51.

Wencker D, Chandra M, Nguyen K, Miao W, Garantziotis S, Factor SM, Shirani J, Armstrong RC & Kitsis RN. A mechanistic role for cardiac myocyte apoptosis in heart failure. J Clin Invest. 2003;111(10):1497–504

Yuan J. Apoptosis Pathway Description. Revised November 2010. www.Cellsignal.com

Yue TL, Ma XL, Wang X, Romanic AM, Liu GL, Louden C, Gu JL, Kumar S, Poste G , Ruffolo RR Jr & Feuerstein GZ. Possible involvement of stress-activated protein kinase signaling pathway and Fas receptor expression in prevention of ischemia/reperfusion-induced cardiomyocyte apoptosis by carvedilol. Circ Res. 1998;82(2): 166–74.

2

Dobutamine-Induced Mechanical Alternans

Akihiro Hirashiki and Toyoaki Murohara
Nagoya Graduate School of Medicine
Japan

1. Introduction

We investigated the relationship between the occurrence of dobutamine-induced mechanical alternans (MA) and prognosis in ambulatory patients with idiopathic dilated cardiomyopathy (IDCM).

Recent American College of Cardiology and American Heart Association guidelines for the management of heart failure have emphasized the need for earlier identification and therapy for patients at high risk of systolic dysfunction, as well as for those with symptomatic heart failure.

MA, a condition characterized by beat-to-beat oscillation in the strength of cardiac muscle contraction at a constant heart rate, has been observed in patients with severe heart failure and in animal models of this condition.

Although MA is rare under resting conditions in individuals with controlled heart failure, at higher heart rates it is more prevalent and likely to be sustained, as exemplified by pacing-induced MA or dobutamine-induced MA. However, few studies have addressed the clinical implications of dobutamine-induced MA in patients with heart failure. We therefore prospectively examined the prognostic value of dobutamine- and pacing- induced MA in ambulatory patients with IDCM in sinus rhythm.(1)

2. Methods

2.1 Patient population

We studied 90 patients with IDCM (mean age, 50 years; range, 20 to 76 years) and an New York Heart Association (NYHA) functional class of I or II. Thirty-eight of the patients had previously been admitted to hospital because of heart failure with dyspnea on exertion, palpitations, or peripheral edema, whereas the remaining 52 were asymptomatic and were identified on the basis of electrocardiogram abnormalities detected at annual health checkups. All patients had normal sinus rhythms. IDCM was defined by the presence of both a reduced left ventricular (LV) ejection fraction (<50%, as determined by contrast left ventriculography) and a dilated LV cavity.

2.2 Cardiac catheterization

All patients initially underwent routine diagnostic left and right heart catheterization. A 6F fluid-filled pigtail catheter with a high-fidelity micromanometer was advanced into the left ventricle through the right radial artery to measure LV pressure. Right atrial pacing was initiated at 80 beats per minute (bpm) and was increased in increments of 10 bpm. We selected steady-state LV pressure data for at least 2 min at the baseline and at each pacing rate for analysis.(2) We calculated the maximum first derivative of LV pressure (LV dP/dt_{max}) as an index of contractility. To evaluate LV isovolumic relaxation, we computed the pressure half-time ($T_{1/2}$) directly, as previously described.(3) The peak pacing rate was defined as the heart rate at which second-degree atrioventricular block occurred. After the hemodynamic values had returned to baseline, dobutamine was infused intravenously at incremental doses of 5, 10, and 15 µg kg^{-1} b.w. min^{-1} and hemodynamic measurements were performed at the end of each 5-min infusion period. MA was diagnosed if the pressure difference between the strong and weak beats was ≥4 mm Hg continuously in the analyzed LV pressure data, as previously described.(4)

2.3 Quantitative RT-PCR analysis
Quantitative reverse transcription (RT) and polymerase chain reaction (PCR) analysis of the mRNAs for sarcoplasmic reticulum Ca^{2+}-ATPase (SERCA2a), ryanodine receptor 2, phospholamban, calsequestrin, and the Na$^+$-Ca^{2+} exchanger was performed as previously described.(5) The amount of each mRNA was normalized against the corresponding amount of glyceraldehyde-3-phosphate dehydrogenase (GAPDH) mRNA.

2.4 Follow-up
We prospectively followed up all patients for the occurrence of primary events, which were defined as cardiac death (death from worsening heart failure or sudden death), unscheduled hospital readmission for worsening heart failure, or receipt of an implantable cardioverter defibrillator (ICD) because of life-threatening arrhythmia.

3.Results

3.1 Classification of IDCM patients on the basis of MA
To identify on the basis of the classification by hemodynamic response to pacing or dobutamine stress testing, patients were classified into three groups: those who exhibited neither pacing- nor dobutamine-induced MA (n = 60, group N), those who manifested only pacing-induced MA (n = 20, group P), and those who developed both pacing- and dobutamine-induced MA (n = 10, group D). All patients who did not develop pacing-induced MA also did not exhibit dobutamine-induced MA. LV pressure waveforms during atrial pacing at 120 bpm or after dobutamine infusion at 10 µg kg^{-1} min^{-1} are shown for representative patients from each group (Fig. 1).

3.2 Baseline clinical data
There were no significant differences in age and sex among the three groups of patients (Table 1). All patients were classified as NYHA functional class I or II at the time of cardiac catheterization. The LV ejection fraction (LVEF) in groups P and D was significantly lower than that in group N. There were also no significant differences in plasma brain natriuretic peptide (BNP) or norepinephrine levels among the three groups.

3.3 Abundance of Ca^{2+}-handling protein mRNAs in endomyocardial biopsy specimens
The amounts of Ca^{2+}-handling protein mRNAs in endomyocardial biopsy specimens were determined by using quantitative RT-PCR and were normalized against that of GAPDH

mRNA (Table 2). The abundance of phospholamban mRNA was significantly lower in group D than in group P. The SERCA2a/phospholamban mRNA ratio was significantly higher in group D than in groups N and P.

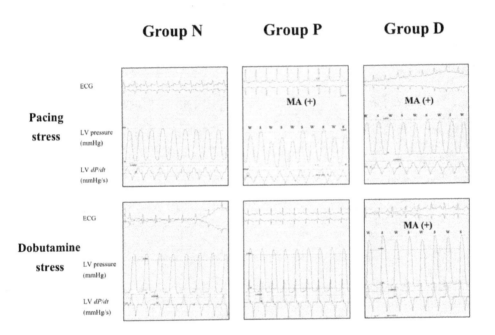

Fig. 1. LV pressure waveforms during atrial pacing at 120 bpm and after infusion of dobutamine at a dose of 10 µg kg⁻¹ min⁻¹ in representative patients of three study groups. The traces represent the lead II electrocardiogram (ECG), LV pressure, and LV dP/dt. Both LV dP/dt_{max} and LV dP/dt_{min} showed alternating changes with LV pressure. Strong and weak beats are indicated by s and w, respectively.

Characteristic	Group N (n = 60)			Group P (n = 20)			Group D (n = 10)		
Age (years)	51	±	12	50	±	13	45	±	11
Sex (M/F)	44	/	16	16	/	4	6	/	4
NYHA functional class I	32	(53%)		9	(45%)		5	(50%)	
class II	28	(47%)		11	(55%)		5	(50%)	
Medication									
Diuretics	30	(50%)		17*	(85%)		9*	(90%)	
ACE inhibitors or ARBs	42	(70%)		19	(95%)		7	(70%)	
Beta blockers	22	(37%)		10	(50%)		5	(50%)	
PAWP (mmHg)	10.7	±	4.7	14.6	±	6.2*	13.9	±	7.2
Cardiac index (L min^{-1} m^{-2})	3.07	±	0.55	2.83	±	0.58	3.26	±	0.66
LVEF (%)	38.9	±	8.1	32.9	±	9.6*	30.3	±	9.0*
Plasma BNP (pg/mL)	100	±	173	179	±	186	249	±	262
Plasma norepinephrine (pg/mL)	440	±	221	689	±	764	664	±	324

*$P < 0.05$ versus group N. Abbreviations not defined in text: ACE, angiotensin-converting enzyme; ARB, angiotensin-II receptor blocker; PAWP, pulmonary artery wedge pressure.

Table 1. Baseline clinical characteristics of patients in the three study groups

mRNA ratio	Group N			Group P			Group D		
SERCA2a/GAPDH	0.42	±	0.15	0.41	±	0.13	0.43	±	0.13
Phospholamban/GAPDH	0.82	±	0.45	1.01	±	0.13	0.42	±	0.24*
Ryanodine receptor 2/GAPDH	0.50	±	0.19	0.53	±	0.21	0.75	±	0.17
SERCA2a/phospholamban	0.63	±	0.31	0.59	±	0.40	1.32	±	0.95*†
SERCA2a/Na$^+$-Ca^{2+} exchanger	0.57	±	0.79	0.50	±	0.56	0.27	±	0.14

*$P < 0.05$ versus group P, †$P < 0.05$ versus group N.

Table 2. Quantitative RT-PCR analysis of the abundance of Ca^{2+}-handling protein mRNAs in endomyocardial biopsy specimens.

3.4 Follow-up evaluation and event-free survival
Of the 90 patients who were followed up, 4 individuals (4%) experienced cardiac death, 10 (11%) manifested worsening heart failure, and 4 (4%) received ICDs. The probability of event-free survival in group D was significantly lower than that in groups N or P (P = 0.002) (Fig. 2).

3.5 Univariate and multivariate analysis of cardiac events
Univariate analysis revealed that dobutamine-induced MA, pacing-induced MA, NYHA functional class, plasma BNP levels, mitral regurgitation, pulmonary artery wedge pressure, LV end-diastolic volume index, LV end-systolic volume index, LVEF, LV end-diastolic pressure and T½ were significant predictors of cardiac events (Table 3). Then, stepwise multivariate analysis identified dobutamine-induced MA (odds ratio, 4.05; 95% confidence interval, 1.35 to 12.2) as a significant independent predictor of cardiac events (Table 4). Both $T_{1/2}$ (odds ratio, 1.079; 95% confidence interval, 1.003 to 1.161) and plasma BNP level (odds ratio, 1.002; 95% confidence interval, 1.0004 to 1.0038) were also significant independent predictors of cardiac events, but with smaller odds ratios than that of dobutamine-induced MA.

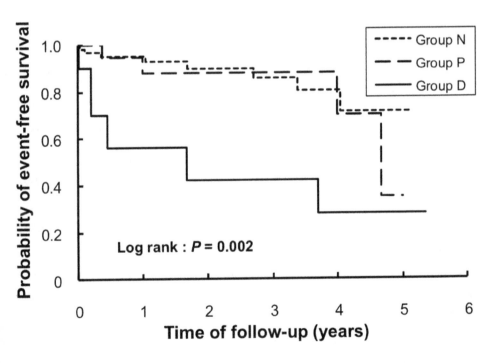

Fig. 2. Kaplan-Meier analysis of the cumulative probability of event-free survival of the 90 IDCM study patients. The probability of event-free survival in group D was significantly lower than that in groups P and N by the log-rank test (P = 0.002).

Parameter	Univariate analysis						
	Event-free group (*n* = 72)			Cardiac-event group (*n* = 18)			*P*
Dobutamine-induced MA (group D/groups P and N)	4	/	68	6	/	12	0.0019
Pacing-induced MA (groups D and P/group N)	20	/	52	10	/	8	0.04
Age (years)	50	±	12	53	±	14	0.34
Sex (M/F)	53	/	19	13	/	5	0.86
Body mass index (kg/m^2)	24.4	±	4.9	22.5	±	2.6	0.15
NYHA functional class	1.3	±	0.5	1.6	±	0.4	0.011
QRS duration (ms)	113	±	27	112	±	22	0.88
Beta blockers	55 (76%)			10 (56%)			0.58
Diuretics	52 (72%)			16 (89%)			0.88
Plasma BNP (pg/mL)	123	±	238	228	±	162	0.0013
eGFR (mL min^{-1} 1.73 m^{-2})	74	±	17	68	±	18	0.089
Plasma norepinephrine (pg/mL)	521	±	452	524	±	292	0.32
Mitral regurgitation	0.56	±	0.64	0.94	±	0.94	0.022
E/E'	15.6	±	8.6	24.2	±	8.4	0.227
PAWP (mmHg)	11.5	±	5.3	13.7	±	6.6	0.044
Cardiac index (L min^{-1} m^{-2})	3.02	±	0.57	3.13	±	0.64	0.85
LVEDVI (mL m^{-2})	73	±	52	115	±	79	0.02
LVESVI (mL m^{-2})	43	±	36	84	±	62	0.018
LVEF (%)	38.2	±	8.7	32.8	±	6.8	0.003
Heart rate (bpm)	76	±	17	75	±	14	0.34
LVEDP (mmHg)	12	±	8	15	±	9	0.019
LVSP (mmHg)	119	±	19	116	±	23	0.62
LV dP/dt_{max} (mmHg/s)	1114	±	263	1160	±	263	0.73
$T_{1/2}$ (ms)	39	±	7	44	±	4.7	0.0086

Table 3. Univariate of predictors of cardiac events.

Parameter	Multivariate analysis			
	β	OR	(95% CI)	P
Dobutamine-induced MA (group D/groups P and N)	1.4	4.05	(1.35–12.2)	0.0126
Plasma BNP (pg/mL)	0.0021	1.002	(1.0004–1.0038)	0.014
$T_{1/2}$ (ms)	0.076	1.079	(1.0033–1.161)	0.041

Table 4. Multivariate analysis of predictors of cardiac events.

4. Discussion

We found that the occurrence of dobutamine-induced MA was a clinical predictor of poor prognosis in ambulatory patients with IDCM in sinus rhythm. Although there was no significant difference in LVEF between patients who manifested only pacing-induced MA and those who developed both pacing- and dobutamine-induced MA, the probability of event-free survival in the latter group was significantly lower than that in the former. Multivariate analysis also revealed that the occurrence of dobutamine-induced MA was a significant independent predictor of cardiac events.

Our study included a group of 90 ambulatory patients with IDCM (mean LVEF of 36.5% and plasma BNP concentration of 132 pg/mL). We sought to investigate whether the hemodynamic response to dobutamine stress testing was associated with prognosis in such patients and could thereby serve as a physiological phenomenon on which risk stratification could be based. Three general mechanisms have been proposed to account for the development of MA: alteration of action potential duration, impaired ventricular relaxation, and abnormal intracellular Ca^{2+} handling.(6) The low relative ratio of phospholamban to SERCA reduces the inhibition of SERCA and increases Ca^{2+}-uptake; this enhances relaxation and contraction in the human atrium. However, humans lacking phospholamban develop lethal IDCM.(7) SERCA2a and ryanodine receptor 2 mRNA levels were similar in all three of our groups, whereas the relative ratio of SERCA to phospholamban was significantly higher in patients with pacing- and dobutamine-induced MA than in those with only pacing-induced MA or with no MA. Our results suggest that an imbalance between phospholamban and SERCA mRNA levels in the abundant Ca^{2+}-handling proteins is associated with dobutamine-induced MA. We also recently found that the amounts of mRNAs for the β_1-adrenergic receptor and SERCA2a in the myocardium were smaller in asymptomatic or mildly symptomatic IDCM patients with reduced adrenergic myocardial contractile reserve than in those with preserved adrenergic contractile reserves.(8) The occurrence of dobutamine-induced MA in our patients in the present study might also reflect abnormal β_1-adrenergic receptor signaling in the myocardium. However, steady-state mRNA levels do not necessarily reflect the corresponding protein levels, in particular because both mRNA and protein synthesis or degradation may be altered in the failing heart.(9, 10) Further studies are needed to elucidate these issues.

In patients with heart failure, dobutamine-induced MA is highly prevalent(4) and mechanical and visible T-wave alternans is detectable under tachycardia or catecholamine exposure.(2, 11) Dobutamine-induced MA may be attributed various factors, including an increase in the heart rate as a result of dobutamine infusion, impaired LV contraction, the influence of preload, and abnormal Ca^{2+} under pathophysiological conditions. Dobutamine is a β-stimulator that increases both heart rate (HR) and LV contraction. The increase in HR, but not that in LV contraction, is likely to be a trigger for the occurrence of dobutamine-induced MA. Therefore, the increased occurrence of dopamine-induced MA in heart failure patients might be related to their poor myocardial contractile reserve

We reported previously that the occurrence of pacing-induced MA is a potentially useful indicator of poor prognosis in patients with mild-to-moderate IDCM in sinus rhythm.(2) Here, we found that, among our ambulatory IDCM patients, those with both pacing- and dobutamine-induced MA had the least favorable clinical course, whereas those with only pacing-induced MA had a moderate clinical course, even though the mean value of baseline LVEF did not differ significantly between these two groups.

Our results show that the occurrence of dobutamine-induced MA is a potentially useful clinical predictor of cardiac events in ambulatory patients with IDCM in sinus rhythm. Recent guidelines for the management of heart failure emphasize the need for earlier identification of and therapy for patients who are at high risk of developing heart failure or who have asymptomatic LV systolic dysfunction.(12) We showed here that the prevalence of cardiac events or cardiac death was higher in patients with dobutamine- and pacing-induced MA than in those without it. Assessment of dobutamine-induced MA in addition to routine clinical evaluation in patients with IDCM may thus contribute to stratification of individuals into low- or high-risk groups.

Our study had several limitations. First, it included only a small number of patients. Second, the identification of pacing- or dobutamine-induced MA requires an invasive examination and time-consuming hemodynamic stress assessment. The current trend in clinical medicine is to find a non-invasive test with prognostic consequences. However, these results of the present study suggested that the hemodynamic phenomenon by dobutamine stress testing might be also potentially useful marker for predicting the occurrence of cardiac events. The fact that such examinations are not amenable to being repeated over time is a potential limitation of their prognostic utility. Whether our findings will also hold for patients with more severe heart failure requires further investigation.

In conclusion, the occurrence of dobutamine-induced MA is a potentially useful clinical predictor of poor prognosis in ambulatory patients with IDCM in sinus rhythm.

5. References

[1] Hirashiki A, Izawa H, Cheng XW, Unno K, Ohshima S, Murohara T. Dobutamine-induced mechanical alternans is a marker of poor prognosis in idiopathic dilated cardiomyopathy. *Clin Exp Pharmacol Physiol* 2010; 37(10):1004–1009.

[2] Hirashiki A, Izawa H, Somura F, Obata K, Kato T, Nishizawa T, Yamada A, Asano H, Ohshima S, Noda A, Iino S, Nagata K, Okumura K, Murohara T, Yokota M. Prognostic value of pacing-induced mechanical alternans in patients with mild-to-moderate idiopathic dilated cardiomyopathy in sinus rhythm. *J Am Coll Cardiol* 2006; 47(7):1382–1389.

[3] Mirsky I. Assessment of diastolic function: suggested methods and future considerations. *Circulation* 1984; 69(4):836–841.

[4] Kodama M, Kato K, Hirono S, Okura Y, Hanawa H, Ito M, Fuse K, Shiono T, Watanabe K, Aizawa Y. Mechanical alternans in patients with chronic heart failure. *J Card Fail* 2001; 7(2):138–145.

[5] Somura F, Izawa H, Iwase M, Takeichi Y, Ishiki R, Nishizawa T, Noda A, Nagata K, Yamada Y, Yokota M. Reduced myocardial sarcoplasmic reticulum Ca(2+)-ATPase mRNA expression and biphasic force-frequency relations in patients with hypertrophic cardiomyopathy. *Circulation* 2001; 104(6):658–663.

[6] Lab MJ, Lee JA. Changes in intracellular calcium during mechanical alternans in isolated ferret ventricular muscle. *Circ Res* 1990; 66(3):585–595.

[7] Haghighi K, Kolokathis F, Pater L, Lynch RA, Asahi M, Gramolini AO, Fan GC, Tsiapras D, Hahn HS, Adamopoulos S, Liggett SB, Dorn GW II, MacLennan DH, Kremastinos DT, Kranias EG. Human phospholamban null results in lethal dilated cardiomyopathy revealing a critical difference between mouse and human. *J Clin Invest* 2003; 111(6):869–876.

[8] Kobayashi M IH, Cheng XW Asano H, Hirashiki A, Unno K, Ohshima S,Yamada T, Murase Y, Kato ST, Obata K, Noda A, Nishizawa T, Isobe S, Nagata K, Matsubara T, Murohara T, Yokota M. Dobutamine stress testing as a diagnostic tool for evaluation of myocardial contractile reserve in asymptomatic or mildly symptomatic patients with dilated cardiomyopathy. *J Am Coll Cardiol Imaging* 2008; (6):718–726.

[9] Linck B, Boknik P, Eschenhagen T, Muller FU, Neumann J, Nose M, Jones LR, Schmitz W, Scholz H. Messenger RNA expression and immunological quantification of phospholamban and SR-Ca(2+)-ATPase in failing and nonfailing human hearts. *Cardiovasc Res* 1996; 31(4):625–632.

[10] Hasenfuss G. Alterations of calcium-regulatory proteins in heart failure. *Cardiovasc Res* 1998; 37(2):279–289.

[11] Kodama M, Kato K, Hirono S, Okura Y, Hanawa H, Yoshida T, Hayashi M, Tachikawa H, Kashimura T, Watanabe K, Aizawa Y. Linkage between mechanical and electrical alternans in patients with chronic heart failure. *J Cardiovasc Electrophysiol* 2004; 15(3):295–299.

[12] Radford MJ, Arnold JM, Bennett SJ, Cinquegrani MP, Cleland JG, Havranek EP, Heidenreich PA, Rutherford JD, Spertus JA, Stevenson LW, Goff DC, Grover FL, Malenka DJ, Peterson ED, Redberg RF. ACC/AHA key data elements and definitions for measuring the clinical management and outcomes of patients with chronic heart failure: a report of the American College of Cardiology/American Heart Association Task Force on Clinical Data Standards

(Writing Committee to Develop Heart Failure Clinical Data Standards): developed in collaboration with the American College of Chest Physicians and the International Society for Heart and Lung Transplantation: endorsed by the Heart Failure Society of America. *Circulation* 2005; 112(12):1888–1916.

3

MicroRNAs Telltale Effects on Signaling Networks in Cardiomyopathy

Manveen K. Gupta[2], Zhong-Hui Duan[1],
Sadashiva S. Karnik[2] and Sathyamangla V. Naga Prasad[2]
[1]Department of Computer Sciences, University of Akron, Akron, OH,
[2]Department of Molecular Cardiology, Lerner Research Institute,
Cleveland Clinic, Cleveland, OH,
USA

1. Introduction

MicroRNAs (miRNAs) are single-stranded, highly conserved, short non-coding RNAs (~ 22 nucleotides) regulating target gene expression by base pairing with specific sequences of target mRNAs (Ambros, 2004). miRNAs negatively regulate gene expression post-transcriptionally by suppressing translation and/or inducing mRNA degradation. Bioinfomatically, it is estimated that human genome may contain approximately 1000 miRNAs (Bartel, 2004; Berezikov et al., 2005; Griffiths-Jones et al., 2008) and consistently, additional miRNAs are continually being identified (Griffiths-Jones et al., 2006). miRNAs modulate the expression of target proteins in a non-canonical manner by binding to specific sequences regulating functional networks. Consequentially, a single miRNA might target hundreds of distinct genes or alternatively expression of a single coding gene can be regulated by many different miRNAs (Lewis et al., 2005; Miranda et al., 2006). Recent studies show the important role of miRNAs in the regulation of a variety of physiological functions ranging from stem cell differentiation to cardiac muscle development and stress (Krichevsky et al. 2006; Chen et al., 2006; Zhao et al., 2005; Pedersen et al., 2007; Kloosterman et al., 2007; Felli et al., 2005; Tay et al., 2008). Furthermore, aberrant expression of miRNAs has been found in various diseases including cancer, diabetes and cardiac hypertrophy/failure.

The binding specificity of miRNAs depend on complementary base pairing of ~ 7 nucleotide seed sequence region at the 5' end of the miRNA with the corresponding mRNA target. Another caveat that needs to be considered in the miRNA regulation is the miRNA sequences outside the 7 nucleotide seed region which pairs with the mRNA that may also play a role in determining the strength/efficacy of regulating the target mRNA. The binding of miRNAs to their cognate target mRNAs commonly results in decreased expression of target genes through translational repression or mRNA degradation (Fig. 1). Conversely, decreased expression of miRNAs will lead to increased target gene expression (Gregory et al., 2008).

This realm of knowledge has allowed for studies on miRNAs on their tissue specificity and disease specificity but critically little information is available with regards to temporal or spatial expression profiles of miRNAs in the heart. By and large studies have used micro-array analysis to identify altered miRNAs to define signature of altered miRNAs in a specific cardiac phenotype. As miRNAs target multiple proteins, these signatures have been used to predict the array of molecules altered. Over time sophisticated computational approaches have been developed that has lead to identification of previously unrecognized targets within disease pathways of interest (Ivanovska and Cleary, 2008; Gusev et al., 2007). Among the computational tools the most commonly used target prediction algorithms include DIANA-microT (Kiriakidou et al., 2004), miRanda (Griffiths-Jones et al., 2006), TargetScan (Lewis et al., 2003), TargetScanS (Lewis et al., 2005), PicTar (Krek et al., 2005) and PITA (Kertesz et al., 2007). These algorithms rely on criteria like conservation among species, seed complementarity, thermo-stability of miRNA-mRNA hybrids, delta G of target mRNA binding site, and multiple miRNA binding sites in the 3'UTR (cooperativity) to predict targets (Bartel, 2009; Cacchiarelli et al., 2008; Ivanovska and Cleary, 2008; Gusev et al., 2007). Thus, use of these algorithms provide hundreds of targets indicating that miRNA alteration in expression could have wide ranging effects on molecules belonging to multiple signaling pathways. It is important to note that target prediction with these algorithms remains challenging but these are the tools currently available in field to provide a window into understanding the role of miRNAs. These predicted targets can then be used as a platform for identifying signaling pathways and networks that are altered manifesting in the phenotype. Critically these bioinformatic tools are evolving with the field and are pivotal to understanding the global role of miRNAs in cardiomyopathy. Although miRNA regulation adds another layer of complexity to the already complex etiology, understanding the regulation could provide novel therapeutic strategies due to miRNAs ability to target multiple molecules. In this regard, the focus of our article is to provide an overview of altered miRNAs in cardiac stress and the available tools that could be used to understand their global implications.

2. miRNA generation

2.1 Genome distribution, miRNA processing and nuclear export

miRNAs are encoded by their own genes which are an integral part of cell's genetic make up and are evolutionarily conserved (Ambros, 2004; Bartel, 2004). miRNAs can be transcribed as polycistronic primary transcripts or as individual transcripts from intergenic regions, exon sequences of non-coding strand or intronic sequences (Kim and Nam, 2006; Altuvia, et al., 2005) (Fig. 1). Intronic miRNAs are generally transcribed coincidentally with the gene and excised by the splicing machinery from the larger gene transcript in which they are embedded (Rodriguez et al., 2004). Indeed, intronic miRNAs may represent a simple way for a protein-coding gene to regulate other protein-coding genes in a non-canonical manner. miRNAs are transcribed by the RNA polymerase II as a primary transcript several kilobases long characterized by stem-loop hairpin structures called pri-miRNAs that are 5' capped and a poly (A) to stabilize these pre-miRNAs similar to that of the traditional mRNAs (Lee et al., 2004). The generated pre-miRNA is processed in the nucleus and exported out through a regulated process. The stem-loop structures of pre-miRNAs are recognized by Drosha (a double-stranded specific RNase III) and its partner DGCR8 (a double stranded RNA binding protein) that cleave at the hair-pin base to release ~ 70-90 nucleotide stem-loop pri-miRNA precursor (Lee et al., 2003, 2004). In addition to this classical pathway, recent studies have identified alternate pathway wherein intronic pre-miRNA precursors "mirtrons" uses the cellular splicing machinery to bypass Drosha mediated processing (Ruby et al., 2007; Okamura et al., 2007) . The cleaved stem-loop pre-miRNA hairpins are exported into the cytoplasm by the exportin-5 (a Ran-GTP-dependent nuclear transport receptor) (Yi et al., 2003). The interaction of exportin-5 with the pre-miRNA 'minihelix motif' (~14 nucleotide stem and a short 30 nucleotide overhang) is thought to stabilize the pre-miRNAs (Yi et al., 2003; Filipowicz, 2005) manifesting in efficient transport.

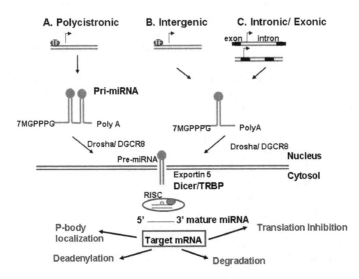

Fig. 1. MicroRNA (miRNA) genomic organization, biogenesis and function
Genomic distribution of miRNA genes. TF: transcription factor. (A) Clusters throughout the genome transcribed as polycistronic primary transcripts and subsequently cleaved into multiple miRNAs; (B) intergenic regions transcribed as independent transcriptional units; (C) intronic sequences of protein-coding or -non-coding transcription units or exonic sequences (black cylinders) of non-coding genes. Primary miRNAs(pri-miRNAs) transiently have a 7- methylguanosine (7mGpppG) cap and a poly(A) tail. The pri-miRNA is processed into a precursor miRNA (pre-miRNA) stem-loop of 60 nucleotides (nt) in length by the nuclear RNase III enzyme Drosha and its partner DiGeorge syndrome critical region gene 8 (DGCR8). Exportin-5 actively transports pre-miRNA into the cytosol, where it is processed by the Dicer RNaseIII enzyme, together with its partner TAR (HIV) RNA binding protein (TRBP), into mature, 22 nt-long double strand miRNAs. The RNA strand (in red) is recruited as a single-stranded molecule into the RNA-induced silencing (RISC) effector complex and assembled through processes that are dependent on Dicer and other double strand RNA binding domain proteins, as well as on members of the Argonaute family. Mature miRNAs then guide the RISC complex to the 3' untranslated regions (3'-UTR) of the complementary messenger RNA (mRNA) targets and repress their expression by several mechanisms: repression of mRNA translation, destabilization of mRNA transcripts through cleavage, de-adenylation, and localization in the processing body (P-body), where the miRNA-targeted mRNA can be sequestered from the translational machinery and degraded or stored for subsequent use. Nuclear localization of mature miRNAs has also been described and is a novel mechanism of action for miRNAs.

2.2 Generation of mature miRNA, activation and target recognition

The pre-miRNA is processed into a mature miRNA of ~22 nucleotides long by another double stranded RNase III called the Dicer (Hutvagner et al., 2001). Single stranded RNA is assembled into a RNA-inducing silencing complex (RISC) with the help of Dicer, TAR (HIV) RNA binding protein (TRBP), and dsRNA-binding proteins of the argonaute (AGO) family (Chapman and Carrington, 2007; Filipowicz, 2005; Schwarz et al., 2003; MacRae et al., 2008; Okamura et al., 2004). Additional factors have also been isolated and implicated (Chapman and Carrington, 2007; Filipowicz, 2005; Schwarz et al., 2003; MacRae et al., 2008; Okamura et al., 2004) to be a part of RISC complex bringing about miRNA-mediated silencing of gene expression that could be either a translational repression or degradation of mRNA. miRNAs recognize their target mRNAs through specific interaction of the 5' end 'seed' region (2–8 nt from the 5' end) and the complementary sequences of conserved target mRNAs (Bartel, 2004). Since only a few miRNAs have perfect complementarity to the target mRNAs leading to degradation, majority of the miRNAs have imperfect match resulting in translational repression (Nilsen, 2007). Another caveat in the miRNA silencing dynamics is the ability of multiple miRNAs to bind to the same mRNA initiating translational repression with different potencies. Repressed mRNAs are sequestered from translational machinery, degraded or stored for subsequent use in large macroscopic cytoplasmic foci, named processing bodies (P-bodies) upon silencing by miRNAs. The P-bodies contain a wide range of enzymes involved in RNA turnover, including de-capping enzymes, de-adenylases and exonucleases (Eulalio et al., 2007). In addition to their cytoplasmic role, miRNAs with nuclear localization sequence have been identified demonstrating their role in transcriptional control of gene expression (Chapman and Carrington, 2007; Volpe et al., 2002; Zilberman, et al., 2003; Aravin et al., 2007; Yu et al., 2008; Hwang et al., 2007; Calin et al., 2007).

3. miRNAs and cardiac development

3.1 miRNA expression in cardiac development

Studies have shown that miRNA mediated fine tuning leads to critical cell lineage commitment and embryonic tissue development (Latronico, et al., 2007; Farh et al., 2005; Ivey et al., 2008). Consistent with the role of miRNA in development, deletion of Dicer leads to embryonic lethality resulting from defects in cardiogenesis due to deficiencies in miRNAs biogenesis (Giraldez et al., 2006; Ebert et al., 2007). In tune with complex process of cardiogenesis many miRNAs are shown to be involved and the selection of miRNAs enriched during the differentiation of mouse embryonic stem cells to cardiomyocytes are detailed in Table 1 (Lakshmipathy et al., 2007; Thum et al., 2007). Significant increase in miRNA expression with development shows that miRNAs play an important role in early embryonic patterning and orchestrating organogenesis (Ivey et al., 2008). Expression pattern of miRNA-1 and -133 show that these two miRNAs play a key role in skeletal muscle proliferation and differentiation (Chen et al., 2006). Specifically, miRNA-1 promotes myogenesis by targeting histone deacetylase (HDAC4), a transcriptional repressor while miRNA-133 enhances myoblast proliferation by repressing serum response factor (SRF) (Zhao et al., 2005, 2007; Kwon et al., 2005; Niu et al., 2007). In this context, loss of function of miRNA-1 in Drosophila results in embryonic/larval lethality due to altered sarcomeric gene expression and increased number of undifferentiated muscle progenitors (Kwon et al., 2005). Where as miRNA-1 gain of function results in embryonic lethality due to insufficient numbers of cardioblasts indicating that cardiogenesis and differentiation is a spatio-temporal process tightly regulated by miRNA-1 mediated by cardiac transcription factor Hand2 (Zhao et al., 2005; Srivastava et al., 1997). Another important component of miRNA expression is the Dicer mediated generation of miRNA during development. Dicer expression during development determines miRNA expression and its regulation. Indeed, Dicer-deficient animals fail to synthesize new miRNAs resulting in embryonic lethality in zebrafish (Giraldez et al., 2005) and mice (Bernstein et al., 2003). More importantly cardiac specific deletion of Dicer results in aberrant cardiac contractile protein expression and severe sarcomere disarray, leading to progressive dilated cardiomyopathy (DCM), failure and postnatal lethality (Chen et al., 2008).

Downregulated miRs		Upregulated miRs		Species
Development	Disease	Development	Disease	
	1, 7d*, 10a/b, 26a/b, 29a/b/c, 30a-3p/a-5p/b/ c/d/e/e*, 30e, 93, 126-5p, 133a/b, 139, 149, 150, 151, 155, 181b, 185, 187, 194, 218, 292-5p, 373, 378, 451, 466, 486	1, 12, 20, 24b, 24, 29a/c, 133, 143, 152, 193, 206a/b, 29c, 30, 208, 298, 335	10b, 15b, 17-5p, 18b, 19a/b, 20b, 21, 23a/b, 24, 25, 27a/b, 29a, 31, 103, 106a, 107, 125b, 126, 127, 140*, 142-3p, 146, 153, 154, 195, 199a/a*/b, 200a, 208, 210, 211, 214, 217, 218, 221, 222, 330, 341, 351, let-7b/c, 424	Mouse
	16, 17-5p, 19b, 22, 23b, 24, 27a, 30a-5p/b/c/e-5p, 107, 126, 130b, 135a, 136, 148a, 150, 182, 186, 192, 199a*, 218, 299-5p, 302b*, 302c*, 325, 339, 342, 452/ *, 494, 495, 497, 499, 507, 512-5p, 515-5p, 520d*/h, 520, 523, 526b/b*, 378,7	1, 20, 21, 26a, 92, 127, 129, 130a, 199b, 200a, 335, 424	1, 7a/b/c/d/e/f, 10b, 17-3p, 21, 23, 24, 26a, 28, 29a/b/c, 32, 34b, 98, 106b, 125a/b, 126*, 129/-3p, 130a, 132, 195, 196a, 199a/b, 200c, 204, 205, 208, 210, 211, 212, 213, 214, 215, 292-3p, 294, 295, 296, 297, 300, 302a, 320, 322, 330, 331, 333, 340, 341, 343, 365, 367, 372, 373, 377, 381, 382, 423, 424, 429, 432, 500, 520c, 525*	Human

Upregulated (enriched) miRNA during mouse cardiac development as shown by Srivastava and colleagues. Data about altered miRNAs in heart failure and animal models of heart disease originate from different results published earlier. Note that in some cases results were not consistent between the different laboratories.

Table 1. Summary of regulated microRNAs (miRNAs) in cardiac development and disease.

3.2 Regulation of miRNA transcription

Understanding transcriptional regulation of miRNAs is critical as expression of miRNAs is a major determinant of miRNA dependent regulatory mechanisms. As miRNAs are transcribed like other genes, they are regulated by transcription factors and expression of transcription factors determines the miRNA expression. SRF is a cardiac enriched transcription factor that regulates sarcomere organization in the heart and SRF expression follows a restrictive pattern during development (Olson and Schneider, 2003; Niu et al., 2007; Barron et al., 2005). SRF expression is very important as multiple SRF binding sites have been identified in promoters of genes regulating contractility, cell movement, and growth signaling (Sun et al., 2006; Zhang et al., 2005). Consistent with the role of SRF in cardiac development, several miRNAs have been identified to contain SRF binding sites in their promoter including miRNA-1-1, -1-2, -21, -206, -214, -133 and others (Niu et al., 2007). In addition, studies have unequivocally have shown that miRNA-1-1, -1-2 and -133 are regulated by SRF transcription factor alone or in conjunction with co-factors like GATA5, MyoD, Nkx 2.5 or MEF2 (Fig. 2) (Zhao et al., 2005; Chen et al., 2006; Niu et al., 2007; Rao et al., 2006; Xiao et al., 2007). It is important to note that the outlined co-factors of SRF by themselves can act as transcriptional regulators in their own right increasing complexity of regulation. For example, MEF2 along with MyoD is known to regulate miRNA-1-2/133a-1 in myotomes during embryogenesis and all skeletal fibers in adulthood (Liu et al., 2007).

3.3 miRNA expression patterns

miRNA expression is greatly enriched in a tissue/cell-specific manner indicating unique signature patterns for each type. This enrichment and signature pattern suggests that miRNAs play a critical role in regulating and maintaining the specific cellular phenotype which is of essence in an organ with diverse cell/tissue types contributing to effective functioning. In this regard, heart as an organ contains many "non-cardiomyocyte" cell types like endothelial cells, smooth muscle cells and fibroblasts and each of which have distinct function in the heart. Consistently, differential enrichment of miRNAs are observed in cardiomyocyte versus cardiac fibroblasts indicating important role in cellular specificity (Landgraf et al., 2007; Kuehbacher et al., 2007; Harris et al., 2008). Although specific miRNA enrichments are being found in different cell types (Kuehbacher et al., 2007; Harris et al., 2008), lot more work needs to be done to determine contribution of miRNAs towards regulation of global networking pathways that defines specific fingerprints for each cell type. The current studies have all been focused on one or two miRNAs (Chen et al., 2006; Gregory et al., 2008; Harris et al., 2008) which by themselves may not be sufficient to determine a cellular phenotype indicating requirement of more comprehensive studies on specific miRNAs signature for cellular phenotype.

4. miRNAs and cardiac disease

The heart is responsive to physiological stimuli or pathological stress and accordingly undergoes remodeling to meet the demand (Catalucci et al., 2008). Following stress, the heart undergoes extensive remodeling in the form of physiological or pathological hypertrophy defined as an augmentation of ventricular mass due to increased cardiomyocyte size. Cardiac hypertrophy is characterized by initial compensatory mechanisms that adapt the heart towards sustaining the cardiac output. However, this process is only an initial 'adaptive' response and chronic exposure to stress eventually leads to impaired function that, in many cases, progresses to failure. This maladaptive change is accompanied by alterations in the underlying molecular map including a switch in the gene expression program leading to reexpression of fetal genes (Catalucci et al., 2008; Thum et al., 2007). The involvement of miRNAs in this pathological process has been recognized and is thought to be integral 'switch' in the gene expression program. Intense efforts have been put into identifying miRNAs altered in pathology and evolving signature of deregulated miRNAs identified cardiac disease is detailed in Table 2.

4.1 Myocardial hypertrophy, remodeling, and heart failure

Cardiac remodeling is characterized by structural alterations of myocardial tissue, modification of the extracellular matrix, and reshaping of left ventricle geometry and performance (Catalucci et al., 2008; Dash et al., 2001). The presence of chronic stress results in deleterious remodeling.

microRNA	Experiment	Phenotype
miRNA-1-2	Mouse knockout	Cardiac septal defects, hyperplasia and delay between atrial an ventricular repolarizations (PR interval) was shortened (Zhao et al.,2007)
miRNA-1	Neonatal cardiomyocyte	Inhibits FBS/endothelin/isoproterenol overexpression mediated hypertrophy (Ikeda et al., 2009)
miRNA-21	TAC and isoproterenol induced hypertrophy	Upregulated in compensatory hypertrophy and reduced in decompensation (Sayed et al., 2008)
	Neonatal cardiomyocyte overexpression	Outgrowths in the cardiomyocytes accompanied by connections via gap junctions (Sayed et al., 2008)
	Transgenic cardiomyocyte-specific expression	No specific phenotype indicating minimal role for miRNA21 in cardiomyocytes (Thum et al., 2008)
	Cardiac fibroblast overexpression	Anti-apoptotic (Thum et al., 2008)
miRNA-23a	Antagomir infusion using minipumps	Isoproterenol-induced cardiac hypertrophy is attenuated with miRNA23a antagomirs (Lin et al., 2009)
	Neonatal cardiomyocyte overexpression	Induces hypertrophy (van Rooij et al., 2006;, Lin et al., 200955)
miRNA-23b	Neonatal cardiomyocyte overexpression	Induces hypertrophy (van Rooij et al., 2006)
miRNA-24	Antagomir infusion using minipumps / Neonatal cardiomyocyte overexpression	Isoproterenol-induced cardiac hypertrophy is not altered (Lin et al., 2009) / Induces hypertrophy (van Rooij et al., 2006)
miRNA-27	Antagomir infusion using minipumps	Isoproterenol-induced cardiac hypertrophy is not attenuated (Lin et al., 2009)
miRNA-92	miRNA inhibitor treatment of neonatal cardiomyocytes	Minimal effect on fetal gene expression (Sucharov et al., 2008)
miRNA-100	miRNA mimic treatment of neonatal cardiomyocytes	Results in re-expression of fetal genes (Sucharov et al., 2008)
miRNA-129	Neonatal cardiomyocyte transfection	Induces hypertrophy (Thum et al., 2007)
miRNA-133	Neonatal cardiomyocyte transfection	Inhibited hypertrophy (Care et al., 2007)
	Antagomir infusion using minipumps	Induces cardiac hypertrophy (Care et al., 2007)
	Double knockout of miRNA-133-a/b	Embryonic myocyte proliferation, septal defects, and surviving adults have severe dilated cardiomyopathy (Liu et al., 2008)
	Transgenic cardiomyocyte specific expression	Inhibitor of cardiomyocyte proliferation (Liu et al., 2008)
	Transgenic cardiomyocyte-specific expression subjected to TAC	Cardiac hypertrophy is not inhibited, but decreases myocardial fibrosis and cardiomyocyte apoptosis (Matkovich et al., 2010)
miRNA-195	Neonatal cardiomyocyte overexpression	Induces hypertrophy (van Rooij et al., 2006)
	Transgenic cardiomyocyte specific expression	Induces cardiac hypertrophy and dilated cardiomyopathy (van Rooij et al., 2006)
miRNA-199a	Neonatal cardiomyocyte overexpression	Cardiomyocyte enlargement (van Rooij et al., 2006)]
miRNA-208	Knockout mice subjected to TAC or bred to mouse model of hypertrophy	No hypertrophic response in both the cases [van Rooij et al., 2007)
miRNA-214	Neonatal cardiomyocyte overexpression	Cardiomyocyte hypertrophy (van Rooij et al., 2006)
	Transgenic cardiomyocyte specific expression	No phenotype (van Rooij et al., 2006)

Table 2. miRNAs experimentally determined to play a role in cardiac hypertrophy/ cardiomyopathy

Multiple studies have been carried out to reveal important roles of miRNAs in cardiac hypertrophy and heart failure. Studies have found that a unique set of miRNAs are upregulated, downregulated or unaltered during the adaptive response of the heart to stress stimuli (Latronico et al., 2007). Furthermore, unique subset of miRNAs are known to be altered within the various etiologies of heart failure indicating significant role of miRNAs in these disease states (Sucharo et al., 2008). Consistent with the reexpression of fetal gene program, a high degree of similarity has been found between the miRNA expression pattern occurring in failing human hearts and those observed in the 12- 14 week-old hearts (Thum et al., 2007). Approximately, 80% of the analyzed miRNAs are similarly altered in failing adult and fetal human hearts compared to non-failing hearts. Multiple miRNAs have been implicated in cardiomyocyte hypertrophy and studies have consistently found upregulation of miRNA-21, -23a, -23b, -24, -195, -199a and miR-214 and downregulation of miRNA-1, -7, - 133 and 378 (Naga Prasad and Karnik, 2010). Many of these miRNAs have been tested for hypertrophic response in neonatal cardiomyocytes. Concordant data from human and mice samples indicate that miRNAs may be involved in common pathway mediating hypertrophic response (Thum et al., 2007; van Rooij et al., 2006; Chen et al., 2008; Ikeda et al., 2007; Tatsuguchi et al., 2007; Sayed et al., 2007; Cheng et al., 2007) .

Among the miRNAs altered in various cardiac etiologies, some of them have been studied indepth and these include miRNA-1, -21, -133 and -208. It is well known that miRNA-1 is downregulated with a week of transverse aortic banding and its expression is inversely correlated with cardiac hypertrophy (Table 2) (Sayed et al., 2007; Catalucci et al., 2008; Ikeda et al., 2009, Naga Prasad et al., 2009 after al., 2009)). Similarly, Care et al., observed impaired expression of both miR-1 and miR-133 in patients with hypertrophic cardiomyopathy and atrial dilatation as well as in 3 different murine models of cardiac hypertrophy (Catalucci et al., 2008). In vitro cellular overexpression of miRNA-133 resulted in suppression of protein synthesis and block in hypertrophic response. Contrastingly, utilization of a decoy for miRNA-133 resulted in cellular hypertrophy and in vivo administration resulted in significant myocardial hypertrophy associated with reexpression of the fetal gene program (Catalucci et al., 2008). Some of targets of miRNA-133 have been validated and many are still being validated to provide evidence of miRNA-133 targeting multiple molecules to bring about hypertrophic response. miRNA-133 is encoded by 133a-1 and –2 and deletion of individual miRNA have no obvious cardiac abnormalities but combined deletion results in severe cardiac malformations with embryonic and post-natal lethality (Care et al., 2007). In contrast, overexpression of miRNA-133a results in embryonic lethality (E 15.5) caused by ventricular septal defected and impaired cardiomyocyte proliferation resulting in thinning of ventricular walls unable to meet hemodynamic needs (Care et al., 2007). These studies reveal that miRNA-133 plays a key role in myocardial development, hypertrophy and function. miRNA-208 is unique as it is a cardiac-specific miRNA encoded within the intron of α-myosin heavy chain (α-MHC) gene. miR-208 knockout mice are viable and do not show any obvious cardiac phenotype, but they fail to undergo stress-induced cardiac remodeling, hypertrophic growth, and α-MHC upregulation following transverse aortic constriction (Table 2) (van Rooij et al., 2007). It is believed that miRNA-208 regulation of this process involves α-MHC alterations balancing α-MHC.

While miRNA-208 mediates cardiac function by cardiomyocyte specific expression, miRNA-21 regulates cardiac function by its expression in both myocytes as well as cardiac fibroblasts. Recent studies (Thum et al., 2008) have shown progressive upregulation of miR-21 during late stages of heart failure, with an expression profile restricted exclusively to cardiac fibroblasts (Table 2). Upregulation of miR-21 was shown to be responsible for increased extracellular signal-regulated kinase (ERK) signaling through inhibition of its target, spry1 (sprouty 1), an inhibitor of the ERK/extracellular signal-regulated kinase pathway. These studies suggest that miRNA-21 expression results in increased fibroblast survival and reduced interstitial fibrosis independent of cardiomyocyte loss that may provide protective effects (Thum et al., 2008). Likewise, it has been (van Rooij et al., 2008) recently demonstrated that downregulation of the fibroblast-enriched miRNA-29 family in fibrotic areas surrounding a cardiac infarct is responsible for the regulation of mRNAs that encode a multitude of proteins involved in fibrosis such as collagens, fibrillins, and elastins. In addition to these miRNAs, we have recently shown that 8 miRNAs are differentially expressed in human dilated cardiomyopathy (DCM) (Naga Prasad et al., 2009). The miRNA-1, -29b, -7, and -378 were significantly down-regulated in the DCM samples compared with non-failing controls. In contrast, miRNA-214, -342, -125b and -181b were significantly upregulated in DCM compared with non-failing controls. These studies identified miRNA-7 and -378 as novel miRNAs which are significantly downregulated during end stage cardiac dysfunction whose role in cardiac pathology remains to be determined.

4.2 Arrhythmia
One of the well known contributing factors for heart failure are the changes in ion channel function and expression leading to electrophysiological remodeling in both atria and

ventricles. Although the role of miRNAs with regard to arrhythmia is not yet well established, recent evidence supports their role in the induction of arrhythmia. Expression of miRNA-1 by viral transduction following myocardial infarction in rat resulted in significant enlargement of the QRS complex, prolongation of the QT interval, and an increased incidence of arrhythmias (Yang et al., 2007). Conversely, a low incidence of fatal arrhythmias was obtained when antisense for miRNA-1 was used. These studies further identified that miRNA-1 targets GJA1 (connexin 43) and KCNJ2 a critical K+ channel subunit both of which are required for maintenance of membrane potential. Consistently, miRNA-1 and -2 double knockout mice that survived until birth had high incidence of electrophysiological abnormalities resulting in sudden death (Zhao et al., 2007). In addition to miRNA-1, miRNA-133 has been implicated in contributing towards cardiac disease by altering electrophysiological remodeling. In particular, downregulation of miRNA-133 in hypertrophic hearts has been associated with an increase in ion channels HCN2/HCN4 which when upregulated, enhance automaticity and the development of arrhythmia (Luo et al., 2008). Moreover, in a model of diabetic cardiomyopathy, overexpression of miR-133 has been shown to downregulate the ERG (ether a-go-go-related gene) with consequent QT prolongation responsible for arrhythmias (Xiao et al., 2007). Although only two miRNAs have been extensively studied with regards to arrhythmia, it is only matter of time that more miRNAs will be found to play a critical contributing role in complex electrophysiological remodeling that may cause heart failure and sudden death.

5. Cardiac microRNA targets

5.1 Identification of microRNA targets

To comprehensively understand the miRNA function and potential therapeutic use in heart disease, identification and validation of miRNA targets is of fundamental importance. A large number of bioinformatic methods have been developed to predict miRNA targets based on the assumption that the 5'-nucleotides of miRNAs are most critical for target recognition (Lai, 2002; Lewis et al., 2003). Such methods easily result in the prediction of hundreds of potential miRNA targets which are difficult to validate using conventional means. Target accessibility is an important factor for miRNA target repression as nearly all the miRNA binding sites reside in the 3'-UTRs of target mRNA that is located in the unstable regions of mRNA structure calculated on the basis of free energy predictions and RNA structure (Zhao et al., 2005; Lee et al., 2002). Although various target prediction algorithms use the sequence complimentarity as a major determinant, newer tools are being developed as our understanding of the miRNA biology improves. In addition to the previous tools a novel miRNA target identification algorithms are being developed that also include target accessibility by evaluation of energy states of sequences flanking the miRNA target (Lewis et al., 2003; Lai, 2002). Such a tool has become a necessity as previous prediction algorithms seem to have higher levels of false positives. In this context, however it remains to be determined whether this stringent approach may identify less false-positive targets without missing others (Bruneau, 2005). A potential relationship between altered miRNA expression and changes in messenger RNA expression profiles in failing human left ventricles has recently been explored (Thum et al., 2007). Computational prediction identified multiple potential target genes with at least one binding site for highly upregulated miRNAs during heart failure. In contrast, transcriptome analysis conducted in parallel showed that theoretically predicted target genes were upregulated, demonstrating no obvious preponderance of gene repression (Thum et al., 2007). This obvious disconnect could be because the analysis was carried out at transcriptome level and not at a proteome level. It is potentially possible that the target proteins are significantly altered in response to miRNA alterations. The observed increase in miRNA transcripts could be due to feed back mechanism of reduced protein levels of the respective target proteins. These observations bring to focus our incomplete understanding of mRNA targeting by miRNA and we still have lot more to learn with regards to determining the underlying mechanisms regulating these processes. However, simultaneous use of current prediction algorithms and proteomic analysis should be able to provide a realistic idea on the target proteins. An important caveat that needs consideration is the sensitivity of proteome analysis which may still miss out on proteins altered at lower potency by miRNAs.

5.2 MicroRNA targets in cardiac disease

Despite the shortcomings of the tools available to accurately predict the targets, various studies have used traditional and non-traditional tools to verify and validate the targets of miRNAs. In many cases the targets have been identified in the knock-out or overexpression system which provides validity to the targets and it is further strengthened by the function of the target protein. We quote some of the examples below that provide a view point the way studies are currently being carried to unequivocally show that a specific protein is a miRNA target. Targeted deletion of miR-1-2 in mice causes 50% lethality mainly because of ventricular wall defects (Zhao et al., 2007) along with arrhythmias leading to sudden death. This has been linked to upregulation of Irx5, which is a target of miR-1 (Zhao et al., 2007). Conversely, it is also known that miRNA-1 expression resulted in repression of target KCNJ2 and GJA1 channels that code for the main potassium channel subunit Kir2.1 and connexin (Yang et al., 2007). This to a certain degree explains higher degree of arrhythmias found in patients with coronary artery disease where miRNA-1 expression is elevated and similar elevation is observed in mice following myocardial infarction. In contrast to these findings our studies in end-stage dilated cardiomyopathy and studies by others on aortic stenosis have found reduction in miRNA-1 expression (Naga Prasad et al., 2009). A preview of these studies show varied expression pattern of miRNA-1 based on the variations of diseases, biopsy locations, technical differences, or altered cellular composition of the biopsies. This indicates a need for appreciation of the differences so that in future a much more representative pattern develops for each of the altered miRNAs. In this context, miRNA-1 targets have been very well summarized that includes Ras GTPase-activating protein (RasGAP), cyclin-dependent kinase 9 (Cdk9), Ras homolog enriched in brain (Rheb), and fibronectin (Latronico et al., 2007).

On a similar note, miRNA-133 targets have also been well studied and they have been identified using in vitro and in vivo techniques (Care et al., 2007). They include Cdc42 (implicated in cytoskeletal modifications during cardiac remodelling), Rho-A (a GTP–GDP-binding molecule, also critical for hypertrophy), and NELF-A/WHSC2 (a nuclear factor involved in heart genesis). While Rho-A and Cdc42 have already been established as fundamental factors for cell growth, cytoskeletal reorganization, and regulation of contractility in cardiomyocytes, (Brown et al., 2006; Ke et al., 2004) the role of NELF-A/WHSC2 in cardiac hypertrophy is yet to be defined. Transduction of cardiomyocytes both in vitro and in vivo with an adenoviral vector containing a Whsc2 transgene resulted in protein synthesis inhibition, but induced the fetal gene program and upregulation of Rho-A, (Care et al., 2007) supporting the postulation that WHSC2 could play a selective role in hypertrophy. In addition

to targeting molecules modulating cardiac hypertrophy, miRNA-133 also targets molecules regulating cardiac conductance. In the diabetic heart, upregulation of miR-133 expression results in downregulation of protein expression of the ether-a-go-go-related gene (ERG), encoding the rapid delayed rectifier potassium channel (Xiao et al., 2007) .
The studies on miRNA-133 targets are interesting suggesting a lot needs to be understood in terms of alteration of these miRNAs in stress results in a unique pathological phenotype. Such a view is further supported by studies on miRNA-208 which is expressed specifically in the cardiomyocytes (van Rooij et al., 2007). A major target of miRNA-208 is thrap1 [thyroid hormone receptor (THR)-associated protein 1] and reduction in the expression of miRNA-208 results in loss of negative regulation on THRAP-1 (van Rooij et al., 2007). The resulting increase in THRAP 1 protein affects the THR-regulated expression of α-MHC and β-MHC, which are inversely regulated through a positive and negative thyroid hormone response element on their promoters. This shift in expression is thought to be the underlying factor for the blunted response to pressure overload in miR-208 knockout mice. In this context, our studies have shown that miRNA-7 is significantly down-regulated in end-stage human heart failure and upon TAC in mice and consistently its targets ERBB2 (epidermal growth factor receptor 2) and COL1A (Collagen 1) are upregulated (Naga Prasad et al., 2009). The above discussed studies are only a representative window on plethora of studies identifying targets for various miRNAs altered in conditions of cardiac stress. These studies have been discussed with an aim to provides a bird eye view of the complexity in regulation of target protein expression by miRNAs and to appreciate the diverse effects miRNA alteration can have in a pathology accounting for the phenotype.

6. Specific molecules and network pathways altered in cardiac disease

In this section we will specifically discuss the study initiated by our group to uncover the specific set of molecules and pathways altered during end stage human heart failure. Our published study comprehensively showed alterations in eight miRNAs which are significantly altered in heart failure out of which two new miRNAs that are yet to be implicated in cardiac pathophysiology. We have built signaling pathway networks using predicted targets for the miRNAs and identified nodal molecules that control these networks. Genome-wide profiling of miRNAs was performed using custom-designed miRNA microarray followed by validation on an independent set of samples. To gain an unbiased global perspective on regulation by altered miRNAs, predicted targets of eight miRNAs were analyzed using the Ingenuity Pathways Analysis network algorithm to build signaling networks and identify nodal molecules. The majority of nodal molecules identified in our analysis were targets of altered miRNAs and well known regulators of cardiovascular signaling. A heart failure gene expression data base was used to analyze changes in the expression patterns for these target nodal molecules (Naga Prasad et al., 2009). Indeed, expression of nodal molecules was altered in heart failure and inversely correlated to miRNA changes validating our analysis. Importantly, using network analysis we were successful in identification of a limited number of key functional targets that may regulate expression of the myriad proteins in heart failure and could be potential therapeutic targets. Furthermore, we have been able to independently see these 2 new miRNAs mir-7 and -378 in TAC mice hearts (Naga Prasad et al., 2009). We have shown miRNA-7 and -378 to be downregulated in the end stage human heart failure and targets of miRNA-7, ERBB2 and Col1A to be upregulated. miRNA-7-1 is encoded by the intron-1 of the HNRNPk gene. Similarly, we found miRNA-378 target SLC2A to be upregulated. Out of 1785 predicated targets, 1716 could be mapped to signaling networks in the IPATM, and 995 predicated targets were found to be network-eligible. The 995 network-eligible candidates mapped to 43 networks that are predicted to be involved in the cross-talk with the peripheral molecules bridging different networks. A representative network with NFkB, a known mediator in cardiac dysfunction (Naga Prasad et al., 2009) as a central node, is shown in Fig. 2 wherein the members that network with NFkB are targets for the miRNAs 1, 29b, 125b, 181b 214, 342, and 378. As individual miRNA acts on each target, the net effect on the node would be the collective influence of all the members connected to the central node, NFkB (Fig. 2) Based on this consideration, we predicted that the complete NFkB regulatory signaling network (Fig. 2) would be significantly down-regulated in DCM since molecules in this network are predicted targets for up-regulated miRNAs 125b, 181b, 214, and 243.

To directly evaluate whether nodal molecules are potential targets for altered miRNAs, immunoblotting studies in the end-stage human heart failure samples revealed an inverse co-relation with the level of respective miRNAs (Fig. 3). Immunoblotting showed ERBB2, HDAC4, COL1, MMP2, and TIMP2 were significantly up-regulated in human DCM (Fig. 3) and were inversely correlated to the down-regulation of their respective miRNAs. In contrast, STAT3 and E2F3 are down-regulated, consistent with the observation of up-regulation of their respective miRNAs suggesting that expression of these molecules may be regulated by miRNAs. Interestingly, we did not observe changes in expression levels of RB1 or EZH2 (Fig. 4) despite being predicted targets for miRNAs consistent with our data.

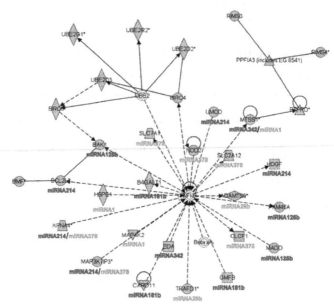

Fig. 2. A representative network showing NF-κB as high connectivity node: The hub is the center of the web of signaling connections and NF-κB is connected to nearly all the molecules in the network. Altered miRNAs in end-stage heart failure are overlaid with their respective predicted targets. miRNA represented in green are downregulated and in red are upregulated in end-stage human dilated cardiomyopathy. Importantly, NF-κB is not a predicted target to any of the altered miRNAs in DCM, yet it could be regulated by alterations in miRNA targets.

7. miRNA databases and computational tools

In recent years, many miRNA database systems have been developed and each of the databases has unique capabilities as they distinguish themselves by the types of data collected, the organization principles, and sources of the data contents. Therefore, it is important for researchers to use all of them to make an informed decision regarding execution of their experimental plan. These databases provide valuable resources to the research community towards understanding the functions of miRNAs in gene regulation. Critically, these databases contain miRNA sequences, annotations and nomenclature, miRNA targets and their relationships, as well as in some cases miRNA expression profiles in different cell types and tissues.

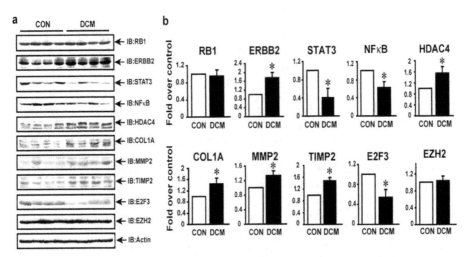

Fig. 3. Immunoblotting in end stage human heart failure *a*, Western immunoblotting analysis was carried out on nonfailinghuman hearts (*CON*, controls; *n*=8), and hearts from patients diagnosed with DCM (*n*=8). 170 microgram of myocardial lysate was resolved with SDS-polyacrylamide gel and immunoblotted (*IB*) with respective antibodies. The blots were stripped and re-probed multiple times with various antibodies, including beta-actin antibody that was used to ensure equal loading. *b*, densitometric analysis in the DCM samples is represented as fold over nonfailing controls.*, $p < 0.001$ control *versus* DCM.

miRBase (Griffiths-Jones et al., 2008) and Rfam (Gardner et al.,) are two major databases containing miRNA sequences and their annotations. miRBase database is an online repository for miRNA sequences and annotations that provides naming service for new miRNA genes isolated by researchers prior to publication. As of April 2011, miRBase contains 16772 mRNA entries from 153 species. Each entry represents a predicted hairpin portion of a miRNA transcript with information on the location and sequence of the mature miRNA as well as functional information/references. In this regard, Rfam database contains information about non-coding RNA families and annotations for family of RNA genes. As of June 2011, Rfam contains 1973 RNA families annotating over 2,756,313 regions in 1,723 unique species. Each family in Rfam is represented by multiple sequence alignments, its consensus secondary structures, and the associated probabilistic covariance models. In addition, Rfam coordinates a community annotation system providing access through Wikipedia allowing researchers to update entries and create families in the database.

An essential aspect of the functional analysis of miRNAs is the annotation of their targets. Increasing number of miRNA target genes are being identified and confirmed experimentally and simultaneously numerous target prediction algorithms are being developed to enhance the certainty of prediction. miRNA target prediction data base TargetScan (Lewis et al., 2003) predicts miRNA targets in mammals by searching for the presence of conserved 8-mer and 7-mer sites that match the seed region of the miRNA. The criteria for prediction and ranking include stringent seed sequence base pairing, untranslated region (UTR) context, the degree of target sequence conservation across the range of species and finally the thermodynamic stability of the predicted pairings. In addition to TargetScan, there are also several other miRNA target prediction algorithms like PicTar (Lall et al., 2006), MiRanda (John et al., 2004) , EMBL (Stark et al., 2005). They all adopt similar criteria (of rigorous seed pairing, site number, site type and context, likelihood of preferential conservation, and predicted site accessibility) for the target prediction. Historically, during the early phases of target prediction algorithm development, the predicted targets would vary remarkably with many non-overlapping predictions. But with time, utilization of similar criteria has significantly reduced the discrepancies with many overlaps of predicted targets. Such cross-references across the data bases for the miRNA targets is provided by miRecords. This computational tool provides an integrated view of experimentally validated miRNA targets and displays predicted targets generated by 11 established miRNA target prediction programs.

Since targets for many miRNAs are being identified, there is an ongoing simultaneous effort to develop databases that exclusively provides information on validated miRNA targets like TarBase (Sethupathy et al., 2006) and miRTarBase. TarBase database collects manually curated and experimentally supported miRNA targets in animal species, plants and viruses. It includes more than 1300 targets and each target is described by the miRNA it binds, the experiments that tested this relationship and the link to citation. Database miRTarBase (Hsu et al.,) curates 3576 experimentally validated microRNA-target interactions between 657 microRNAs and 2297 target genes among 17 species. In order to provide a disease perspective on the role of miRNA and their targets in pathology, a unique database miR2Disease [miR2Disease] has been generated. miR2Disease (Jiang et al., 2009) documents 1939 curated miRNA-disease relationships between 299 human miRNAs and 94 human diseases. Each entry in the database contains information on the miRNA ID, the disease name, validated targets, expression patterns of the miRNA, a brief description of the miRNA-disease relationship and citation.

Another important issue the readers need to appreciate is that despite the knowledge that there may be 1000 potential miRNA genes in the human genome, all of them have not yet been experimentally validated. These miRNA encoding gene predictions come from the sequence based curation of the genome to determine whether a specific DNA sequence characteristically fits the requirement for encoding a miRNA. RepTar (Elefant et al.,) is one such database that curates genome-wide predicted miRNAs of human and mouse. Furthermore, it can also predict cellular targets of human and mouse viral miRNAs. In addition to the miRNA sequence and target databases, a growing number of entries have been recorded at gene expression databases such as Gene Expression Omnibus (GEO) (Barrett et al.,) at NCBI and ArrayExpress (Brazma et al., 2006) Archive at EBI.

Although we are a long way away from validating all the predicted targets of altered miRNAs in heart failure, the predicted targets provide us a window to assess the global signaling pathways that could potentially be altered by the miRNAs in the heart failure. We have used this idea to build signaling networks of predicted targets of miRNAs altered in human heart failure which involves the role of miRNA target interaction with the biological pathways which ultimately generate the phenotype. A well known web-based tool is the Ingenuity Pathway Analysis (IPA) which is commonly used to model, analyze, and understand biological data derived from mRNA/miRNA gene expression arrays, SNP microarrays, proteomics, as well as small scale experiments. The core of IPA is its knowledge database on genes, proteins, chemicals, and molecular relationships. The database contains highly structured information about molecular interactions and functional annotations as well as contextual details of the biological interactions. IPA provides modules that can be used to integrate data at multiple levels to obtain insight into the molecular interactions, cellular phenotypes and disease processes of the biological system like heart failure. The main analysis modules include 1) IPA Core Analysis for identifying signaling and metabolic pathways, molecular networks, and biological processes that are related to the biological data; 2) IPA-Metabolomics for extracting biological insight into cell physiology and metabolism; 3) IPA-Tox for analyzing toxicity of candidate compounds; and 4) IPA-Biomarker for identifying the most promising and relevant biomarker candidates within experimental datasets. In addition, IPA's Path Designer provides researchers with help for transforming customized networks/pathways into pathway graphics for easy representation. It is well known historically that as the field evolves, so also the tools and miRNA target filter in the IPA analysis is one such evolution. miRNA Target Filter was introduced in the recent version of IPA (IPA 9.0) that allows researcher to examine both predicted and experimentally confirmed miRNA targets. Furthermore, it prioritizes targets based on related biological context and allows visualization of molecular interactions between miRNAs, their targets and other related molecules. IPA uses TargetScan database for predicted targets and TarBase for experimentally confirmed targets.

8. miRNAs as therapeutic targets

The current evidence from multiple studies show that miRNAs are altered with cardiac stress and genetic manipulation shows that miRNAs may actively contribute towards the deleterious cardiac phenotype. The regulation of cardiac phenotype by miRNAs, indicates that miRNAs can be used in therapeutic strategies to ameliorate deleterious outcomes. Since miRNAs are RNAs, they can be manipulated using the existing antisense and gene therapy approaches in vivo. Modified antisense oligonucleotides targeting the mature miRNA sequence, antimiRs, can reduce the levels of pathogenic or aberrantly expressed miRNAs (Krutzfeldt et al., 2005). Conversely, miRNA mimics can elevate the levels of miRNAs with beneficial outcomes (Xiao et al., 2007). Since miRNAs typically act as inhibitors of gene expression, the effect of adding specific miRNA mimics to a system is to decrease the expression of the mRNAs controlled by the miRNA. Conversely, the effect of inhibitors of specific miRNAs is to relieve the inhibition of the genes normally targeted by the miRNA. Thus, the primary effect of a miRNA inhibitor is activation of gene expression and a miRNA mimic is suppression of gene expression.

8.1 Antisense miRNA oligonucleotides and miRNA mimics

Disease condition is contributed by upregulation or downregulation of miRNAs. In conditions of upregulation specific reduction of the miRNA would be therapeutically desirable. One of the efficient ways to inhibit miRNAs would be the use of chemically modified single-stranded reverse complement oligonucleotides. The synthetic reverse complement oligonucleotide approach affects miRNA levels by (1) binding the mature miRNA within the RISC and acting as a competitive inhibitor; (2) binding to the pre-miRNA and preventing its processing or entry into the RISC; (3) interfering with the processing or export of the pre- or pri-miRNA from the nucleus. In any case, the net result is a reduction in the concentration of a specific miRNA-programmed RISC. This approach is similar in concept to traditional antisense targeting of mRNAs, except the number of targeting sites for a miRNA is very limited. Although conceptually comparable, only a handful of modifications have been achieved for inhibition of miRNAs. Such a technique has been effectively used to knock down let-7 in Drosophila (Hutvagner, Simard et al. 2004) while miRNA-122 was the first mammalian miRNA to be targeted for liver (Krutzfeldt et al., 2005). In this context, miRNA-133 (Altuvia et al., 2005) and miRNA-29 (van Rooij et al., 2008) have been effectively used to alter cardiac phenotype suggesting that this specific technique would be a viable option for therapeutic strategy. More recently, the technique of modifying the oligonucleotides with 2'O-methoxyethyl phosphorothioate is being extensively used as it seems to provide long term stability for the administered oligos thus extending the beneficial effects in vivo.

Anti-sense oligos can be used in conditions of targeting upregulated miRNAs and in conditions where reduction in miRNA level causes a disease state, beneficial therapeutic approach would be to increase its concentration. Instead of delivering the single-stranded oligonucleotide equivalent of the mature miRNA, an increase in the effective concentration of a reduced miRNA can be achieved through the use of synthetic RNA duplexes in which 1 strand is identical to the native miRNA. In this case, short double stranded oligonucleotides are designed in which 1 strand is the mature miRNA sequence (guide strand) and a complimentary or partially complementary stand is complexed with the mature miRNA sequence (passenger strand). The double stranded structure is required for recognition and loading into the RISC (Martinez et al., 2002). The only caveat in this kind of the design is to make sure that the passenger strand is eliminated and does not act as a new miRNA that may complicate the interpretation. Alternatively, approaches similar to that undertaken with siRNA using bioinformatic and chemical modification can be used and provides attractive means to elevate miRNA levels.

8.2 Therapeutic targeting of miRNA and challenges

Despite the ability to manipulate miRNAs in vivo to provide unique opportunities therapeutically, miRNA-based therapeutics pose challenges that are different from those associated with classic drugs. One of the major stumbling blocks for miRNA targeting is the issue of specificity. While specificity for a single cellular target is vital in classic drugs, miRNAs have numerous molecular targets raising the possibility that targeting of a miRNA may perturb multiple cellular functions both deleterious as well as beneficial. Since miRNAs are new set of molecules that are being targeted, better understanding of pharmacokinetics, biodistribution, and cell penetration is required to develop these as therapeutics. It is known that native nucleic acids are rapidly degraded by a variety of nucleases and phosphodiesterases in blood. Furthermore, biological environments and requirement of chemical modifications on the synthetic nucleotide derivatives may alter miRNA biophysical properties reducing the efficiency of therapeutic function. In this regards, several modifications that increase the stability of the oligonucleotides, including phosphorothioate, 2'-O-methyl, and 2'-fluoro substitutions can be effectively put to use in developing therapeutic strategies (Soutschek et al., 2004).

8.3 Methods of Delivery

In addition to efforts on developing miRNAs that are stable by modification, intense efforts are also ongoing to identify agents capable of targeted delivery of nucleic acids to tissues and cells. Delivery approaches can be broadly divided into 2 categories, conjugation and formulation. Conjugation strategies include direct attachment of targeting and cell-penetrating peptides, antibodies, and other bioactive molecules to the oligonucleotide. Formulation approaches vary broadly and include complex lipid emulsions from natural sources, synthetic liposomes, polyplexes, polymers and nanoparticles. To enter mammalian cells, the reverse-complement oligonucleotide needs to cross the lipid bilayer of the cell membrane and can be achieved by packaging the oligonucleotide into liposomes or nanoparticles that facilitates endocytosis. Alternatively, the oligonucleotide can be linked to a lipophilic moiety or receptor ligand, such as cholesterol that seems to greatly enhance cellular uptake (Soutschek et al., 2004). Despite significant advances in systemic delivery technology, most nucleic acid delivery agents developed to date have demonstrated efficacy in delivery to the liver. Therefore, effective delivery approaches especially to the heart would be a great stepping stone in the direction towards use of synthetic nucleic acids as therapeutics for cardiovascular disease. Interestingly, heart failure affords a unique opportunity to expand the potential for local delivery through the use of catheters providing additional level of sophistication.

9. Conclusions

It is remarkable to consider that miRNAs were first shown to function in mammals less than a decade ago, and the concept of miRNA manipulation in vivo to regulate disease-related processes is already becoming a feasible future therapeutic approach. Moreover, the rapidly expanding number of miRNAs makes it likely that the relatively few miRNAs studied to date represent only a subset of the miRNAs of interest in human disease. Given the established involvement of miRNAs in many facets of heart disease, it becomes pertinent to understand the underlying basis for its contributing role before taking on miRNA based human trials. Understanding the role of miRNAs in regulating various targets is the weakest link in this chain of fast moving area of miRNA that needs effort and resources. We believe the efforts are needed simultaneously in the direction of indepth contemporary proteomics along with assessment of miRNAs providing platform for linking miRNA to target protein expression which are the ultimate determinants of the phenotype. Therefore, identifying and validating miRNA targets are of paramount importance and establishment of the miRNA targets will provide a sound foundation for development of global signaling networks. Understanding the global regulation of networks by a miRNA rather than a specific target would be a more feasible approach to understand the overall function of miRNAs in development and disease conditions as a single miRNA could target both synergistic as well as antagonistic pathways. Appreciation of this unique regulation by miRNAs in physiology as well as pathology is the incentive to develop tools and technology to better understand the role of miRNAs in effecting global change rather than specific molecules in a given pathway.

10. Acknowledgement

This work was supported in part by Department of Molecular Cardiology Startup Funds, LRI, Cleveland Clinic Foundation NIH RO1 HL089473 (S.V.NP), RO1 HL083243 (S.S.K) and AHA 10POST3610049 (M.K.G).

11. References

Altuvia, Y., P. Landgraf, et al. (2005). "Clustering and conservation patterns of human microRNAs." *Nucleic Acids Res* 33(8): 2697-706.

Ambros, V. (2004). "The functions of animal microRNAs." *Nature* 431(7006): 350-5.

Aravin, A. A., G. J. Hannon, et al. (2007). "The Piwi-piRNA pathway provides an adaptive defense in the transposon arms race." *Science* 318(5851): 761-4.

Barrett, T., D. B. Troup, et al. "NCBI GEO: archive for functional genomics data sets--10 years on." *Nucleic Acids Res* 39(Database issue): D1005-10.

Barron, M. R., N. S. Belaguli, et al. (2005). "Serum response factor, an enriched cardiac mesoderm obligatory factor, is a downstream gene target for Tbx genes." *J Biol Chem* 280(12): 11816-28.

Bartel, D. P. (2004). "MicroRNAs: genomics, biogenesis, mechanism, and function." *Cell* 116(2): 281-97.

Bartel, D. P. (2009). "MicroRNAs: target recognition and regulatory functions." *Cell* 136(2): 215-33.

Berezikov, E., V. Guryev, et al. (2005). "Phylogenetic shadowing and computational identification of human microRNA genes." *Cell* 120(1): 21-4.

Bernstein, E., S. Y. Kim, et al. (2003). "Dicer is essential for mouse development." *Nat Genet* 35(3): 215-7.

Brazma, A., M. Kapushesky, et al. (2006). "Data storage and analysis in ArrayExpress." *Methods Enzymol* 411: 370-86.

Brown, J. H., D. P. Del Re, et al. (2006). "The Rac and Rho hall of fame: a decade of hypertrophic signaling hits." *Circ Res* 98(6): 730-42.

Bruneau, B. G. (2005). "Developmental biology: tiny brakes for a growing heart." *Nature* 436(7048): 181-2.

Cacchiarelli, D., D. Santoni, et al. (2008). "MicroRNAs as prime players in a combinatorial view of evolution." *RNA Biol* 5(3): 120-122.

Calin, G. A., C. G. Liu, et al. (2007). "Ultraconserved regions encoding ncRNAs are altered in human leukemias and carcinomas." *Cancer Cell* 12(3): 215-29.

Care, A., D. Catalucci, et al. (2007). "MicroRNA-133 controls cardiac hypertrophy." *Nat Med* 13(5): 613-8.

Catalucci, D., M. V. Latronico, et al. (2008). "Physiological myocardial hypertrophy: how and why?" *Front Biosci* 13: 312-24.

Chapman, E. J. and J. C. Carrington (2007). "Specialization and evolution of endogenous small RNA pathways." *Nat Rev Genet* 8(11): 884-96.

Chen, J. F., E. M. Mandel, et al. (2006). "The role of microRNA-1 and microRNA-133 in skeletal muscle proliferation and differentiation." *Nat Genet* 38(2): 228-33.

Chen, J. F., E. P. Murchison, et al. (2008). "Targeted deletion of Dicer in the heart leads to dilated cardiomyopathy and heart failure." *Proc Natl Acad Sci U S A* 105(6): 2111-6.

Cheng, Y., R. Ji, et al. (2007). "MicroRNAs are aberrantly expressed in hypertrophic heart: do they play a role in cardiac hypertrophy?" *Am J Pathol* 170(6): 1831-40.

Dash, R., V. Kadambi, et al. (2001). "Interactions between phospholamban and beta-adrenergic drive may lead to cardiomyopathy and early mortality." *Circulation* 103(6): 889-96.

Ebert, M. S., J. R. Neilson, et al. (2007). "MicroRNA sponges: competitive inhibitors of small RNAs in mammalian cells." *Nat Methods* 4(9): 721-6.

Elefant, N., A. Berger, et al. "RepTar: a database of predicted cellular targets of host and viral miRNAs." *Nucleic Acids Res* 39(Database issue): D188-94.

Eulalio, A., I. Behm-Ansmant, et al. (2007). "P-body formation is a consequence, not the cause, of RNA-mediated gene silencing." *Mol Cell Biol* 27(11): 3970-81.

Farh, K. K., A. Grimson, et al. (2005). "The widespread impact of mammalian MicroRNAs on mRNA repression and evolution." *Science* 310(5755): 1817-21.

Felli, N., L. Fontana, et al. (2005). "MicroRNAs 221 and 222 inhibit normal erythropoiesis and erythroleukemic cell growth via kit receptor down-modulation." *Proc Natl Acad Sci U S A* 102(50): 18081-6.

Filipowicz, W. (2005). "RNAi: the nuts and bolts of the RISC machine." *Cell* 122(1): 17-20.

Gardner, P. P., J. Daub, et al. "Rfam: Wikipedia, clans and the "decimal" release." *Nucleic Acids Res* 39(Database issue): D141-5.

Giraldez, A. J., R. M. Cinalli, et al. (2005). "MicroRNAs regulate brain morphogenesis in zebrafish." *Science* 308(5723): 833-8.

Giraldez, A. J., Y. Mishima, et al. (2006). "Zebrafish MiR-430 promotes deadenylation and clearance of maternal mRNAs." *Science* 312(5770): 75-9.

Gregory, P. A., A. G. Bert, et al. (2008). "The miR-200 family and miR-205 regulate epithelial to mesenchymal transition by targeting ZEB1 and SIP1." *Nat Cell Biol* 10(5): 593-601.

Griffiths-Jones, S., R. J. Grocock, et al. (2006). "miRBase: microRNA sequences, targets and gene nomenclature." *Nucleic Acids Res* 34(Database issue): D140-4.

Griffiths-Jones, S., H. K. Saini, et al. (2008). "miRBase: tools for microRNA genomics." *Nucleic Acids Res* 36(Database issue): D154-8.

Gusev, Y., T. D. Schmittgen, et al. (2007). "Computational analysis of biological functions and pathways collectively targeted by co-expressed microRNAs in cancer." *BMC Bioinformatics* 8 Suppl 7: S16.

Harris, T. A., M. Yamakuchi, et al. (2008). "MicroRNA-126 regulates endothelial expression of vascular cell adhesion molecule 1." *Proc Natl Acad Sci U S A* 105(5): 1516-21.

Hsu, S. D., F. M. Lin, et al. "miRTarBase: a database curates experimentally validated microRNA-target interactions." *Nucleic Acids Res* 39(Database issue): D163-9.

Hutvagner, G., J. McLachlan, et al. (2001). "A cellular function for the RNA-interference enzyme Dicer in the maturation of the let-7 small temporal RNA." *Science* 293(5531): 834-8.

Hutvagner, G., M. J. Simard, et al. (2004). "Sequence-specific inhibition of small RNA function." *PLoS Biol* 2(4): E98.

Hwang, H. W., E. A. Wentzel, et al. (2007). "A hexanucleotide element directs microRNA nuclear import." *Science* 315(5808): 97-100.

Ikeda, S., A. He, et al. (2009). "MicroRNA-1 negatively regulates expression of the hypertrophy-associated calmodulin and Mef2a genes." *Mol Cell Biol* 29(8): 2193-204.

Ikeda, S., S. W. Kong, et al. (2007). "Altered microRNA expression in human heart disease." *Physiol Genomics* 31(3): 367-73.

Ivanovska, I. and M. A. Cleary (2008). "Combinatorial microRNAs: working together to make a difference." *Cell Cycle* 7(20): 3137-42.

Ivey, K. N., A. Muth, et al. (2008). "MicroRNA regulation of cell lineages in mouse and human embryonic stem cells." *Cell Stem Cell* 2(3): 219-29.

Jiang, Q., Y. Wang, et al. (2009). "miR2Disease: a manually curated database for microRNA deregulation in human disease." *Nucleic Acids Res* 37(Database issue): D98-104.

John, B., A. J. Enright, et al. (2004). "Human MicroRNA targets." *PLoS Biol* 2(11): e363.

Ke, Y., L. Wang, et al. (2004). "Intracellular localization and functional effects of P21-activated kinase-1 (Pak1) in cardiac myocytes." *Circ Res* 94(2): 194-200.

Kertesz, M., N. Iovino, et al. (2007). "The role of site accessibility in microRNA target recognition." *Nat Genet* 39(10): 1278-84.

Kim, V. N. and J. W. Nam (2006). "Genomics of microRNA." *Trends Genet* 22(3): 165-73.

Kiriakidou, M., P. T. Nelson, et al. (2004). "A combined computational-experimental approach predicts human microRNA targets." *Genes Dev* 18(10): 1165-78.

Kloosterman, W. P., A. K. Lagendijk, et al. (2007). "Targeted inhibition of miRNA maturation with morpholinos reveals a role for miR-375 in pancreatic islet development." *PLoS Biol* 5(8): e203.

Krek, A., D. Grun, et al. (2005). "Combinatorial microRNA target predictions." *Nat Genet* 37(5): 495-500.

Krichevsky, A. M., K. C. Sonntag, et al. (2006). "Specific microRNAs modulate embryonic stem cell-derived neurogenesis." *Stem Cells* 24(4): 857-64.

Krutzfeldt, J., N. Rajewsky, et al. (2005). "Silencing of microRNAs in vivo with 'antagomirs'." *Nature* 438(7068): 685-9.

Kuehbacher, A., C. Urbich, et al. (2007). "Role of Dicer and Drosha for endothelial microRNA expression and angiogenesis." *Circ Res* 101(1): 59-68.

Kwon, C., Z. Han, et al. (2005). "MicroRNA1 influences cardiac differentiation in Drosophila and regulates Notch signaling." *Proc Natl Acad Sci U S A* 102(52): 18986-91.

Lai, E. C. (2002). "Micro RNAs are complementary to 3' UTR sequence motifs that mediate negative post-transcriptional regulation." *Nat Genet* 30(4): 363-4.

Lakshmipathy, U., B. Love, et al. (2007). "MicroRNA expression pattern of undifferentiated and differentiated human embryonic stem cells." *Stem Cells Dev* 16(6): 1003-16.

Lall, S., D. Grun, et al. (2006). "A genome-wide map of conserved microRNA targets in C. elegans." *Curr Biol* 16(5): 460-71.

Landgraf, P., M. Rusu, et al. (2007). "A mammalian microRNA expression atlas based on small RNA library sequencing." *Cell* 129(7): 1401-14.

Latronico, M. V., D. Catalucci, et al. (2007). "Emerging role of microRNAs in cardiovascular biology." *Circ Res* 101(12): 1225-36.

Lee, N. S., T. Dohjima, et al. (2002). "Expression of small interfering RNAs targeted against HIV-1 rev transcripts in human cells." *Nat Biotechnol* 20(5): 500-5.

Lee, Y., C. Ahn, et al. (2003). "The nuclear RNase III Drosha initiates microRNA processing." *Nature* 425(6956): 415-9.

Lee, Y., M. Kim, et al. (2004). "MicroRNA genes are transcribed by RNA polymerase II." *EMBO J* 23(20): 4051-60.

Lewis, B. P., C. B. Burge, et al. (2005). "Conserved seed pairing, often flanked by adenosines, indicates that thousands of human genes are microRNA targets." *Cell* 120(1): 15-20.

Lewis, B. P., I. H. Shih, et al. (2003). "Prediction of mammalian microRNA targets." *Cell* 115(7): 787-98.

Liu, N., A. H. Williams, et al. (2007). "An intragenic MEF2-dependent enhancer directs muscle-specific expression of microRNAs 1 and 133." *Proc Natl Acad Sci U S A* 104(52): 20844-9.

Luo, X., H. Lin, et al. (2008). "Down-regulation of miR-1/miR-133 contributes to re-expression of pacemaker channel genes HCN2 and HCN4 in hypertrophic heart." *J Biol Chem* 283(29): 20045-52.

MacRae, I. J., E. Ma, et al. (2008). "In vitro reconstitution of the human RISC-loading complex." *Proc Natl Acad Sci U S A* 105(2): 512-7.

Martinez, J., A. Patkaniowska, et al. (2002). "Single-stranded antisense siRNAs guide target RNA cleavage in RNAi." *Cell* 110(5): 563-74.

Miranda, K. C., T. Huynh, et al. (2006). "A pattern-based method for the identification of MicroRNA binding sites and their corresponding heteroduplexes." *Cell* 126(6): 1203-17.

Naga Prasad, S. V., Z. H. Duan, et al. (2009). "Unique microRNA profile in end-stage heart failure indicates alterations in specific cardiovascular signaling networks." *J Biol Chem* 284(40): 27487-99.

Naga Prasad and Karnik SS (2010). "MicroRNAs--regulators of signaling networks in dilated cardiomyopathy."*J Cardiovasc Transl Res*. 3(3):225-34.

Nilsen, T. W. (2007). "Mechanisms of microRNA-mediated gene regulation in animal cells." *Trends Genet* 23(5): 243-9.

Niu, Z., A. Li, et al. (2007). "Serum response factor micromanaging cardiogenesis." *Curr Opin Cell Biol* 19(6): 618-27.

Okamura, K., J. W. Hagen, et al. (2007). "The mirtron pathway generates microRNA-class regulatory RNAs in Drosophila." *Cell* 130(1): 89-100.

Okamura, K., A. Ishizuka, et al. (2004). "Distinct roles for Argonaute proteins in small RNA-directed RNA cleavage pathways." *Genes Dev* 18(14): 1655-66.

Olson, E. N. and M. D. Schneider (2003). "Sizing up the heart: development redux in disease." *Genes Dev* 17(16): 1937-56.

Pedersen, I. M., G. Cheng, et al. (2007). "Interferon modulation of cellular microRNAs as an antiviral mechanism." *Nature* 449(7164): 919-22.

Rao, P. K., R. M. Kumar, et al. (2006). "Myogenic factors that regulate expression of muscle-specific microRNAs." *Proc Natl Acad Sci U S A* 103(23): 8721-6.

Rodriguez, A., S. Griffiths-Jones, et al. (2004). "Identification of mammalian microRNA host genes and transcription units." *Genome Res* 14(10A): 1902-10.

Ruby, J. G., C. H. Jan, et al. (2007). "Intronic microRNA precursors that bypass Drosha processing." *Nature* 448(7149): 83-6.

Sayed, D., C. Hong, et al. (2007). "MicroRNAs play an essential role in the development of cardiac hypertrophy." *Circ Res* 100(3): 416-24.

Schwarz, D. S., G. Hutvagner, et al. (2003). "Asymmetry in the assembly of the RNAi enzyme complex." *Cell* 115(2): 199-208.

Sethupathy, P., B. Corda, et al. (2006). "TarBase: A comprehensive database of experimentally supported animal microRNA targets." *RNA* 12(2): 192-7.

Soutschek, J., A. Akinc, et al. (2004). "Therapeutic silencing of an endogenous gene by systemic administration of modified siRNAs." *Nature* 432(7014): 173-8.

Srivastava, D., T. Thomas, et al. (1997). "Regulation of cardiac mesodermal and neural crest development by the bHLH transcription factor, dHAND." *Nat Genet* 16(2): 154-60.

Stark, A., J. Brennecke, et al. (2005). "Animal MicroRNAs confer robustness to gene expression and have a significant impact on 3'UTR evolution." *Cell* 123(6): 1133-46.

Sucharov, C., M. R. Bristow, et al. (2008). "miRNA expression in the failing human heart: functional correlates." *J Mol Cell Cardiol* 45(2): 185-92.

Sun, Q., G. Chen, et al. (2006). "Defining the mammalian CArGome." *Genome Res* 16(2): 197-207.

Tatsuguchi, M., H. Y. Seok, et al. (2007). "Expression of microRNAs is dynamically regulated during cardiomyocyte hypertrophy." *J Mol Cell Cardiol* 42(6): 1137-41.

Tay, Y. M., W. L. Tam, et al. (2008). "MicroRNA-134 modulates the differentiation of mouse embryonic stem cells, where it causes post-transcriptional attenuation of Nanog and LRH1." *Stem Cells* 26(1): 17-29.

Thum, T., P. Galuppo, et al. (2007). "MicroRNAs in the human heart: a clue to fetal gene reprogramming in heart failure." *Circulation* 116(3): 258-67.

Thum, T., C. Gross, et al. (2008). "MicroRNA-21 contributes to myocardial disease by stimulating MAP kinase signalling in fibroblasts." *Nature* 456(7224): 980-4.

van Rooij, E., L. B. Sutherland, et al. (2006). "A signature pattern of stress-responsive microRNAs that can evoke cardiac hypertrophy and heart failure." *Proc Natl Acad Sci U S A* 103(48): 18255-60.

van Rooij, E., L. B. Sutherland, et al. (2007). "Control of stress-dependent cardiac growth and gene expression by a microRNA." *Science* 316(5824): 575-9.

van Rooij, E., L. B. Sutherland, et al. (2008). "Dysregulation of microRNAs after myocardial infarction reveals a role of miR-29 in cardiac fibrosis." *Proc Natl Acad Sci U S A* 105(35): 13027-32.

Volpe, T. A., C. Kidner, et al. (2002). "Regulation of heterochromatic silencing and histone H3 lysine-9 methylation by RNAi." *Science* 297(5588): 1833-7.

Xiao, J., X. Luo, et al. (2007). "MicroRNA miR-133 represses HERG K+ channel expression contributing to QT prolongation in diabetic hearts." *J Biol Chem* 282(17): 12363-7.

Yang, B., H. Lin, et al. (2007). "The muscle-specific microRNA miR-1 regulates cardiac arrhythmogenic potential by targeting GJA1 and KCNJ2." *Nat Med* 13(4): 486-91.

Yi, R., Y. Qin, et al. (2003). "Exportin-5 mediates the nuclear export of pre-microRNAs and short hairpin RNAs." *Genes Dev* 17(24): 3011-6.

Yu, W., D. Gius, et al. (2008). "Epigenetic silencing of tumour suppressor gene p15 by its antisense RNA." *Nature* 451(7175): 202-6.

Zhang, S. X., E. Garcia-Gras, et al. (2005). "Identification of direct serum-response factor gene targets during Me2SO-induced P19 cardiac cell differentiation." *J Biol Chem* 280(19): 19115-26.

Zhao, Y., J. F. Ransom, et al. (2007). "Dysregulation of cardiogenesis, cardiac conduction, and cell cycle in mice lacking miRNA-1-2." *Cell* 129(2): 303-17.

Zhao, Y., E. Samal, et al. (2005). "Serum response factor regulates a muscle-specific microRNA that targets Hand2 during cardiogenesis." *Nature* 436(7048): 214-20.

Zilberman, D., X. Cao, et al. (2003). "ARGONAUTE4 control of locus-specific siRNA accumulation and DNA and histone methylation." *Science* 299(5607): 716-9.

4

Intercellular Connections in the Heart: The Intercalated Disc

Maegen A. Ackermann, Li-Yen R. Hu and
Aikaterini Kontrogianni-Konstantopoulos
Department of Biochemistry and Molecular Biology, University of Maryland,
School of Medicine, Baltimore, MD,
USA

1. Introduction

Proper cardiac function requires the synchronous mechanical and electrical activity of individual cardiomyocytes to ensure the coordinated excitation and contractile performance of the heart, as an organ. The intercalated disc (ID), a unique membrane structure forming at the edges of mammalian cardiomyocytes (Li and Radice, 2010), fulfills this role by allowing the transmission of mechanical and electrical activity between neighboring cells; (reviewed in Delmar and McKenna, 2010; Noorman et al., 2009).

1.1 A brief history of the ID

The ID was first depicted in 1866 by Karl Josef Ebhert *et al.* as "verdichtungsstreifen", which literally translates to "compression strips", but was later referred to as a homogeneous "cementing material" found at the ends of cardiac myocytes (Saphir and Karsner, 1924). A decade later, Engelman described the heart as a continuous syncytium, while a century later Weidmann suggested the presence of "membrane areas of synchronicity", characterized by low resistance that allows the transmission of electrical potential (Engelmann, 1875; Weidmann, 1952).

The idea of a continuous region connecting two cells was challenged in the mid 1950's by several groups who used electron microscopy to show that cardiac cells are separated from one another by a specialized extension of the sarcoplasm oriented transversely with respect to the cell's boundaries (Sjostrand and Andersson, 1954; Van Breemen, 1953). Since the middle of the 20th century, we have significantly advanced our understanding of the structure and composition of the ID. Accordingly, the ID was found to be a highly organized structure composed of three main junctional complexes; the gap junctions, which enable the propagation of electrical stimuli throughout heart cells, the adherens junctions, and the desmosomes, which provide mechanical coupling and stability to cardiomyocytes, respectively. The advent of electron microscopy in the 1950's to 1970's further provided detailed visualizations of the regions connecting two cardiomyocytes (Fawcett and McNutt, 1969; McNutt et al., 1970; Muir, 1957; Rayns et al., 1969; Sjostrand and Andersson, 1954; Van Breemen, 1953). Recently, novel cellular isolation techniques combined with scanning or transmission electron microscopy (SEM and TEM, respectively) have yielded three-dimensional images of the ID (Hoyt et al., 1989; Shimada et al., 2004; Tandler et al., 2006), showing that in the mammalian ventricular heart, IDs are arranged both transversely and longitudinally in a stairwell like fashion with steps and risers. Transverse or plicate segments, resembling the steps, run in a zigzag arrangement with finger-like micro-projections, and contain mainly adherens junctions and desmosomes with smaller regions of gap junction plaques. Longitudinal or interplicate segments resemble the risers and contain mainly desmosomes and larger areas of gap junction plaques. The many folds and projections found within this region, increase the surface area of the ID, providing the cardiac cells with superior intercellular communication.

1.2 Spatiotemporal distribution of ID components

During cardiomyocyte development and maturation, major changes occur in structures associated with the ID. Studies using human myocardium showed that during embryonic development adherens junction and desmosomal organization follows that of gap junctions (Pieperhoff and Franke, 2007). However, during postnatal development proteins of the adherens and gap junctions appear to orient themselves at IDs simultaneously (Peters et al., 1994). Moreover, *in vivo* studies of lower mammals (including rodent, bovine and canine) have shown that at embryonic stages and postnatal day 1, components of gap junctions, desmosomes and adherens junctions are uniformly distributed throughout the sarcolemma, mutually exclusive from one another (Angst et al., 1997; Hirschy et al., 2006). However, at later postnatal stages (days 6-20), proteins of the adherens junctions and desmosomes begin to concentrate towards the termini of cardiomyocytes, leaving proteins of gap junctions uniformly distributed at the plasma membrane. By postnatal day 90, all components of the three junctions are segregated and organized at IDs. These findings were also supported by *in vitro* studies using primary cultures of rat and mouse cardiomyocytes (Geisler et al., 2010; Kostin et al., 1999). Interestingly, the latter further demonstrated that when individual cardiocytes are allowed to make contact in culture, proteins of the adherens junctions are the first to assemble and "mark" the location of the developing ID, closely followed by desmosomal proteins and finally proteins of gap junctions (Geisler et al., 2010; Kostin et al., 1999). Supporting this, the organization of adherens junctions and desmosomes is independent of gap junctions; however, gap junction organization requires that of adherens junctions and desmosomes (Gutstein et al., 2003; Wei et al., 2005). Taken together, these observations suggest that proteins necessary for mechanical coupling, i.e. components of adherens junctions and desmosomes, create the appropriate environment for proteins mediating electro-chemical coupling, i.e. those associated with gap junctions.

1.3 Organization of the ID

Gap junctions mediate the direct communication between neighboring cells by forming a low resistance pathway for the transmission of signals and electrical current (Rohr, 2004). A gap junction is composed of twelve connexin proteins, with connexin-43 being the most prominent in mammalian cardiomyocytes, along with low amounts of connexin-45 and 40 (Beyer et al., 1987; Vozzi et al., 1999). Each cardiomyocyte contributes six connexin molecules to form a hemi-channel, or a connexon; two connexons join to form a pore or gap junction channel, which is isolated from the extracellular space and connects the cytosol of two neighboring cells (Sohl and Willecke, 2004). These channels are responsible for the occurrence of synchronous contractions throughout the heart (Sohl and Willecke, 2004).

Consequently, in the absence of connexin-43 channels, normal propagation of contraction is disrupted, and lethal arrhythmias develop (Gutstein et al., 2001a; Gutstein et al., 2001b).

Adherens junctions facilitate the transmission of contractile force from one cell to the next and are crucial in maintaining mechanical strength uniformly across the heart (Tepass et al., 2000). They are mainly composed of transmembrane cadherins and cytosolic catenins (Niessen, 2007). N-cadherin, the main cardiac isoform, is a transmembrane protein, with extracellular and intracellular components (Niessen, 2007). Its extracellular portion forms homodimers bringing together the membranes of two opposing cells, while its intracellular segment forms a complex with various members of the catenin family (α-, β-, γ- and p120) present in the cytosol, which in turn are linked to the actin cytoskeleton (Bass-Zubek et al., 2009). Consequently, adherens junctions serve as anchors between the extracellular space and the actin cytoskeleton (Noorman et al., 2009).

Desmosomes provide structural support to cardiomyocytes, which are subjected to strong contractile stress (Delmar, 2004). Desmosomes, similar to adherens junctions, are composed of intercellular and intracellular components (Rayns et al., 1969). The intercellular component consists of desmosomal cadherins, desmocollin and desmoglein, which form a hetero-complex within the extracellular space joining together two bordering cells (Green and Simpson, 2007), while the intracellular component consists of proteins of the armadillo/catenin (plakoglobin and plakophilin) and plakin (desmoplakin) families (Bass-Zubek et al., 2009). Desmoplakin directly interacts with intermediate filaments to stabilize the desmosomal structure. Importantly, a high incidence of mutations within genes encoding desmosomal proteins has been linked to the development of arrhythmogenic right ventricular cardiomyopathy (ARVC).

Although, the ID has been traditionally described to contain three distinct structures (i.e. gap junctions, adherens junctions and desmosomes), recent technological advancements indicate that they are more interwined than originally proposed (Delmar and McKenna, 2010). Consistent with this, adherens junctions and desmosomes are intimately associated in the *"area composita"* where proteins from both structures are present (Borrmann et al., 2006; Franke et al., 2006). Similarly, proteins of the adherens and gap junctions have been shown to interact directly (Delmar, 2004). Taken together, these observations suggest that the ID is actually a single functional unit where macromolecular complexes interact to maintain structural integrity and synchronous contraction throughout the heart.

Bridging the gap between the ID and the sarcomeric cytoskeleton is a newly defined region termed the transitional junction. This area is rich in structural proteins, including spectrin, ankyrin-G, α-actinin and the NH_2-terminal region of titin, which typically localizes to the Z-disc (Bennett et al., 2006). The transitional junction is suggested to connect the ID with the contractile apparatus, mediating the transmission of force between adjacent cardiocytes.

The high degree of complexity and organization of junctions at the ID suggests a tight interplay between mechanical and electrical activities. Disruption of either mechanical or electrical coupling leads to irregular conduction of electrical impulses and deterioration of cardiac function, subsequently resulting in the development of cardiac arrhythmias. Various mutations in genes encoding for ID proteins have been causatively linked to these complex disorders, many of which manifest themselves as ARVC; (recently reviewed in Protonotarios et al., 2011).

There are ~200 known proteins that are associated with the ID (Dowling et al., 2008; Estigoy et al., 2009; Geisler et al., 2007; Lin et al.; Kargacin et al., 2006; Satomi-Kobayashi et al., 2009;

Schroen et al., 2007; Seeger et al., 2010). Herein, we provide a summation of the current knowledge on the junctional structures present in the ID, focusing on their most prominent and influential components, and how these relate to each other and the sarcomeric cytoskeleton in normal and disease states.

2. Gap junctions

Gap junctions were first described by Revel and Karnovsky in 1967, as "hexagonal arrays" that localize to the ID and mediate the electrical and metabolic coupling of adjacent cardiomyocytes by allowing the diffusion of small molecules (<1000 Da) (Elfgang et al., 1995; Ravel and Karnovsky, 1967). At gap junctions, the distance between opposing membranes is ~3 nm (Fig. 1; Perkins et al., 1997). Gap junction plaques can contain from a few up to 200,000 connexon channels (Evans et al., 2006).

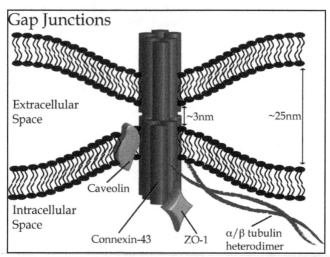

Fig. 1. Gap junctions in ventricular cardiomyocytes are composed of two homo-hexameric hemi-channels. forming a channel or a connexon. Each hemi-channel consists of six connexin-43 monomers (shown in dark purple), allowing the transmission of electrical current and small signalling molecules from adjoining cardiomyocytes. Zona Occludens-1 (ZO-1) (depicted in light purple) interacts directly with connexin-43. In addition, the connexin-43 complex interacts with members of the caveolin family (shown in light grey) that target gap junctions to lipid rafts, and cytosolic α/β tubulin heterodimers (shown in dark grey) that link gap junctions to the microtubular network.

2.1 Structural organization of connexons: Connexin-43

Connexin-43: The human connexin super-family is composed of at least twenty-one members. Connexin-43 is the predominant form expressed in the human heart, while connexins 40 and 45 are present in lower amounts (reviewed in Sohl and Willecke, 2004). Connexin-43 is a four-pass transmembrane protein that contains a cytoplasmic loop and two extracellular loops (Fig. 2A). Notably, both its NH_2- and COOH- termini are located in the cytosol (reviewed in Sohl and Willecke, 2004). Three conserved cysteine residues, located in the extracellular loops, have been implicated in disulfide bond formation between neighboring connexins of adjacent cells, and contribute to the development of a tight seal that prevents the exchange of materials with the extracellular matrix (Unger et al., 1999). Consistent with this, a constitutive connexin-43 null murine model is embryonic lethal (Reaume et al., 1995), while a cardiac-specific knock-out model exhibits sudden cardiac death by 2 months of age (Gutstein et al., 2001a; Gutstein et al., 2001b).

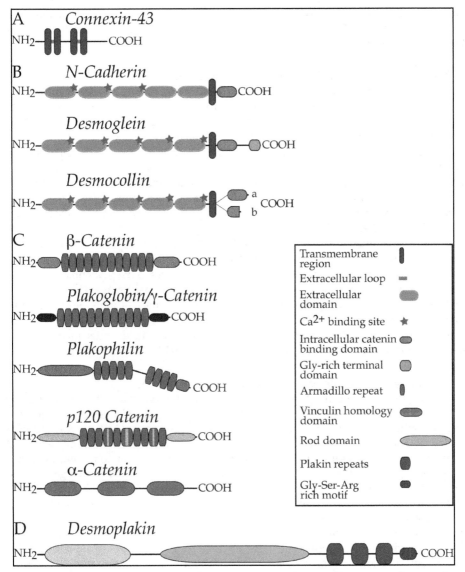

Fig. 2. Schematic representation of the domain structure of major ID proteins. Grey ovals denote protein specific domains.

NMR studies have demonstrated the presence of short, flexible α-helical segments in the cytoplasmic loop and the COOH-terminus of connexin-43, which provide binding sites for several proteins and mediate gating of the connexon (Duffy et al., 2002; reviewed in Gonzalez et al., 2007). Consequently, connexons can exist in a closed or open conformation; at high Ca^{2+} concentrations (i.e. 1.8 mM), they tend to adapt a closed conformation, however, in the absence of Ca^{2+} they exist in an open state (Thimm et al., 2005). Importantly, the gating of connexons is regulated by additional factors, including pH, levels of Mg^{2+}, voltage as well as the phosphorylation status of connexins (please see below; Bukauskas and Verselis, 2004; Delmar, 2004; Ek et al., 1994; Ek-Vitorin et al., 1996; Gonzalez et al., 2007; Matsuda et al., 2010).

2.2 Propagation of electrical stimulation throughout the heart

The propagation of electrical stimulation is the driving force for heart contraction. It originates at the sinoatrial (SA) node, traverses through the atria, crosses the atrioventricular (AV) node and propagates through the bundle of His and the Purkinje fibers before it activates the ventricles. The coordinated contraction of the atria and ventricles is achieved by conduction of the electrical impulse at variable speeds, mediated by the different forms of connexins, which confer to gap junction plaques distinct electrophysiological properties. As such, connexin-45 is preferentially expressed in the SA and AV nodes, but co-expressed with connexin-43 in the bundle of His and the Purkinje fibers. Conversely, connexin-43 is primarily present in the ventricles, but also co-expressed with connexin-40 in the atria; (reviewed in Severs et al., 2008).

Conferring low conductance in a single homotypic channel, connexin-45 is distributed at SA node in a sparse and scattered pattern that ensures poor coupling between adjacent cardiocytes. Similarly at the AV node, connexin-45 contributes to the sequential activation of the atria and ventricles reducing the occurrence of arrhythmias; (reviewed in Severs et al., 2008). On the contrary, the rapid propagation of electrical signals through the Purkinje fibers is mediated by gap junctions mainly consisting of connexins 43 and 40, which confer relatively large conductance, and to a lesser extent connexin-45, thus maintaining the regular contractions of the heart (Gonzalez et al., 2007; Kirchhoff et al., 1998).

2.3 Phosphorylation regulates the permeability of connexons

Several kinases modulate the function of connexons. Although a complete listing of all identified kinases is beyond the scope of this chapter, we will refer to major ones, highlighting their roles during normalcy and stress. Connexin-43 is a substrate of Src tyrosine kinase, which phosphorylates Tyr-265 to disrupt its interaction with ZO-1 (discussed below, Toyfuku et al., 2001), and suppress gap junction communication in the failing heart (Giepmans et al., 2001a; Toyofuku et al., 2001). Similarly, mitogen-activated protein kinase (MAPK) phosphorylates connexin-43 at Ser-255, Ser-279 and Ser-282 to repress gap junction communication (Warn-Cramer et al., 1998; Warn-Cramer et al., 1996). Conversely, phosphorylation of Ser-365 by protein kinase A (PKA) promotes gap junction assembly and communication (Burghardt et al., 1995; Solan et al., 2007; TenBroek et al., 2001). Although several isozymes of protein kinase C (PKC) phosphorylate connexin-43 in diverse cell types and tissues, PKCε is the only isoform that phosphorylates it at the ID (Bowling et al., 2001; Doble et al., 2000; Lampe et al., 2000; Lin et al., 2003; Saez et al., 1997). Consistent with this, PKCε suppresses gap junction communication in the ischemic heart through phosphorylation of connexin-43 at Ser-368 (Ek-Vitorin et al., 2006; Hund et al., 2007; Hund et al., 2008).

Several phosphorylation sites (i.e. Ser-306 and Ser-325/Ser-328/Ser-330) on connexin-43 are non- or de-phosphorylated in ischemic and hypertrophic hearts (Lampe et al., 2006; Procida et al., 2009). The absence of phosphorylation at these sites has been suggested to correlate with reduced cardiac conductance (Lampe et al., 2006; Procida et al., 2009). In agreement with this, transgenic mice in which Ser-325/Ser-328/Ser-300 were substituted by glutamic acid (phosphomimetic residue) were less susceptible to arrhythmia. Yet, the kinase(s) that is responsible for these phosphorylation events remain(s) to be identified. Importantly, Ser-325/Ser-328/Ser-330 are substrates of casein kinase 1 (CK1) in normal rat kidney cells (Cooper and Lampe, 2002), however, its role in cardiac muscle remains to be defined. Moreover, Ca^{2+}/Calmodulin-dependent protein kinase II (CaMKII) is capable of phosphorylating many Ser residues on connexin-43 *in vitro*, including Ser-306, Ser-325, Ser-328 and Ser-330 (Huang et al., 2011), however the physiological significance of these results requires further investigation.

The phosphatases acting upon and regulating the activities of connexin-43 have been also long sought after. Receptor protein tyrosine phosphatase μ (RPTPμ) has been suggested to dephosphorylate Tyr residues present in connexin-43 in lung cells (Giepmans et al., 2003), however, its physiological relevance in the myocardium remains to be established. Moreover, serine/threonine phosphatase type 1 and type 2A (PP1 and PP2A, respectively) have been implicated in the dephosphorylation of connexin-43 (Ai and Pogwizd, 2005; Duthe et al., 2001; Jeyaraman et al., 2003). For instance, PP1, but not PP2A, modulates the phosphorylation status of Ser-368 (Jeyaraman et al., 2003). Conversely, PP2A exists in a complex with connexin-43 in homogenates prepared from patients suffering from dilated cardiomyopathy (DCM) or idiopathic dilated cardiomyopathy (IDCM), as well as from a non-ischemic heart failure rabbit model (Ai and Pogwizd, 2005; Ai et al., 2011). Consistent with this, application of specific PP2A inhibitors prevented uncoupling of cardiocytes in the rabbit failing heart (Ai and Pogwizd, 2005).

2.4 Connexin-43 interacts with ZO-1, caveolins and microtubules at the ID

Zona occludens-1: Zona occludens-1 (ZO-1) interacts with connexin-43 in cardiac myocytes via its PDZ2 domain that directly binds to the last five residues present in the COOH-terminus of connexin-43 (Giepmans and Moolenaar, 1998; Giepmans et al., 2001a; Toyofuku et al., 1998). Interestingly though, their interaction is not abolished in a transgenic murine model that expresses a truncated form of connexin-43 that is missing the last 124 amino acid residues (Maass et al., 2007), suggesting that additional domains contribute to binding.

The interaction of ZO-1 and connexin-43 mainly takes place at the periphery of the gap junctional plaque (Hunter et al., 2005; Zhu et al., 2005). Notably, their binding is suppressed in the presence of Src (Sorgen et al., 2004; Toyofuku et al., 2001). A number of early studies suggested that ZO-1 targets or retains connexin-43 to the ID, while others proposed that it regulates the size of gap junctions or the internalization of connexin-43 (Barker et al., 2002; Hunter et al., 2005; Rhett et al., 2011; Toyofuku et al., 1998). Intriguingly, recent studies from failing human hearts have provided conflicting results. Bruce *et al.* reported that in hearts of DCM and IDCM patients, ZO-1 interacts more extensively with connexin-43 compared to healthy ones (Bruce et al., 2008), whereas Laing *et al.* and Kostin, described diminished colocalization of connexin-43 and ZO-1 in hearts from patients with DCM, ischaemic cardiomyopathy and end-stage heart failure (Kostin, 2007; Laing et al., 2007). In support of this, transgenic mice lacking ZO-1 are embryonic lethal, exhibiting cardiac developmental challanges (Katsuno et al., 2008; Xu et al., 2008). Recently, Rhett *et al.* proposed a model, whereby ZO-1 interacts with connexin-43 to inhibit the incorporation of additional connexons into gap junctional plaques (Rhett et al., 2011).

Caveolin-1: Caveolins are the main scaffolding components of caveolae in lipid rafts, and have been found to interact with connexin-43 in different cell types (Langlois et al., 2008; Liu et al., 2010; Schubert et al., 2002). While the caveolin scaffolding domain along with the COOH-terminus of caveolin-1 are sufficient to support binding to connexin-43, the respective interacting region of the latter has yet to be defined (Schubert et al., 2002). Contrary to epithelial cells, the interaction between caveolins and connexin-43 in the myocardium is less understood. Along these lines, caveolin-3, which is specifically expressed in heart and skeletal muscle (Tang et al., 1996), has been shown to interact with connexin-43 in a yeast-two-hybrid study and confirmed by co-immunoprecipitation assays using heart homogenates (Liu et al., 2010). As caveolin-3 is present at the sarcolemma, but not the ID, the physiological relevance of this interaction remains to be examined (Abi-Char et al., 2007; Yarbrough et al., 2002). Moreover, a murine model lacking caveolin develop DCM at early stages (Zhao, 2002).

Microtubules: First characterized as binding partners of connexin-43 in RAT-1 cells and other fibroblast and epithelial cell lines, α/β-tubulins have been shown to specifically interact with the tubulin-binding motif present in the COOH-terminus of connexin-43 (Giepmans et al., 2001a; Giepmans et al., 2001b). Immunofluorescence studies and live-cell imaging further demonstrated that connexin-43 co-localizes with tubulins along microtubule tracks, as it traverses from the Golgi apparatus to other membranes (Giepmans et al., 2001b; Lauf et al., 2002; Shaw et al., 2007). To date, only a handful of studies have described the interaction between tubulins and connexin-43 in the heart. Accordingly, a recent study by Smyth *et al.* proposed that EB1, a microtubule plus-end tracking protein, is required to deliver connexin-43 to the ID (Smyth et al., 2010). Consistent with this, disruption of the interaction between EB1 and microtubules (e.g. during ischemia) significantly decreases the surface expression of connexin-43 at the ID (Smyth et al., 2010).

3. Adherens junctions

Adherens junctions are specialized structures necessary for cell-cell adhesion that provide uniform mechanical strength to the heart. Unlike gap junctions where membranes remain relatively close, opposing membranes at adherens junctions are separated by ~20 nm (Niessen, 2007). Adherens junctions frequently alternate with gap junctions along the sarcolemma at the ID, and are typically oriented perpendicular to the long axis of cardiomyocytes, optimizing the transmission of mechanical force (Hoyt et al., 1989). In addition, they can be found with desmosomes at the *area composita*. Functional adherens junctions require two main anchor points, one within the extracellular space where cadherins from adjacent cells tightly interact in a homophillic manner, and the other within the cytoplasmic region linking the adherens junction complex to the actin cytoskeleton through direct interactions with members of the catenin family (Fig. 3; reviewed in Niessen, 2007; Noorman et al., 2009).

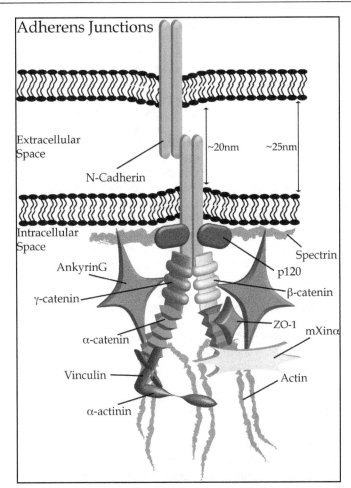

Fig. 3. Adherens Junctions connect neighbouring cardiomyocytes through homophilic dimers of N-cadherin. Connections within the intracellular space link N-cadherin to the actin cytoskeleton (depicted in grey), via additional adherens junction proteins (shown in hues of teal), ie. p120 catenin, β-catenin, α-catenin and mXinα. Proteins not traditionally considered as components of adherens junctions, but localizing to the ID are shown in grey. Proteins of other ID structures, ZO-1 (gap junctions) and γ-catenin (desmosomes), are depicted in light purple and gold, respectively.

3.1 N-cadherin

N-Cadherin: Cadherins are a super-family of transmembrane glycoproteins that mediate Ca^{2+}-dependent adhesion between neighbouring cells. In the early 1980s, N-cadherin was identified as a major component of the myocardium, that localizes to the ID (Volk and Geiger, 1984). Five extracellular domains are present in N-cadherin, with the first three possessing Ca^{2+} binding sites; each domain is composed of up to ~110 amino acids (Fig. 2B). The extreme NH_2-terminus of N-cadherin contains a highly conserved ligand recognition site composed of repeating motifs of His-Ala-Val residues, necessary for homophilic dimer formation (Nose et al., 1990). Two cadherin monomers, one from each adjacent myocyte, form a Ca^{2+}-dependent, zipper-like homodimer (Takeichi, 1994). Although Ca^{2+} is necessary for maintaining cadherin homodimers, it does not mediate their initial interaction (Nagaraj et al., 1996). Following the extensive extracellular domain, N-cadherin contains a single-pass transmembrane region and a short cytoplasmic segment that associates with the actin cytoskeleton via proteins of the catenin family (Ozawa et al., 1990).

The importance of N-cadherin in the stability of IDs is evidenced in various animal models. A murine systemic knock-out model of N-cadherin resulted in embryonic lethality due to improper development of the heart tube among other abnormalities, despite the development of primitive myocardial tissue (Radice et al., 1997). Interestingly, isolated murine myocytes from the same model were able to weakly contract and aggregate in culture (Radice et al., 1997). Taken together, these results suggested that N-cadherin is critical for embryonic development of the heart and other tissues, however it is not required for electrical coupling and cell adhesion at this stage. Moreover, in a murine conditional cardiac-specific knock-out model where N-cadherin was deleted in 6-10 week old mice, sudden death occurred after ~2 months (Li et al., 2005). A significant decrease in the expression levels of gap junction proteins was also observed in this model, which was accompanied by the development of dilated cardiomyopathy and impaired left ventricular function (Li et al., 2005). In addition, the amounts of other proteins at ID were reduced, including plakoglobin and α-, β-, and p120 catenins, resulting in dissolution of the ID structure (Kostetskii et al., 2005; Li et al., 2005). Similarly, mice overexpressing N-cadherin developed early onset dilated cardiomyopathy (Ferreira-Cornwell et al., 2002), and N-cadherin/connexin-43 compound heterozygous mice were prone to cardiac arrhythmias (Li et al., 2008). Collectively, these studies suggested that N-cadherin is necessary for the maintenance and stabilization of the ID, while its absence may lead to the development of heart failure and ultimately death.

3.2 Proteins of the catenin family

Within adherens junctions, N-cadherin associates with the actin cytoskeletal network through direct interactions mediated by members of the catenin/armadillo family; these include β-, α-, p120 and γ-catenin (also called plakoglobin). β- and p120 catenin bind directly to the cytoplsmic domain of N-cadherin, whereas α-catenin links the actin cytoskeleton to N-cadherin, via its direct interactions with both components (reviewed in Aho et al., 1999; Butz and Larue, 1995; Niessen, 2007).

β-Catenin: β-Catenin, like other members of the catenin/armadillo family, is characterized by a series of central domains, referred to as armadillo (arm) repeats, each composed of 42 amino acids, that form an elongated superhelix when repeated in tandem (Huber et al., 1997). β-Catenin contains twelve arm repeats (Fig. 2C; Peifer et al., 1994); deletion mutagenesis has mapped the binding site for N-cadherin to the central repeat region of β-catenin (Hulsken et al., 1994). Flanking the arm repeats are small, ~100 amino acids long, NH_2- and COOH- termini that mediate the regulatory functions of β-catenin.

p120 Catenin: p120 Catenin shares a similar organization with β-catenin, and a ~22% identity within the arm repeats region (Peifer et al., 1994; Reynolds et al., 1992). Alternative splicing gives rise to four similar p120 catenin isoforms (Keirsebilck et al., 1998). Each isoform is composed of ten arm repeats that are responsible for their direct interaction with the COOH-terminus of cadherins (Fig. 2C; Daniel and Reynolds, 1995; Finnemann et al., 1997; Reynolds et al., 1992; Shibamoto et al., 1995; Staddon et al., 1995; Thoreson et al., 2000). p120 catenin does not interact with α-catenin or the actin cytoskeleton (Daniel and Reynolds, 1995), suggesting a novel, yet unidentified, function within adherens junctions.

α-Catenin: α-Catenin is a subfamily of proteins that differs significantly in both primary sequence and structural organization from the other members of the traditional catenin/armadillo family (reviewed in Kobielak and Fuchs, 2004). Instead of arm repeats, α-catenin contains three vinculin homology (VH) domains, therefore sharing considerable homology with vinculin (Fig. 2C; Rudiger, 1998). Of the main α-catenin isoforms, αT-catenin is the most prominent in the mammalian heart and localizes to the ID (Janssens et al., 2001). Through its most NH_2-terminal VH domain, α-catenin dimerizes and interacts directly with β- and γ-catenin (Koslov et al., 1997; Pokutta and Weis, 2000), while through its middle VH domain supports binding to vinculin and α-actinin, both of which are present within the transitional junction of the ICD (McGregor et al., 1994; Weiss et al., 1998). Similar to vinculin, α-catenin associates with filamentous actin through its last VH domain and its COOH-terminus (Rimm et al., 1995). In addition, its COOH-terminus interacts with ZO-1, which is also complexed with connexin-43 at gap junctions (Imamura et al., 1999; Talhouk et al., 2008). Taken together, these observations indicate that α-catenin functions as an intracellular adhesion protein.

It is well established that β- and p120 catenins play essential roles in diverse signaling pathways, including modulation of cell-cell adhesion; (reviewed in Anastasiadis and Reynolds, 2000; Niessen, 2007). Recently, α-catenin was also implicated in the regulation of cell adhesion and proliferation (reviewed in Kobielak and Fuchs, 2004). Although many of their suggested signaling roles originate from studies in non-cardiac cells, it is presumed that catenins may have similar regulatory activities at the ID of cardiomyocytes. In support of this, transgenic mice lacking either β- or α-catenin result in detrimental effects on the longevity of the animals, with phenotypes ranging from embryonic lethality to the development of early onset DCM (Haegel et al., 1995; Piven et al., 2011; Sheikh et al., 2006). Future studies are necessary to continue addressing this question.

4. Desmosomes

Similar to adherens junctions, desmosomes are also symmetrical protein complexes with intercellular elements connecting adjacent cells, and intracellular components associating with intermediate filaments. First identified as adhesive structures of epithelial cells by Giulio Bizzozero in the late 19th century, the term desmosomes was initially coined in 1920 by Josef Schaffer from the Greek words "desmo" and "soma" meaning bond or fastening and body, respectively; (reviewed in Delva et al., 2009). In the middle of the 20th century, desmosomes were identified as a major component of the cardiac ID (Fawcett and McNutt, 1969; Grimley and Edwards, 1960; Muir, 1957; Sjostrand and Andersson, 1954), where its main function is to provide structural support to neighboring cardiomyocytes (reviewed in Delmar and McKenna, 2010; Delva et al., 2009; Thomason et al., 2010). Desmosomes bring apposing cells within 20-35 nm of each other (Noorman et al., 2009), and are typically found in close proximity to gap junctions, although recent studies indicate that they are also present next to adherens junctions within the *area composita*. They consist of proteins from three families: the desmosomal cadherins, the catenin/armadillo family and the plakins (Fig. 4).

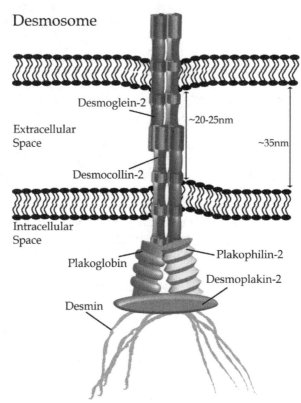

Fig. 4. Desmosomes connect neighbouring cardiomyocytes through heterophilic dimers of desmocollin-2 and desmoglein-2 (shown in hues of orange) forming within the extracellular space. Interactions with plakophilin-2, plakoglobin (a.k.a. γ-catenin) and desmoplakin-1 (depicted in hues of gold and orange) link the desmosomal complex to the intermediate filament protein desmin (shown in gray) in cardiomyocytes.

4.1 Desmosomal cadherins

Desmosomal cadherins are a superfamily of Ca^{2+}-dependent adhesion molecules, which form dimers to make up the core of desmosomal junctions (Dusek et al., 2007). Desmogleins and desmocollins, the two main types of desmosomal cadherins, possess several isoforms (4 and 3 respectively in humans, Green and Simpson, 2007; Lorimer et al., 1994; Schmelz et al., 1986) with desmoglein-2 and desmocollin-2 being the main isoforms expressed in mammalian cardiomyocytes (Garrod and Chidgey, 2008).

Desmoglein and Desmocollin: These classical cadherins are highly homologous; desmogleins and desmocollins share ~30% identity with each other and with other members of the cadherin family (Garrod et al., 2002). Much of their homology is found within their extracellular domains. They possess five extracellular domains or cadherin repeats of ~110 ımino acids and are separated by Ca^{2+} binding motifs, which are necessary for dimerization (Fig 2B; Pokutta and Weis, 2007). A single-pass transmembrane domain and an intracellular ınchoring segment follow the extracellular domains (Green and Simpson, 2007; Kowalczyk ət al., 1999). Within their intracellular regions, desmogleins and desmocollins possess a ːadherin-like sequence capable of binding catenins, or in the case of desmosomal cadherins, ɔlakoglobin (Mathur et al., 1994). Desmoglein and desmocollin differ significantly within their COOH-termini, however. In ɔarticular, the COOH-terminal region of desmoglein contains a proline-rich linker region, a ɜeries of short (~29 amino acids long) repeats and a glycine-rich terminal domain (Garrod ınd Chidgey, 2008; Holthofer et al., 2007), which likely mediates weak interactions with ɔther desmosomal proteins (Kami et al., 2009). Conversely, alternative splicing within the COOH-terminus of desmocollin gives rise to two forms (Collins et al., 1991; Parker et al., 1991); the "b" or shorter form does not contain the traditional catenin-binding domain, however, the longer "a" form possesses a normal catenin-binding domain and has been ɜhown to bind plakoglobin with high affinity (Troyanovsky et al., 1993). Many studies suggest that both desmoglein and desmocollin are necessary for desmosomal formation (Getsios et al., 2004; Marcozzi et al., 1998; Tselepis et al., 1998). However, it is unclear if homophilic or heterophilic interactions maintain desmosomal adhesion. Although heterophilic complexes between desmoglein-2 and desmocollin-2 have been reported, it has been suggested that homophilic interactions between desmogleins mediate complex formation (Heupel et al., 2008; Syed et al., 2002; Waschke et al., 2005). Nonetheless, the importance of both desmoglein and desmocollin in cardiac function is further evidenced by the numerous mutations identified in their respective genes that lead to cardiomyopathies, mainly manifested as ARVC. Consistent with this, mice harbouring a mutation resulting in a truncated form of desmoglein-2 develop ARVC (Krusche et al., 2011), while a systemic knockout mouse model of desmoglein-2 is embryonic lethal (Eshkind et al., 2002).

4.2 Proteins of the catenin/armadillo family

Desmosomal cadherins form cytoplasmic connections with intermediate filaments in part through proteins of the armadillo family. Armadillo proteins include plakoglobin (also called γ-catenin) and plakophilin, which are found at desmosomal structures (Cowin et al., 1986; Hatzfeld, 2005; Hatzfeld, 2007; Mertens et al., 1996; Mertens et al., 1999; Peifer et al., 1992), in addition to β-catenin, α–catenin and p120 catenin, which are mainly associated with adherens junctions (Hatzfeld, 2005; Hatzfeld, 2007). In addition to facilitating the anchoring of desmosomes to intermediate filaments, desmosomal armadillo proteins function in diverse signal transduction pathways.

Plakoglobin: Plakoglobin contains 12 arm repeats, which share 65% identity with the ones present in β-catenin, and are flanked by Pro-Lys-Gly rich NH$_2$- and COOH-terminal domains (Fig. 2C; Garrod and Chidgey, 2008; Huber et al., 1997; Peifer et al., 1992). Mutation analysis suggested that plakoglobin interacts with desmosomal cadherins through its NH$_2$-terminal domain as well as the arm repeats near its COOH-terminus (Chitaev et al., 1996; Wahl et al., 1996). Although the Pro-Lys-Gly motif interacts with both desmosomal and adherens junction cadherins, it has a higher affinity for desmoglein supporting plakoglobin's mainly desmosomal localization (Chitaev et al., 1996; Choi et al., 2009). Moreover, through its central arm repeats plakoglobin interacts with desmoplakin, which in turn binds to intermediate filaments.

Plakophilin: Plakophilins undergo alternative splicing giving rise to four products, referred to as plakophilin 1-4; (reviewed in Bass-Zubek et al., 2009), with plakophilin-2 being the most prominent form in mammalian cardiomyocytes (Mertens et al., 1996). Plakophilins contain 9 arm repeats flanked by an NH_2-terminal head and a short COOH-terminal region (Fig. 2C; Bass-Zubek et al., 2009). In addition, plakophilins 1-3 possess a flexible insertion between repeats 5 and 6, which introduces a major bend to their overall structure (Choi and Weis, 2005). Plakophilins bind to several desmosomal proteins through their NH_2-terminal regions, including desmocollin, desmoplakin and plakoglobin as well as actin and the intermediate filament proteins keratin and desmin (Hofmann et al., 2000). Notably, plakophilin-2 also interacts with ankyrin-G at the ID, a sodium channel anchoring protein and with connexin-43 (Sato et al., 2011). Consequently, loss of plakophilin-2 leads to a decrease in the level of the α-subunit of the sodium channel ($Na_v1.5$) at the membrane, which results in slow propagation of the action potential in cardiocytes (Sato et al., 2009). In addition to ankyrin-G, plakophilin-2 interacts with $PKC\alpha$, which is necessary for phosphorylation and recruitment of desmoplakin to newly forming desmosomes in the developing heart and during repair of myocardial injury (reviewed in Garrod and Chidgey, 2008). Thus, through its multiple interactions, plakophilin-2 may serve as a scaffold to contribute to adhesion and signalling at the ID by facilitating the lateral interaction between desmosomes and adherens junctions (Kowalczyk et al., 1999).

The critical roles of both plakoglobin and plakophilin-2 in desmosomal assembly and maintenance is evidenced by the severe phenotypes that relevant transgenic mice models exhibit and the different forms of heart disease associated with mutations in their respective genes (please see Tables 1 and 2). Consistent with this, both plakoglobin and plakophilin-2 null mice show premature death during embryogenesis because of myocardial fragility (Bierkamp et al., 1996; Grossmann et al., 2004; Ruiz et al., 1996). Similarly, cardiac-specific knockout of plakoglobin results in progressive development of cardiac dysfunction (Li et al., 2011).

4.3 Plakins

Desmoplakin: Plakins are large multi-domain proteins that mediate the interaction of intermediate filaments (desmin in heart) with desmosomes. Desmoplakin, the main plakin protein expressed in heart, is characterized by a central α-helical coiled-coil rod domain, which is flanked by globular NH_2- and COOH-termini (Fig. 2D; Franke et al., 1982). Through its coiled-coil region, desmoplakin has been suggested to form homodimers (Kowalczyk et al., 1994), while its NH_2-terminal region binds to plakoglobins and plakophilins, targeting them to desmosomes (Bornslaeger et al., 1996; Bornslaeger et al., 2001; Holthofer et al., 2007; Kowalczyk et al., 1999). Its COOH-terminal tail is composed of three plakin-repeat domains and a Gly-Ser-Arg rich motif; both shown to mediate binding to desmin (Choi et al., 2002; Getsios et al., 2004). Interestingly, mice lacking desmoplakin exhibit embryonic lethality characterized by reduced number of desmosomes with residual structures separated from intermediate filaments (Gallicano et al., 1998). These results, along with the various desmoplakin mutations associated with human genetic disorders (please see below) support a strong role for desmoplakin in the assembly and interlinking of desmosomes to desmin intermediate filaments in cardiomyocytes.

	Major Proteins	References	Animal Models	Phenotype	References
Gap Junctions	Connexin-43	Beyer et al., 1987	Systemic KO	Embryonic lethal	Reaume et al., 1995
			Cardiac Specific KO	Sudden cardiac death ~2 months	Gutstein et al., 2001b
	ZO-1	Giepmans et al., 1998; Toyofuku et al., 1998	Systemic KO	Embryonic lethal	Xu et al., 2008; Katsuno et al., 2008
	Caveolin	Schubert et al., 2002	Systemic KO	Development of DCM	Zhao et al., 2002
	Microtubule	Shaw et al., 2007	N/A	N/A	N/A
Adherens Junctions	N-Cadherin	Volk et al., 1984	Systemic KO	Embryonic lethal	Radice et al., 1997
			Cardiac specific KO	Sudden cardiac death ~2 months	Li et al., 2005; Kostetskii et al., 2005
			Dual heterozygote with connexin-43	Develop arythmias	Li et al., 2008
	β-catenin	Butz et al., 1995	Systemic KO	Embryonic lethal	Haegel et al., 1995
			Cardiac specific KO	Low survival rate	Piven et al., 2011
	α-catenin	Butz et al., 1995	Cardiac specific KO	Development of DCM	Piven et al., 2011; Sheikh et al., 2006
	P120 catenin	Aho et al., 1999	N/A	N/A	N/A
Desmosomes	Desmocollin-2	Lorimer et al., 1994	N/A	N/A	N/A
	Desmoglein-2	Schmelz et al., 1986	Transgenic lacking extracellular domains	Develop ARVC	Krusche et al., 2011
			Systemic KO	Embryonic lethal	Eshkind et al., 2002
	Plakoglobin	Peifer et al., 1992; Cowin et al., 1986	Systemic KO	Embryonic lethal	Bierkamp et al., 1996; Ruiz et al., 1996
			Cardiac Specific KO	Premature death due to cardiac dysfunction	Li et al., 2011
	Plakophilin-2	Mertens et al., 1996; Mertens et al., 1999	Systemic KO	Embryonic lethal	Grossmann et al., 2004
	Desmoplakin	Franke et al., 1982	Systemic KO	Embryonic lethal	Gallicano et al., 1998; Uzumcu et al., 2006
			Tetraploid rescue of systemic KO	Embryonic lethal	Gallicano et al., 2001
			Val30Met & Gln90Arg cardiac specific mutations	Embryonic lethal	Yang et al., 2006

Table 1. Listing of major proteins found at the ID and associated animal models with appropriate references; DCM: Dilated Cardiomyopathy, N/A: not applicable, and KO: knock-out.

Gene Product	Mutations	Disease	References
Plakophilin-2	Arg79Stop Arg735Stop IVSAS10, G-C, -1 (nt 2146) IVS12, G-A, +1 (nt 2489)	ARVC	Gerull et al., 2004
Desmocollin-2	1bp deletion, 1430C 1bp deletion, 1841G 2bp deletion, 2687GA IVS5AS, A-G, -2 (nt 631)	ARVC	Syrris et al, 2006 Simpson et al. , 2009
Desmoglein-2	Arg45Gln Arg48His Val56Met Asn266Ser Glu331Lys Trp305Stop Cys506Tyr Gly811Cys IVS12AS, A-G, -2 (nt 1881)	ARVC	Awad et al., 2006 Pilichou et al., 2006 Syrris et al., 2007 Posch et al., 2008
Plakoglobin	3bp deletion, 118GCA Ser39Lys40insSer	ARVC	McKoy et al., 2000
	2bp deletion, 2157TG	Naxos disease	Asimaki et al., 2007
Desmoplakin	Val30Met Ser299Arg Lys959Met Arg1255Lys Arg1267X Arg1775Ile Arg2834His Gly2375Arg 2034insA Arg1934Stop 1bp deletion, 7901G IVS, G-A, +1 (nt 423)	ARVC/ Carvajal syndrome	Norgett et al., 2000 Rampazzo et al., 2002 Norman et al., 2005 Yang et al., 2006 Uzumcu et al., 2006 Bolling et al., 2010 Bauce et al., 2010

Table 2. Listing of mutations found in desmosomal genes that have been causally linked to the development of ARVC or variations of it; bp: base pair, IVS or AVSAS: denotes a splice site mutation, IVS: intervening sequence, AS: acceptor splice site, nt: nucleotide, ins: insertion.

5. ID proteins in human heart disease

Arrhythmogenic Right Ventricular Cardiomyopathy (ARVC) is a progressive disease characterized by loss of the right ventricular myocardium, and at advanced stages of the left ventricular myocardium as well, accompanied by fibro-fatty tissue infiltration and replacement. Its clinical manifestations include ventricular arrhythmias, syncope, heart failure and sudden cardiac death (Delmar and McKenna, 2010; Estigoy et al., 2009; Lombardi and Marian, 2011). ARVC has an estimated prevalence of 1 in 5,000 (Sen-Chowdhry et al., 2010), although in some regions (e.g. northern Italy) it reaches 1 in 2,000 (Thiene et al., 2007). Genetic studies have indicated that ~50% of the diagnosed ARVC cases are familial, with an autosomal dominant inheritance (Marcus et al., 1982). Accordingly, a number of mutations have been identified in the genes that encode cardiac desmosomal proteins, and thus ARVC is also referred to as "a disease of the desmosome" (Li and Radice, 2010). These mutations not only affect the number, structural integrity and proper localization of desmosomes, but also of gap junctions, resulting in impaired intercellular conductance and thus development of arrhythmias. To date, five desmosomal genes have been identified that carry inherited mutations causing different variations of ARVC, including: plakophilin-2, desmocollin-2, desmoglein-2, plakoglobin and desmoplakin. Table 2 includes a comprehensive list of mutations identified to date in these five desmosomal genes; for updated listing please refer to: http://www.ncbi.nlm.nih.gov/omim.

More than 70% of the identified desmosomal mutations associated with the development of familial ARVC are present in the gene encoding plakophilin-2 (Gerull et al., 2004; Sen-Chowdhry et al., 2010; van Tintelen et al., 2007). These account for ~20% of diagnosed ARVC cases, while mutations in the genes encoding desmocollin-2 (Simpson et al., 2009; Syrris et al., 2006) and desmoglein-2 (Awad et al., 2006; Posch et al., 2008; Syrris et al., 2006) account for ~10-15% of cases each (Lombardi and Marian, 2011; Pilichou et al., 2006).

Plakoglobin was the first desmosomal protein to be causally associated with a cardiocutaneous subtype of ARVC, known as Naxos disease, which was first characterized by Protonotarios *et al.* (Protonotarios et al., 1986). Genetic studies of patients from the Greek island Naxos, where the syndrome took its name from, revealed a homozygous two-base-pairs deletion (2157-2158delGT) in the gene encoding plakoglobin that was inherited in an autosomal recessive manner (McKoy et al., 2000). In addition to developing ARVC, these individuals also suffered from palmoplantar keratoderma and woolly hair. Recently though, a variation of the Naxos syndrome was diagnosed in a German family that carried a dominantly inherited mutation in the plakoglobin gene (Ser39Lys40insSer) that caused ARVC without the accompanying cutaneous abnormalities (Asimaki et al., 2007). Importantly, the reduced expression or complete absence of plakoglobin from the ID of ARVC patients is a consistent feature, making it a valuable marker for its diagnosis, which still remains problematic with many cases being un- or misdiagnosed.

Mutations in the gene encoding desmoplakin have been identified as the underlying cause of a variation of Naxos disease, referred to as Carvajal syndrome that is also characterized by woolly hair, palmoplantar keratoderma and cardiac disease (Kaplan et al., 2004a; Kaplan et al., 2004b; Norman et al., 2005; Rampazzo et al., 2002; Saffitz, 2009; Yang et al., 2006; Bauce et al., 2010; Bolling et al., 2010; Norgett et al., 2000; Uzumcu et al., 2006). Notably, cardiac disease is presented as a generalized hypertrophy and dilation, involving both the right and left ventricles, and accompanied by focal ventricular aneurysms without any apparent fibro-fatty tissue replacement (Kaplan et al., 2004a; Yang et al., 2006). A major feature of the

Carvajal syndrome is the virtual absence of desmoplakin in the affected hearts, indicating that the missense or nonsense mutations identified result in truncated and/or unstable forms of the protein (Norman et al., 2005; Rampazzo et al., 2002).

Alterations in the amounts, localization and functional properties of desmosomal proteins not only affect intercellular adhesion, but also promote remodelling of gap junctions by leading to abnormal expression and distribution of gap junctional proteins, and primarily connexin-43, which in turn induces defects in the electrochemical coupling of neighbouring cardiocytes and leads to the development of severe arrhythmias (Kaplan et al., 2004a; Pieperhoff et al., 2008; Saffitz, 2009). On the contrary, changes in gap junctions do not affect the structural integrity or proper function of desmosomes and adherens junctions, and thus mechanical coupling of adjacent cardiocytes is not disrupted (Delmar and McKenna, 2010; Li and Radice, 2010; Noorman et al., 2009).

A number of mutations have also been identified in the gene encoding connexin-43, which are associated with the development of oculodentodigital dysplasia (ODDD) that is frequently accompanied by hair and skin defects, too (Kelly et al., 2006). Some of these mutations have been further linked to the development of cardiac disturbances. In such patients, the expression levels of connexin-43, and thus the number of gap junctions, are moderately decreased (Manias et al., 2008); however, cardiac conduction is not affected. Thus, sole mutations in the gene encoding connexin-43 cannot be the primary inducers of electrical or mechanical defects underlying arrhythmogenesis. Interestingly, neither loss- nor gain-of-function mutations have been identified in proteins of adherens junctions that are causally associated with the development of cardiac disease. A plausible explanation is that dysfunctional adherens junctions may be detrimental to the developing myocardium and thus may result in embryonic lethality. Consistent with this, a constitutive null model of N-cadherin was embryonic lethal, while a developmental and cardiac tissue specific model developed dilated cardiomyopathy and died 2 months following excision of the gene, due to mechanical and electrical abnormalities (Li et al., 2005; Radice et al., 1997); for review of available animal models of N-cadherin and their phenotypic characterization, please refer to (Li et al., 2006).

6. Concluding remarks: The intercalated disc is a single functional unit

Although traditionally depicted as a composition of three separate units, data from the last decade suggest that the ID of cardiomyocytes is in fact a single functional unit. Several studies have begun to describe *area composita* as a hybrid between proteins of adherens junctions and desmosomes that form a single anchoring unit (Delmar, 2004; Franke et al., 2006; Pieperhoff and Franke, 2007; Saffitz, 2005). Consistent with this, plakophilin-2 and desmoglein, which typically localize to desmosomes, interact with β- or α-catenin and p120 catenin, respectively, present in adherens junctions (Chen et al., 2002; Goossens et al., 2007). Similarly, molecular linkages between desmosomes and gap junctions have also been identified (Rohr, 2007; Saffitz, 2005). As such, desmocollin-2 directly interacts with connexin-43 (Gehmlich et al., 2011). Taken together, these studies clearly suggest that there is a three-way exchange and cross-talk of junctional proteins, supporting the idea of the ID being a single functional unit.

During the last decade, there have been significant advancements concerning the structural composition of the ID. A plethora of new proteins has been identified as integral or peripheral components of the ID that directly or indirectly contributes to the mechanical and electrical coupling of neighbouring cardiocytes. The challenge of the future lies in the characterization of the precise roles that these proteins play to ensure the synchronous contraction of the myocardium. A combination of sophisticated molecular, genetic and cellular approaches will be needed to address this unequivocally important question.

7. Acknowledgments

Our research has been supported by grants to A.K.K. through the National Institutes of Health (R21 HL106197) and the American Heart Association (GRNT 3780035), to M.A.A from the National Institutes of Health (F32 AR058079) and to L.-Y.R.H. from the National Institutes of Health (Training Grant 2T32AR7592-16).

8. References

Abi-Char J., Maguy A., Coulombe A., Balse E., Ratajczak P., Samuel J.L., Nattel S., Hatem S.N. (2007) Membrane cholesterol modulates Kv1.5 potassium channel distribution and function in rat cardiomyocytes. J Physiol 582:1205-17.

Aho S., Rothenberger K., Uitto J. (1999) Human p120ctn catenin: tissue-specific expression of isoforms and molecular interactions with BP180/type XVII collagen. J Cell Biochem 73:390-9.

Ai X., Pogwizd S.M. (2005) Connexin 43 downregulation and dephosphorylation in nonischemic heart failure is associated with enhanced colocalized protein phosphatase type 2A. Circ Res 96:54-63.

Ai X., Jiang A., Ke Y., Solaro R.J., Pogwizd S.M. (2011) Enhanced activation of p21-activated kinase 1 in heart failure contributes to dephosphorylation of connexin 43. Cardiovasc Res, In Press.

Anastasiadis P.Z., Reynolds A.B. (2000) The p120 catenin family: complex roles in adhesion, signaling and cancer. J Cell Sci 113 (Pt 8):1319-1334.

Angst B.D., Khan L.U., Severs N.J., Whitely K., Rothery S., Thompson R.P., Magee A.I., Gourdie R.G. (1997) Dissociated spatial patterning of gap junctions and cell adhesion junctions during postnatal differentiation of ventricular myocardium. Circ Res 80:88-94.

Asimaki A., Syrris P., Wichter T., Matthias P., Saffitz J.E., McKenna W.J. (2007) A novel dominant mutation in plakoglobin causes arrhythmogenic right ventricular cardiomyopathy. Am J Hum Genet 81:964-73.

Awad M.M., Dalal D., Cho E., Amat-Alarcon N., James C., Tichnell C., Tucker A., Russell S.D., Bluemke D.A., Dietz H.C., Calkins H., Judge D.P. (2006) DSG2 mutations contribute to arrhythmogenic right ventricular dysplasia/cardiomyopathy. Am J Hum Genet 79:136-42.

Barker R.J., Price R.L., Gourdie R.G. (2002) Increased association of ZO-1 with connexin43 during remodeling of cardiac gap junctions. Circ Res 90:317-24.

Bass-Zubek A.E., Godsel L.M., Delmar M., Green K.J. (2009) Plakophilins: multifunctional scaffolds for adhesion and signaling. Curr Opin Cell Biol 21:708-716.

Bauce B., Nava A., Beffagna G., Basso C., Lorenzon A., Smaniotto G., De Bortoli M., Rigato I., Mazzotti E., Steriotis A., Marra M.P., Towbin J.A., Thiene G., Danieli G.A., Rampazzo A. (2010) Multiple mutations in desmosomal proteins encoding genes in arrhythmogenic right ventricular cardiomyopathy/dysplasia. Heart Rhythm 7:22-9.

Bennett P.M., Maggs A.M., Baines A.J., Pinder J.C. (2006) The transitional junction: a new functional subcellular domain at the intercalated disc. Mol Biol Cell 17:2091-2100.

Beyer E.C., Paul D.L., Goodenough D.A. (1987) Connexin43: a protein from rat heart homologous to a gap junction protein from liver. J Cell Biol 105:2621-9.

Bierkamp C., McLaughlin K.J., Schwarz H., Huber O., Kemler R. (1996) Embryonic heart and skin defects in mice lacking plakoglobin. Dev Biol 180:780-5.

Bolling M.C., Veenstra M.J., Jonkman M.F., Diercks G.F., Curry C.J., Fisher J., Pas H.H., Bruckner A.L. (2010) Lethal acantholytic epidermolysis bullosa due to a novel homozygous deletion in DSP: expanding the phenotype and implications for desmoplakin function in skin and heart. Br J Dermatol 162:1388-94.

Bornslaeger E.A., Corcoran C.M., Stappenbeck T.S., Green K.J. (1996) Breaking the connection: displacement of the desmosomal plaque protein desmoplakin from cell-cell interfaces disrupts anchorage of intermediate filament bundles and alters intercellular junction assembly. J Cell Biol 134:985-1001.

Bornslaeger E.A., Godsel L.M., Corcoran C.M., Park J.K., Hatzfeld M., Kowalczyk A.P., Green K.J. (2001) Plakophilin 1 interferes with plakoglobin binding to desmoplakin, yet together with plakoglobin promotes clustering of desmosomal plaque complexes at cell-cell borders. J Cell Sci 114:727-38.

Borrmann C.M., Grund C., Kuhn C., Hofmann I., Pieperhoff S., Franke W.W. (2006) The area composita of adhering junctions connecting heart muscle cells of vertebrates. II. Colocalizations of desmosomal and fascia adhaerens molecules in the intercalated disk. Eur J Cell Biol 85:469-85.

Bowling N., Huang X., Sandusky G.E., Fouts R.L., Mintze K., Esterman M., Allen P.D., Maddi R., McCall E., Vlahos C.J. (2001) Protein kinase C-alpha and -epsilon modulate connexin-43 phosphorylation in human heart. J Mol Cell Cardiol 33:789-98.

Bruce A.F., Rothery S., Dupont E., Severs N.J. (2008) Gap junction remodelling in human heart failure is associated with increased interaction of connexin43 with ZO-1. Cardiovasc Res 77:757-65.

Bukauskas F.F., Verselis V.K. (2004) Gap junction channel gating. Biochim Biophys Acta 1662:42-60.

Burghardt R.C., Barhoumi R., Sewall T.C., Bowen J.A. (1995) Cyclic AMP induces rapid increases in gap junction permeability and changes in the cellular distribution of connexin43. J Membr Biol 148:243-53.

Butz S., Larue L. (1995) Expression of catenins during mouse embryonic development and in adult tissues. Cell Adhes Commun 3:337-52.

Chen X., Bonne S., Hatzfeld M., van Roy F., Green K.J. (2002) Protein binding and functional characterization of plakophilin 2. Evidence for its diverse roles in desmosomes and beta -catenin signaling. J Biol Chem 277:10512-22.

Chitaev N.A., Leube R.E., Troyanovsky R.B., Eshkind L.G., Franke W.W., Troyanovsky S.M. (1996) The binding of plakoglobin to desmosomal cadherins: patterns of binding sites and topogenic potential. J Cell Biol 133:359-69.

Choi H.J., Weis W.I. (2005) Structure of the armadillo repeat domain of plakophilin 1. J Mol Biol 346:367-76.

Choi H.J., Gross J.C., Pokutta S., Weis W.I. (2009) Interactions of plakoglobin and beta-catenin with desmosomal cadherins: basis of selective exclusion of alpha- and beta-catenin from desmosomes. J Biol Chem 284:31776-88.

Choi H.J., Park-Snyder S., Pascoe L.T., Green K.J., Weis W.I. (2002) Structures of two intermediate filament-binding fragments of desmoplakin reveal a unique repeat motif structure. Nat Struct Biol 9:612-20.

Collins J.E., Legan P.K., Kenny T.P., MacGarvie J., Holton J.L., Garrod D.R. (1991) Cloning and sequence analysis of desmosomal glycoproteins 2 and 3 (desmocollins): cadherin-like desmosomal adhesion molecules with heterogeneous cytoplasmic domains. J Cell Biol 113:381-91.

Cooper C.D., Lampe P.D. (2002) Casein kinase 1 regulates connexin-43 gap junction assembly. J Biol Chem 277:44962-8.

Cowin P., Kapprell H.P., Franke W.W., Tamkun J., Hynes R.O. (1986) Plakoglobin: a protein common to different kinds of intercellular adhering junctions. Cell 46:1063-73.

Daniel J.M., Reynolds A.B. (1995) The tyrosine kinase substrate p120cas binds directly to E-cadherin but not to the adenomatous polyposis coli protein or alpha-catenin. Mol Cell Biol 15:4819-24.

Delmar M. (2004) The intercalated disk as a single functional unit. HRTHM 1:12-13.

Delmar M., McKenna W.J. (2010) The cardiac desmosome and arrhythmogenic cardiomyopathies: from gene to disease. Circ Res 107:700-714.

Delva E., Tucker D.K., Kowalczyk A.P. (2009) The desmosome. Cold Spring Harbor perspectives in biology 1:a002543.

Doble B.W., Ping P., Kardami E. (2000) The epsilon subtype of protein kinase C is required for cardiomyocyte connexin-43 phosphorylation. Circ Res 86:293-301.

Dowling J.J., Gibbs E., Russell M., Goldman D., Minarcik J., Golden J.A., Feldman E.L. (2008) Kindlin-2 is an essential component of intercalated discs and is required for vertebrate cardiac structure and function. Circ Res 102:423-431.

Duffy H.S., Sorgen P.L., Girvin M.E., O'Donnell P., Coombs W., Taffet S.M., Delmar M., Spray D.C. (2002) pH-dependent intramolecular binding and structure involving Cx43 cytoplasmic domains. J Biol Chem 277:36706-14.

Dusek R.L., Godsel L.M., Green K.J. (2007) Discriminating roles of desmosomal cadherins: beyond desmosomal adhesion. J Derm Sci 45:7-21.

Duthe F., Plaisance I., Sarrouilhe D., Herve J.C. (2001) Endogenous protein phosphatase 1 runs down gap junctional communication of rat ventricular myocytes. Am J Physiol Cell Physiol 281:C1648-56.

Ek J.F., Delmar M., Perzova R., Taffet S.M. (1994) Role of histidine 95 on pH gating of the cardiac gap junction protein connexin43. Circ Res 74:1058-64.

Ek-Vitorin J.F., King T.J., Heyman N.S., Lampe P.D., Burt J.M. (2006) Selectivity of connexin 43 channels is regulated through protein kinase C-dependent phosphorylation. Circ Res 98:1498-505.

Ek-Vitorin J.F., Calero G., Morley G.E., Coombs W., Taffet S.M., Delmar M. (1996) PH regulation of connexin43: molecular analysis of the gating particle. Biophys J 71:1273-84.

Elfgang C., Eckert R., Lichtenberg-Frate H., Butterweck A., Traub O., Klein R.A., Hulser D.F., Willecke K. (1995) Specific permeability and selective formation of gap junction channels in connexin-transfected HeLa cells. J Cell Biol 129:805-17.

Engelmann T. (1875) Uber die Leitung der Erregung im Herzmuskel. Pfugers Arch Physiol 11.

Eshkind L., Tian Q., Schmidt A., Franke W.W., Windoffer R., Leube R.E. (2002) Loss of desmoglein 2 suggests essential functions for early embryonic development and proliferation of embryonal stem cells. Eur J Cell Biol 81:592-8.

Estigoy C.B., Pontén F., Odeberg J., Herbert B., Guilhaus M., Charleston M., Ho J.W.K., Cameron D., dos Remedios C.G. (2009) Intercalated discs: multiple proteins perform multiple functions in non-failing and failing human hearts. Biophys Rev 1:43-49.

Evans W.H., De Vuyst E., Leybaert L. (2006) The gap junction cellular internet: connexin hemichannels enter the signalling limelight. Biochem J 397:1-14.

Fawcett D.W., McNutt N.S. (1969) The ultrastructure of the cat myocardium. I. Ventricular papillary muscle. J Cell Biol 42:1-45.

Ferreira-Cornwell M.C., Luo Y., Narula N., Lenox J.M., Lieberman M., Radice G.L. (2002) Remodeling the intercalated disc leads to cardiomyopathy in mice misexpressing cadherins in the heart. J Cell Sci 115:1623-1634.

Finnemann S., Mitrik I., Hess M., Otto G., Wedlich D. (1997) Uncoupling of XB/U-cadherin-catenin complex formation from its function in cell-cell adhesion. J Biol Chem 272:11856-62.

Franke W.W., Borrmann C.M., Grund C., Pieperhoff S. (2006) The area composita of adhering junctions connecting heart muscle cells of vertebrates. I. Molecular definition in intercalated disks of cardiomyocytes by immunoelectron microscopy of desmosomal proteins. Eur J Cell Biol 85:69-82.

Franke W.W., Moll R., Schiller D.L., Schmid E., Kartenbeck J., Mueller H. (1982) Desmoplakins of epithelial and myocardial desmosomes are immunologically and biochemically related. Differentiation 23:115-27.

Gallicano G.I., Kouklis P., Bauer C., Yin M., Vasioukhin V., Degenstein L., Fuchs E. (1998) Desmoplakin is required early in development for assembly of desmosomes and cytoskeletal linkage. J Cell Biol 143:2009-22.

Garrod D., Chidgey M. (2008) Desmosome structure, composition and function. Biochim Biophys Acta 1778:572-87.

Garrod D.R., Merritt A.J., Nie Z. (2002) Desmosomal adhesion: structural basis, molecular mechanism and regulation. Mol Membr Biol 19:81-94.

Gehmlich K., Lambiase P.D., Asimaki A., Ciaccio E.J., Ehler E., Syrris P., Saffitz J.E., McKenna W.J. (2011) A novel desmocollin-2 mutation reveals insights into the molecular link between desmosomes and gap junctions. Heart Rhythm 8:711-718.

Geisler S.B., Robinson D., Hauringa M., Raeker M.O., Borisov A.B., Westfall M.V., Russell M.W. (2007) Obscurin-like 1, OBSL1, is a novel cytoskeletal protein related to obscurin. Genomics 89:521-531.

Geisler S.B., Green K.J., Isom L.L., Meshinchi S., Martens J.R., Delmar M., Russell M.W. (2010) Ordered assembly of the adhesive and electrochemical connections within newly formed intercalated disks in primary cultures of adult rat cardiomyocytes. J Biomed Biotechnol 2010:624719.

Gerull B., Heuser A., Wichter T., Paul M., Basson C.T., McDermott D.A., Lerman B.B., Markowitz S.M., Ellinor P.T., MacRae C.A., Peters S., Grossmann K.S., Drenckhahn J., Michely B., Sasse-Klaassen S., Birchmeier W., Dietz R., Breithardt G., Schulze-Bahr E., Thierfelder L. (2004) Mutations in the desmosomal protein plakophilin-2 are common in arrhythmogenic right ventricular cardiomyopathy. Nat Genet 36:1162-4.

Getsios S., Amargo E.V., Dusek R.L., Ishii K., Sheu L., Godsel L.M., Green K.J. (2004) Coordinated expression of desmoglein 1 and desmocollin 1 regulates intercellular adhesion. Differentiation 72:419-33.

Giepmans B.N., Moolenaar W.H. (1998) The gap junction protein connexin43 interacts with the second PDZ domain of the zona occludens-1 protein. Curr Biol 8:931-934.

Giepmans B.N., Verlaan I., Moolenaar W.H. (2001a) Connexin-43 interactions with ZO-1 and alpha- and beta-tubulin. Cell Commun Adhes 8:219-223.

Giepmans B.N., Feiken E., Gebbink M.F., Moolenaar W.H. (2003) Association of connexin43 with a receptor protein tyrosine phosphatase. Cell Commun Adhes 10:201-5.

Giepmans B.N., Verlaan I., Hengeveld T., Janssen H., Calafat J., Falk M.M., Moolenaar W.H. (2001b) Gap junction protein connexin-43 interacts directly with microtubules. Curr Biol 11:1364-1368.

Gonzalez D., Gomez-Hernandez J.M., Barrio L.C. (2007) Molecular basis of voltage dependence of connexin channels: an integrative appraisal. Prog Biophys Mol Biol 94:66-106.

Goossens S., Janssens B., Bonné S., De Rycke R., Braet F., van Hengel J., van Roy F. (2007) A unique and specific interaction between alphaT-catenin and plakophilin-2 in the area composita, the mixed-type junctional structure of cardiac intercalated discs. J Cell Sci 120:2126-2136.

Green K.J., Simpson C.L. (2007) Desmosomes: new perspectives on a classic. J Invest Dermatol 127:2499-515.

Grimley P.M., Edwards G.A. (1960) The ultrastructure of cardiac desnosomes in the toad and their relationship to the intercalated disc. J Biophys Biochem Cytol 8:305-318.

Grossmann K.S., Grund C., Huelsken J., Behrend M., Erdmann B., Franke W.W., Birchmeier W. (2004) Requirement of plakophilin 2 for heart morphogenesis and cardiac junction formation. J Cell Biol 167:149-60.

Gutstein D.E., Liu F.-Y., Meyers M.B., Choo A., Fishman G.I. (2003) The organization of adherens junctions and desmosomes at the cardiac intercalated disc is independent of gap junctions. J Cell Sci 116:875-885.

Gutstein D.E., Morley G.E., Vaidya D., Liu F., Chen F.L., Stuhlmann H., Fishman G.I. (2001a) Heterogeneous expression of Gap junction channels in the heart leads to conduction defects and ventricular dysfunction. Circ 104:1194-9.

Gutstein D.E., Morley G.E., Tamaddon H., Vaidya D., Schneider M.D., Chen J., Chien K.R., Stuhlmann H., Fishman G.I. (2001b) Conduction slowing and sudden arrhythmic death in mice with cardiac-restricted inactivation of connexin43. Circ Res 88:333-9.

Haegel H., Larue L., Ohsugi M., Fedorov L., Herrenknecht K., Kemler R. (1995) Lack of beta-catenin affects mouse development at gastrulation. Development 121:3529-37.

Hatzfeld M. (2005) The p120 family of cell adhesion molecules. Eur J Cell Biol 84:205-14.

Hatzfeld M. (2007) Plakophilins: Multifunctional proteins or just regulators of desmosomal adhesion? Biochim Biophys Acta 1773:69-77.

Heupel W.M., Baumgartner W., Laymann B., Drenckhahn D., Golenhofen N. (2008) Different Ca2+ affinities and functional implications of the two synaptic adhesion molecules cadherin-11 and N-cadherin. Mol Cell Neurosci 37:548-58.

Hirschy A., Schatzmann F., Ehler E., Perriard J.-C. (2006) Establishment of cardiac cytoarchitecture in the developing mouse heart. Dev Biol 289:430-441.

Hofmann I., Mertens C., Brettel M., Nimmrich V., Schnolzer M., Herrmann H. (2000) Interaction of plakophilins with desmoplakin and intermediate filament proteins: an in vitro analysis. J Cell Sci 113 (Pt 13):2471-83.

Holthofer B., Windoffer R., Troyanovsky S., Leube R.E. (2007) Structure and function of desmosomes. Int Rev Cytol 264:65-163.

Hoyt R.H., Cohen M.L., Saffitz J.E. (1989) Distribution and three-dimensional structure of intercellular junctions in canine myocardium. Circ Res 64:563-574.

Huang R.Y.C., Laing J.G., Kanter E.M., Berthoud V.M., Bao M., Rohrs H.W., Townsend R.R., Yamada K.A. (2011) Identification of CaMKII Phosphorylation Sites in Connexin43 by High-Resolution Mass Spectrometry. J Proteome Res 10:1098-1109.

Huber A.H., Nelson W.J., Weis W.I. (1997) Three-dimensional structure of the armadillo repeat region of beta-catenin. Cell 90:871-882.

Hulsken J., Birchmeier W., Behrens J. (1994) E-cadherin and APC compete for the interaction with beta-catenin and the cytoskeleton. J Cell Biol 127:2061-9.

Hund T.J., Lerner D.L., Yamada K.A., Schuessler R.B., Saffitz J.E. (2007) Protein kinase Cepsilon mediates salutary effects on electrical coupling induced by ischemic preconditioning. Heart Rhythm 4:1183-93.

Hund T.J., Decker K.F., Kanter E., Mohler P.J., Boyden P.A., Schuessler R.B., Yamada K.A., Rudy Y. (2008) Role of activated CaMKII in abnormal calcium homeostasis and I(Na) remodeling after myocardial infarction: insights from mathematical modeling. J Mol Cell Cardiol 45:420-8.

Hunter A.W., Barker R.J., Zhu C., Gourdie R.G. (2005) Zonula occludens-1 alters connexin43 gap junction size and organization by influencing channel accretion. Mol Biol Cell 16:5686-98.

Imamura Y., Itoh M., Maeno Y., Tsukita S., Nagafuchi A. (1999) Functional domains of alpha-catenin required for the strong state of cadherin-based cell adhesion. J Cell Biol 144:1311-22.

Janssens B., Goossens S., Staes K., Gilbert B., van Hengel J., Colpaert C., Bruyneel E., Mareel M., van Roy F. (2001) alphaT-catenin: a novel tissue-specific beta-catenin-binding protein mediating strong cell-cell adhesion. J Cell Sci 114:3177-88.

Jeyaraman M., Tanguy S., Fandrich R.R., Lukas A., Kardami E. (2003) Ischemia-induced dephosphorylation of cardiomyocyte connexin-43 is reduced by okadaic acid and calyculin A but not fostriecin. Mol Cell Biochem 242:129-34.

Jung-Ching Lin J., Gustafson-Wagner E.A., Sinn H.W., Choi S., Jaacks S.M., Wang D.-Z., Evans S., Li-Chun Lin J. (2005) Structure, Expression, and Function of a Novel Intercalated Disc Protein, Xin. J Med Sci 25:215-222.

Kami K., Chidgey M., Dafforn T., Overduin M. (2009) The desmoglein-specific cytoplasmic region is intrinsically disordered in solution and interacts with multiple desmosomal protein partners. J Mol Biol 386:531-43.

Kaplan S.R., Gard J.J., Carvajal-Huerta L., Ruiz-Cabezas J.C., Thiene G., Saffitz J.E. (2004a) Structural and molecular pathology of the heart in Carvajal syndrome. Cardiovasc Pathol 13:26-32.

Kaplan S.R., Gard J.J., Protonotarios N., Tsatsopoulou A., Spiliopoulou C., Anastasakis A., Squarcioni C.P., McKenna W.J., Thiene G., Basso C., Brousse N., Fontaine G., Saffitz J.E. (2004b) Remodeling of myocyte gap junctions in arrhythmogenic right ventricular cardiomyopathy due to a deletion in plakoglobin (Naxos disease). Heart Rhythm 1:3-11.

Kargacin G.J., Hunt D., Emmett T., Rokolya A., McMartin G.A., Wirch E., Walsh M.P., Ikebe M., Kargacin M.E. (2006) Localization of telokin at the intercalated discs of cardiac myocytes. Arch Biochem Biophys 456:151-160.

Katsuno T., Umeda K., Matsui T., Hata M., Tamura A., Itoh M., Takeuchi K., Fujimori T., Nabeshima Y., Noda T., Tsukita S. (2008) Deficiency of zonula occludens-1 causes embryonic lethal phenotype associated with defected yolk sac angiogenesis and apoptosis of embryonic cells. Mol Biol Cell 19:2465-75.

Keirsebilck A., Bonne S., Staes K., van Hengel J., Nollet F., Reynolds A., van Roy F. (1998) Molecular cloning of the human p120ctn catenin gene (CTNND1): expression of multiple alternatively spliced isoforms. Genomics 50:129-46.

Kelly S.C., Ratajczak P., Keller M., Purcell S.M., Griffin T., Richard G. (2006) A novel GJA 1 mutation in oculo-dento-digital dysplasia with curly hair and hyperkeratosis. Eur J Dermatol 16:241-5.

Kirchhoff S., Nelles E., Hagendorff A., Kruger O., Traub O., Willecke K. (1998) Reduced cardiac conduction velocity and predisposition to arrhythmias in connexin40-deficient mice. Curr Biol 8:299-302.

Kobielak A., Fuchs E. (2004) Alpha-catenin: at the junction of intercellular adhesion and actin dynamics. Nature Rev 5:614-625.

Koslov E.R., Maupin P., Pradhan D., Morrow J.S., Rimm D.L. (1997) Alpha-catenin can form asymmetric homodimeric complexes and/or heterodimeric complexes with beta-catenin. J Biol Chem 272:27301-6.

Kostetskii I., Li J., Xiong Y., Zhou R., Ferrari V.A., Patel V.V., Molkentin J.D., Radice G.L. (2005) Induced deletion of the N-cadherin gene in the heart leads to dissolution of the intercalated disc structure. Circ Res 96:346-354.

Kostin S. (2007) Zonula occludens-1 and connexin 43 expression in the failing human heart. J Cell Mol Med 11:892-5.

Kostin S., Hein S., Bauer E.P., Schaper J. (1999) Spatiotemporal development and distribution of intercellular junctions in adult rat cardiomyocytes in culture. Circ Res 85:154-167.

Kowalczyk A.P., Stappenbeck T.S., Parry D.A., Palka H.L., Virata M.L., Bornslaeger E.A., Nilles L.A., Green K.J. (1994) Structure and function of desmosomal transmembrane core and plaque molecules. Biophys Chem 50:97-112.

Kowalczyk A.P., Hatzfeld M., Bornslaeger E.A., Kopp D.S., Borgwardt J.E., Corcoran C.M., Settler A., Green K.J. (1999) The head domain of plakophilin-1 binds to desmoplakin and enhances its recruitment to desmosomes. Implications for cutaneous disease. J Biol Chem 274:18145-8.

Krusche C.A., Holthöfer B., Hofe V., van de Sandt A.M., Eshkind L., Bockamp E., Merx M.W., Kant S., Windoffer R., Leube R.E. (2011) Desmoglein 2 mutant mice develop cardiac fibrosis and dilation. Bas Res Cardiol 106:617-633.

Laing J.G., Saffitz J.E., Steinberg T.H., Yamada K.A. (2007) Diminished zonula occludens-1 expression in the failing human heart. Cardiovasc Pathol 16:159-64.

Lampe P.D., Cooper C.D., King T.J., Burt J.M. (2006) Analysis of Connexin43 phosphorylated at S325, S328 and S330 in normoxic and ischemic heart. J Cell Sci 119:3435-42.

Lampe P.D., TenBroek E.M., Burt J.M., Kurata W.E., Johnson R.G., Lau A.F. (2000) Phosphorylation of connexin43 on serine368 by protein kinase C regulates gap junctional communication. J Cell Biol 149:1503-12.

Langlois S., Cowan K.N., Shao Q., Cowan B.J., Laird D.W. (2008) Caveolin-1 and -2 interact with connexin43 and regulate gap junctional intercellular communication in keratinocytes. Mol Biol Cell 19:912-28.

Lauf U., Giepmans B.N., Lopez P., Braconnot S., Chen S.C., Falk M.M. (2002) Dynamic trafficking and delivery of connexons to the plasma membrane and accretion to gap junctions in living cells. Proc Natl Acad Sci U S A 99:10446-51.

Li J., Radice G.L. (2010) A New Perspective on Intercalated Disc Organization: Implications for Heart Disease. Dermatol Res Pract 2010:1-5.

Li J., Patel V.V., Radice G.L. (2006) Dysregulation of cell adhesion proteins and cardiac arrhythmogenesis. Clin Med Res 4:42-52.

Li J., Levin M.D., Xiong Y., Petrenko N., Patel V.V., Radice G.L. (2008) N-cadherin haploinsufficiency affects cardiac gap junctions and arrhythmic susceptibility. J Mol Cell Cardiol 44:597-606.

Li J., Swope D., Raess N., Cheng L., Muller E.J., Radice G.L. (2011) Cardiac tissue-restricted deletion of plakoglobin results in progressive cardiomyopathy and activation of {beta}-catenin signaling. Mol Cell Biol 31:1134-1144.

Li J., Patel V.V., Kostetskii I., Xiong Y., Chu A.F., Jacobson J.T., Yu C., Morley G.E., Molkentin J.D., Radice G.L. (2005) Cardiac-specific loss of N-cadherin leads to alteration in connexins with conduction slowing and arrhythmogenesis. Circ Res 97:474-481.

Lin D., Zhou J., Zelenka P.S., Takemoto D.J. (2003) Protein kinase Cgamma regulation of gap junction activity through caveolin-1-containing lipid rafts. Invest Ophthalmol Vis Sci 44:5259-68.

Liu L., Li Y., Lin J., Liang Q., Sheng X., Wu J., Huang R., Liu S., Li Y. (2010) Connexin43 interacts with Caveolin-3 in the heart. Mol Biol Reports 37:1685-1691.

Lombardi R., Marian A.J. (2011) Molecular genetics and pathogenesis of arrhythmogenic right ventricular cardiomyopathy: a disease of cardiac stem cells. Pediatr Cardiol 32:360-5.

Lorimer J.E., Hall L.S., Clarke J.P., Collins J.E., Fleming T.P., Garrod D.R. (1994) Cloning, sequence analysis and expression pattern of mouse desmocollin 2 (DSC2), a cadherin-like adhesion molecule. Mol Membr Biol 11:229-36.

Maass K., Shibayama J., Chase S.E., Willecke K., Delmar M. (2007) C-terminal truncation of connexin43 changes number, size, and localization of cardiac gap junction plaques. Circ Res 101:1283-91.

Manias J.L., Plante I., Gong X.Q., Shao Q., Churko J., Bai D., Laird D.W. (2008) Fate of connexin43 in cardiac tissue harbouring a disease-linked connexin43 mutant. Cardiovasc Res 80:385-95.

Marcozzi C., Burdett I.D., Buxton R.S., Magee A.I. (1998) Coexpression of both types of desmosomal cadherin and plakoglobin confers strong intercellular adhesion. J Cell Sci 111 (Pt 4):495-509.

Marcus F.I., Fontaine G.H., Guiraudon G., Frank R., Laurenceau J.L., Malergue C., Grosgogeat Y. (1982) Right ventricular dysplasia: a report of 24 adult cases. Circ 65:384-98.

Mathur M., Goodwin L., Cowin P. (1994) Interactions of the cytoplasmic domain of the desmosomal cadherin Dsg1 with plakoglobin. J Biol Chem 269:14075-80.

Matsuda H., Kurata Y., Oka C., Matsuoka S., Noma A. (2010) Magnesium gating of cardiac gap junction channels. Prog Biophys Mol Biol 103:102-10.

McGregor A., Blanchard A.D., Rowe A.J., Critchley D.R. (1994) Identification of the vinculin-binding site in the cytoskeletal protein alpha-actinin. Biochem J 301 (Pt 1):225-33.

McKoy G., Protonotarios N., Crosby A., Tsatsopoulou A., Anastasakis A., Coonar A., Norman M., Baboonian C., Jeffery S., McKenna W.J. (2000) Identification of a deletion in plakoglobin in arrhythmogenic right ventricular cardiomyopathy with palmoplantar keratoderma and woolly hair (Naxos disease). Lancet 355:2119-24.

McNutt D.P., Feldman P.D., Houck J.R., Harwit M. (1970) Far-infrared observations of the night sky: different data. Science 167:1277.

Mertens C., Kuhn C., Franke W.W. (1996) Plakophilins 2a and 2b: constitutive proteins of dual location in the karyoplasm and the desmosomal plaque. J Cell Biol 135:1009-25.

Mertens C., Kuhn C., Moll R., Schwetlick I., Franke W.W. (1999) Desmosomal plakophilin 2 as a differentiation marker in normal and malignant tissues. Differentiation 64:277-90.

Muir A.R. (1957) An electron microscope study of the embryology of the intercalated disc in the heart of the rabbit. J Biophys Biochem Cytol 3:193-202.

Nagaraj R.H., Shipanova I.N., Faust F.M. (1996) Protein cross-linking by the Maillard reaction. Isolation, characterization, and in vivo detection of a lysine-lysine cross-link derived from methylglyoxal. J Biol Chem 271:19338-45.

Niessen C.M. (2007) Tight junctions/adherens junctions: basic structure and function. J Invest Dermatol 127:2525-2532.

Noorman M., van der Heyden M.A.G., van Veen T.A.B., Cox M.G.P.J., Hauer R.N.W., de Bakker J.M.T., van Rijen H.V.M. (2009) Cardiac cell-cell junctions in health and disease: Electrical versus mechanical coupling. J Mol Cell Cardiol 47:23-31.

Norgett E.E., Hatsell S.J., Carvajal-Huerta L., Cabezas J.C., Common J., Purkis P.E., Whittock N., Leigh I.M., Stevens H.P., Kelsell D.P. (2000) Recessive mutation in desmoplakin disrupts desmoplakin-intermediate filament interactions and causes dilated cardiomyopathy, woolly hair and keratoderma. Hum Mol Genet 9:2761-6.

Norman M., Simpson M., Mogensen J., Shaw A., Hughes S., Syrris P., Sen-Chowdhry S., Rowland E., Crosby A., McKenna W.J. (2005) Novel mutation in desmoplakin causes arrhythmogenic left ventricular cardiomyopathy. Circ 112:636-42.

Nose A., Tsuji K., Takeichi M. (1990) Localization of specificity determining sites in cadherin cell adhesion molecules. Cell 61:147-55.

Ozawa M., Ringwald M., Kemler R. (1990) Uvomorulin-catenin complex formation is regulated by a specific domain in the cytoplasmic region of the cell adhesion molecule. Proc Natl Acad Sci U S A 87:4246-50.

Parker A.E., Wheeler G.N., Arnemann J., Pidsley S.C., Ataliotis P., Thomas C.L., Rees D.A., Magee A.I., Buxton R.S. (1991) Desmosomal glycoproteins II and III. Cadherin-like junctional molecules generated by alternative splicing. J Biol Chem 266:10438-45.

Peifer M., Berg S., Reynolds A.B. (1994) A repeating amino acid motif shared by proteins with diverse cellular roles. Cell 76:789-91.

Peifer M., McCrea P.D., Green K.J., Wieschaus E., Gumbiner B.M. (1992) The vertebrate adhesive junction proteins beta-catenin and plakoglobin and the Drosophila segment polarity gene armadillo form a multigene family with similar properties. J Cell Biol 118:681-91.

Perkins G., Goodenough D., Sosinsky G. (1997) Three-dimensional structure of the gap junction connexon. Biophys J 72:533-44.

Peters N.S., Severs N.J., Rothery S.M., Lincoln C., Yacoub M.H., Green C.R. (1994) Spatiotemporal relation between gap junctions and fascia adherens junctions during postnatal development of human ventricular myocardium. Circ 90:713-725.

Pieperhoff S., Franke W.W. (2007) The area composita of adhering junctions connecting heart muscle cells of vertebrates - IV: coalescence and amalgamation of desmosomal and adhaerens junction components - late processes in mammalian heart development. Eur J Cell Biol 86:377-391.

Pieperhoff S., Schumacher H., Franke W.W. (2008) The area composita of adhering junctions connecting heart muscle cells of vertebrates. V. The importance of plakophilin-2 demonstrated by small interference RNA-mediated knockdown in cultured rat cardiomyocytes. Eur J Cell Biol 87:399-411.

Pilichou K., Nava A., Basso C., Beffagna G., Bauce B., Lorenzon A., Frigo G., Vettori A., Valente M., Towbin J., Thiene G., Danieli G.A., Rampazzo A. (2006) Mutations in desmoglein-2 gene are associated with arrhythmogenic right ventricular cardiomyopathy. Circ 113:1171-1179.

Piven O.O., Kostetskii I.E., Macewicz L.L., Kolomiets Y.M., Radice G.L., Lukash L.L. (2011) Requirement for N-cadherin-catenin complex in heart development. Exp Biol Med 236:816-22.

Pokutta S., Weis W.I. (2000) Structure of the dimerization and beta-catenin-binding region of alpha-catenin. Mol Cell 5:533-43.

Pokutta S., Weis W.I. (2007) Structure and mechanism of cadherins and catenins in cell-cell contacts. Annu Rev Cell Dev Biol 23:237-61.

Posch M.G., Posch M.J., Geier C., Erdmann B., Mueller W., Richter A., Ruppert V., Pankuweit S., Maisch B., Perrot A., Buttgereit J., Dietz R., Haverkamp W., Ozcelik C. (2008) A missense variant in desmoglein-2 predisposes to dilated cardiomyopathy. Mol Genet Metab 95:74-80.

Procida K., Jorgensen L., Schmitt N., Delmar M., Taffet S.M., Holstein-Rathlou N.H., Nielsen M.S., Braunstein T.H. (2009) Phosphorylation of connexin43 on serine 306 regulates electrical coupling. Heart Rhythm 6:1632-8.

Protonotarios N., Tsatsopoulou A., Patsourakos P., Alexopoulos D., Gezerlis P., Simitsis S., Scampardonis G. (1986) Cardiac abnormalities in familial palmoplantar keratosis. Br Heart J 56:321-6.

Protonotarios N., Anastasakis A., Antoniades L., Chlouverakis G., Syrris P., Basso C., Asimaki A., Theopistou A., Stefanadis C., Thiene G., McKenna W.J., Tsatsopoulou A. (2011) Arrhythmogenic right ventricular cardiomyopathy/dysplasia on the basis of the revised diagnostic criteria in affected families with desmosomal mutations. Eur Heart J 32(9):1097-104.

Radice G.L., Rayburn H., Matsunami H., Knudsen K.A., Takeichi M., Hynes R.O. (1997) Developmental defects in mouse embryos lacking N-cadherin. Dev Biol 181:64-78.

Rampazzo A., Nava A., Malacrida S., Beffagna G., Bauce B., Rossi V., Zimbello R., Simionati B., Basso C., Thiene G., Towbin J.A., Danieli G.A. (2002) Mutation in human desmoplakin domain binding to plakoglobin causes a dominant form of arrhythmogenic right ventricular cardiomyopathy. Am J Hum Genet 71:1200-6.

Ravel J., Karnovsky M. (1967) Hexagonal array of subunits in intercellular junctions of the mouse heart and liver. J Cell Biol 22:1516-1528.

Rayns D.G., Simpson F.O., Ledingham J.M. (1969) Ultrastructure of desmosomes in mammalian intercalated disc; appearances after lanthanum treatment. J Cell Biol 42:322-326.

Reaume A.G., de Sousa P.A., Kulkarni S., Langille B.L., Zhu D., Davies T.C., Juneja S.C., Kidder G.M., Rossant J. (1995) Cardiac malformation in neonatal mice lacking connexin43. Science 267:1831-4.

Reynolds A.B., Herbert L., Cleveland J.L., Berg S.T., Gaut J.R. (1992) p120, a novel substrate of protein tyrosine kinase receptors and of p60v-src, is related to cadherin-binding factors beta-catenin, plakoglobin and armadillo. Oncogene 7:2439-45.

Rhett J.M., Jourdan J., Gourdie R.G. (2011) Connexin 43 connexon to gap junction transition is regulated by zonula occludens-1. Mol Biol Cell 22:1516-28.

Rimm D.L., Koslov E.R., Kebriaei P., Cianci C.D., Morrow J.S. (1995) Alpha 1(E)-catenin is an actin-binding and -bundling protein mediating the attachment of F-actin to the membrane adhesion complex. Proc Natl Acad Sci U S A 92:8813-7.

Rohr S. (2004) Role of gap junctions in the propagation of the cardiac action potential. Cardiov Res 62:309-322.

Rohr S. (2007) Molecular crosstalk between mechanical and electrical junctions at the intercalated disc. Circulation research 101:637-639.

Rudiger M. (1998) Vinculin and alpha-catenin: shared and unique functions in adherens junctions. Bioessays 20:733-40.

Ruiz P., Brinkmann V., Ledermann B., Behrend M., Grund C., Thalhammer C., Vogel F., Birchmeier C., Gunthert U., Franke W.W., Birchmeier W. (1996) Targeted mutation of plakoglobin in mice reveals essential functions of desmosomes in the embryonic heart. J Cell Biol 135:215-25.

Saez J.C., Nairn A.C., Czernik A.J., Fishman G.I., Spray D.C., Hertzberg E.L. (1997) Phosphorylation of connexin43 and the regulation of neonatal rat cardiac myocyte gap junctions. J Mol Cell Cardiol 29:2131-45.

Saffitz J.E. (2005) Dependence of Electrical Coupling on Mechanical Coupling in Cardiac Myocytes: Insights Gained from Cardiomyopathies Caused by Defects in Cell-Cell Connections. Ann New York Acad Sci 1047:336-344.

Saffitz J.E. (2009) Arrhythmogenic cardiomyopathy and abnormalities of cell-to-cell coupling. Heart Rhythm 6:S62-5.

Saphir O., Karsner H.T. (1924) An Anatomical and Experimental Study of Segmentation of the Myocardium and its Relation to the Intercalated Discs. J Med Res 44:539-556.5.

Sato P.Y., Musa H., Coombs W., Guerrero-Serna G., Patiño G.A., Taffet S.M., Isom L.L., Delmar M. (2009) Loss of plakophilin-2 expression leads to decreased sodium current and slower conduction velocity in cultured cardiac myocytes. Circ Res 105:523-526.

Sato P.Y., Coombs W., Lin X., Nekrasova O., Green K.J., Isom L.L., Taffet S.M., Delmar M. (2011) Interactions between ankyrin-g, plakophilin-2, and connexin43 at the cardiac intercalated disc. Circ Res 109:193-201.

Satomi-Kobayashi S., Ueyama T., Mueller S., Toh R., Masano T., Sakoda T., Rikitake Y., Miyoshi J., Matsubara H., Oh H., Kawashima S., Hirata K.-i., Takai Y. (2009) Deficiency of nectin-2 leads to cardiac fibrosis and dysfunction under chronic pressure overload. Hypertension 54:825-831.

Schmelz M., Duden R., Cowin P., Franke W.W. (1986) A constitutive transmembrane glycoprotein of Mr 165,000 (desmoglein) in epidermal and non-epidermal desmosomes. I. Biochemical identification of the polypeptide. Eur J Cell Biol 42:177-83.

Schroen B., Leenders J.J., van Erk A., Bertrand A.T., van Loon M., van Leeuwen R.E., Kubben N., Duisters R.F., Schellings M.W., Janssen B.J., Debets J.J., Schwake M., Høydal M.A., Heymans S., Saftig P., Pinto Y.M. (2007) Lysosomal integral membrane protein 2 is a novel component of the cardiac intercalated disc and vital for load-induced cardiac myocyte hypertrophy. J Exper Med 204:1227-1235.

Schubert A.-L., Schubert W., Spray D.C., Lisanti M.P. (2002) Connexin family members target to lipid raft domains and interact with caveolin-1. Biochemistry 41:5754-5764.

Seeger T.S., Frank D., Rohr C., Will R., Just S., Grund C., Lyon R., Luedde M., Koegl M., Sheikh F., Rottbauer W., Franke W.W., Katus H.A., Olson E.N., Frey N. (2010) Myozap, a Novel Intercalated Disc Protein, Activates Serum Response Factor-Dependent Signaling and Is Required to Maintain Cardiac Function In Vivo. Circ Res 106:880-890.

Sen-Chowdhry S., Morgan R.D., Chambers J.C., McKenna W.J. (2010) Arrhythmogenic cardiomyopathy: etiology, diagnosis, and treatment. Annu Rev Med 61:233-53.

Severs N.J., Bruce A.F., Dupont E., Rothery S. (2008) Remodelling of gap junctions and connexin expression in diseased myocardium. Cardiovasc Res 80:9-19.

Shaw R.M., Fay A.J., Puthenveedu M.A., von Zastrow M., Jan Y.N., Jan L.Y. (2007) Microtubule plus-end-tracking proteins target gap junctions directly from the cell interior to adherens junctions. Cell 128:547-60.

Sheikh F., Chen Y., Chen Y., Liang X., Hirschy A., Stenbit A.E., Gu Y., Dalton N.D., Yajima T., Lu Y., Knowlton K.U., Peterson K.L., Perriard J.-C., Chen J. (2006) alpha-E-catenin inactivation disrupts the cardiomyocyte adherens junction, resulting in cardiomyopathy and susceptibility to wall rupture. Circ 114:1046-1055.

Shibamoto S., Hayakawa M., Takeuchi K., Hori T., Miyazawa K., Kitamura N., Johnson K.R., Wheelock M.J., Matsuyoshi N., Takeichi M., et al. (1995) Association of p120, a tyrosine kinase substrate, with E-cadherin/catenin complexes. J Cell Biol 128:949-57.

Shimada T., Kawazato H., Yasuda A., Ono N., Sueda K. (2004) Cytoarchitecture and intercalated disks of the working myocardium and the conduction system in the mammalian heart. Anatom Rec 280:940-951.

Simpson M.A., Mansour S., Ahnood D., Kalidas K., Patton M.A., McKenna W.J., Behr E.R., Crosby A.H. (2009) Homozygous mutation of desmocollin-2 in arrhythmogenic right ventricular cardiomyopathy with mild palmoplantar keratoderma and woolly hair. Cardiology 113:28-34.

Sjostrand F.S., Andersson E. (1954) Electron microscopy of the intercalated discs of cardiac muscle tissue. Experientia 10:369-70.

Smyth J.W., Hong T.T., Gao D., Vogan J.M., Jensen B.C., Fong T.S., Simpson P.C., Stainier D.Y., Chi N.C., Shaw R.M. (2010) Limited forward trafficking of connexin 43 reduces cell-cell coupling in stressed human and mouse myocardium. J Clin Invest 120:266-79.

Sohl G., Willecke K. (2004) Gap junctions and the connexin protein family. Cardiovasc Res 62:228-32.

Solan J.L., Marquez-Rosado L., Sorgen P.L., Thornton P.J., Gafken P.R., Lampe P.D. (2007) Phosphorylation at S365 is a gatekeeper event that changes the structure of Cx43 and prevents down-regulation by PKC. J Cell Biol 179:1301-9.

Sorgen P.L., Duffy H.S., Sahoo P., Coombs W., Delmar M., Spray D.C. (2004) Structural changes in the carboxyl terminus of the gap junction protein connexin43 indicates signaling between binding domains for c-Src and zonula occludens-1. J Biol Chem 279:54695-701.

Staddon J.M., Smales C., Schulze C., Esch F.S., Rubin L.L. (1995) p120, a p120-related protein (p100), and the cadherin/catenin complex. J Cell Biol 130:369-81.

Syed S.E., Trinnaman B., Martin S., Major S., Hutchinson J., Magee A.I. (2002) Molecular interactions between desmosomal cadherins. Biochem J 362:317-27.

Syrris P., Ward D., Evans A., Asimaki A., Gandjbakhch E., Sen-Chowdhry S., McKenna W.J. (2006) Arrhythmogenic right ventricular dysplasia/cardiomyopathy associated with mutations in the desmosomal gene desmocollin-2. Am J Hum Genet 79:978-84.

Takeichi M. (1994) The cadherin cell adhesion receptor family: roles in multicellular organization and neurogenesis. Progr Clin Biol Res 390:145-153.

Talhouk R.S., Mroue R., Mokalled M., Abi-Mosleh L., Nehme R., Ismail A., Khalil A., Zaatari M., El-Sabban M.E. (2008) Heterocellular interaction enhances recruitment of alpha and beta-catenins and ZO-2 into functional gap-junction complexes and induces gap junction-dependant differentiation of mammary epithelial cells. Exper Cell Res 314:3275-3291.

Tandler B., Riva L., Loy F., Conti G., Isola R. (2006) High resolution scanning electron microscopy of the intracellular surface of intercalated disks in human heart. Tissue Cell 38:417-420.

Tang Z., Scherer P.E., Okamoto T., Song K., Chu C., Kohtz D.S., Nishimoto I., Lodish H.F., Lisanti M.P. (1996) Molecular cloning of caveolin-3, a novel member of the caveolin gene family expressed predominantly in muscle. J Biol Chem 271:2255-61.

TenBroek E.M., Lampe P.D., Solan J.L., Reynhout J.K., Johnson R.G. (2001) Ser364 of connexin43 and the upregulation of gap junction assembly by cAMP. J Cell Biol 155:1307-18.

Tepass U., Truong K., Godt D., Ikura M., Peifer M. (2000) Cadherins in embryonic and neural morphogenesis. Nat Rev Mol Cell Biol 1:91-100.

Thiene G., Corrado D., Basso C. (2007) Arrhythmogenic right ventricular cardiomyopathy/dysplasia. Orphanet J Rare Dis 2:45.

Thimm J., Mechler A., Lin H., Rhee S., Lal R. (2005) Calcium-dependent open/closed conformations and interfacial energy maps of reconstituted hemichannels. J Biol Chem 280:10646-54.

Thomason H.A., Scothern A., McHarg S., Garrod D.R. (2010) Desmosomes: adhesive strength and signalling in health and disease. Biochem J 429:419-433.

Thoreson M.A., Anastasiadis P.Z., Daniel J.M., Ireton R.C., Wheelock M.J., Johnson K.R., Hummingbird D.K., Reynolds A.B. (2000) Selective uncoupling of p120(ctn) from E-cadherin disrupts strong adhesion. J Cell Biol 148:189-202.

Toyofuku T., Yabuki M., Otsu K., Kuzuya T., Hori M., Tada M. (1998) Direct association of the gap junction protein connexin-43 with ZO-1 in cardiac myocytes. J Biol Chem 273:12725-31.

Toyofuku T., Akamatsu Y., Zhang H., Kuzuya T., Tada M., Hori M. (2001) c-Src regulates the interaction between connexin-43 and ZO-1 in cardiac myocytes. J Biol Chem 276:1780-8.

Troyanovsky S.M., Eshkind L.G., Troyanovsky R.B., Leube R.E., Franke W.W. (1993) Contributions of cytoplasmic domains of desmosomal cadherins to desmosome assembly and intermediate filament anchorage. Cell 72:561-74.

Tselepis C., Chidgey M., North A., Garrod D. (1998) Desmosomal adhesion inhibits invasive behavior. Proc Natl Acad Sci U S A 95:8064-9.

Unger V.M., Kumar N.M., Gilula N.B., Yeager M. (1999) Three-dimensional structure of a recombinant gap junction membrane channel. Science 283:1176-80.

Uzumcu A., Norgett E.E., Dindar A., Uyguner O., Nisli K., Kayserili H., Sahin S.E., Dupont E., Severs N.J., Leigh I.M., Yuksel-Apak M., Kelsell D.P., Wollnik B. (2006) Loss of desmoplakin isoform I causes early onset cardiomyopathy and heart failure in a Naxos-like syndrome. J Med Genet 43:e5.

Van Breemen V. (1953) Intercalated discs in heart muscle studied with the electron microscope. Anatom Rec 117:49-63.

van Tintelen J.P., Hofstra R.M., Wiesfeld A.C., van den Berg M.P., Hauer R.N., Jongbloed J.D. (2007) Molecular genetics of arrhythmogenic right ventricular cardiomyopathy emerging horizon? Curr Opin Cardiol 22:185-192.

Volk T., Geiger B. (1984) A 135-kd membrane protein of intercellular adherens junctions EMBO J 3:2249-2260.

Vozzi C., Dupont E., Coppen S.R., Yeh H.I., Severs N.J. (1999) Chamber-related differences in connexin expression in the human heart. J Mol Cell Cardiol 31:991-1003.

Wahl J.K., Sacco P.A., McGranahan-Sadler T.M., Sauppe L.M., Wheelock M.J., Johnson K.R. (1996) Plakoglobin domains that define its association with the desmosomal cadherins and the classical cadherins: identification of unique and shared domains. J Cell Sci 109 (Pt 5):1143-54.

Warn-Cramer B.J., Cottrell G.T., Burt J.M., Lau A.F. (1998) Regulation of connexin-43 gap junctional intercellular communication by mitogen-activated protein kinase. J Biol Chem 273:9188-96.

Warn-Cramer B.J., Lampe P.D., Kurata W.E., Kanemitsu M.Y., Loo L.W., Eckhart W., Lau A.F. (1996) Characterization of the mitogen-activated protein kinase phosphorylation sites on the connexin-43 gap junction protein. J Biol Chem 271:3779-86.

Waschke J., Bruggeman P., Baumgartner W., Zillikens D., Drenckhahn D. (2005) Pemphigus foliaceus IgG causes dissociation of desmoglein 1-containing junctions without blocking desmoglein 1 transinteraction. J Clin Invest 115:3157-65.

Wei C.-J., Francis R., Xu X., Lo C.W. (2005) Connexin43 associated with an N-cadherin-containing multiprotein complex is required for gap junction formation in NIH3T3 cells. J Biol Chem 280:19925-19936.

Weidmann S. (1952) The electrical constants of Purkinje fibres. J Physiol 118:348-60.

Weiss E.E., Kroemker M., Rudiger A.H., Jockusch B.M., Rudiger M. (1998) Vinculin is part of the cadherin-catenin junctional complex: complex formation between alpha-catenin and vinculin. J Cell Biol 141:755-64.

Xu J., Kausalya P.J., Phua D.C., Ali S.M., Hossain Z., Hunziker W. (2008) Early embryonic lethality of mice lacking ZO-2, but Not ZO-3, reveals critical and nonredundant roles for individual zonula occludens proteins in mammalian development. Mol Cell Biol 28:1669-78.

Yang Z., Bowles N.E., Scherer S.E., Taylor M.D., Kearney D.L., Ge S., Nadvoretskiy V.V., DeFreitas G., Carabello B., Brandon L.I., Godsel L.M., Green K.J., Saffitz J.E., Li H., Danieli G.A., Calkins H., Marcus F., Towbin J.A. (2006) Desmosomal dysfunction due to mutations in desmoplakin causes arrhythmogenic right ventricular dysplasia/cardiomyopathy. Circ Res 99:646-55.

Yarbrough T.L., Lu T., Lee H.C., Shibata E.F. (2002) Localization of cardiac sodium channels in caveolin-rich membrane domains: regulation of sodium current amplitude. Circ Res 90:443-9.

Zhao Y.Y., Liu Y., Stan R. V., Fan L., Gu Y., Dalton N., Chu P.H., Peterson K., Ross J., Chien K.R. (2002) Defects in *caveolin-1* cause dilated cardiomyopathy and pulmonary hypertension in knockout mice. Proc Natl Acad Sci USA 99:11375-80.

Zhu C., Barker R.J., Hunter A.W., Zhang Y., Jourdan J., Gourdie R.G. (2005) Quantitative analysis of ZO-1 colocalization with Cx43 gap junction plaques in cultures of rat neonatal cardiomyocytes. Microsc Microanal 11:244-8.

5

Cardiac Myocytes and Mechanosensation

Byambajav Buyandelger and Ralph Knöll
British Heart Foundation – Centre for Research Excellence,
National Heart & Lung Institute, Imperial College, London,
UK

1. Introduction

Mechanosensation is a fundamental process in biology and may have been developed by the early cells in response to hypo-osmotic stress [1]. With the evolution of different cell types and the appearance of multi-cellular organisms the mechanisms of mechanosensation and the corresponding transmission of signals became more complex and evolved in different cell types differently [2]. Particularly in cardiac myocytes different mechanosensory protein - complexes can be found: i) cell membrane associated ii) intracellular embedded iii) sarcomere related (figure 1). All these various signalosomes are sensitive to different types of mechanical signals. For example, a deformation of the cell membrane may be detected by cell membrane associated signalosomes, such as stretch activated channels (SAC), angiotensin receptors, the caveolae, and integrin mediated signalling. Depending on severity and duration, these events may also be sensed by intermediate filaments (IF) and or even by the sarcomere associated signalosomes. However it is important to differentiate between different types of stresses, such as the normal "stress" (σ) which is physically defined by:

$$\sigma = \frac{F}{A}$$

(where F is the applied force per unit area (A), dimension: N/m^2)
And "shear stress (τ)", where the applied force (F(S) = shear force) acts parallel to the area (A) (dimension: N/m^2):

$$\tau = \frac{F(S)}{A}$$

Other types of physical stresses such as compression and torsion may also occur and are equally important. Distinct from stress is "strain" (ε) which is physically defined by:

$$\varepsilon = \frac{\Delta L}{L}$$

(where L is the initial length and ΔL is the change in length, dimensionless)
Importantly different types of stress do cause strain or any type of deformation, or in other words, strain is the consequence of stress. Cells are able to detect strain via changes in conformation of proteins or macromolecular protein complexes, but the precise molecular mechanisms remains often unclear. In this regard two different models have been

developed to explain mechanosensory behaviour: i) the localized and ii) the decentralized model. The localized model proposes that changes at the cell membrane are sensed immediately and are transmitted from there to other parts of the cell. In contrast the decentralized model proposes that any force applied at the cell surface will cause deformations of elastic cytoskeletal components and as such can be sensed far away from the area of impact. The latter model is also called the "tensegrity" model (derived from: tensional integrity) based on Buckminster Fuller's geodesic dome.

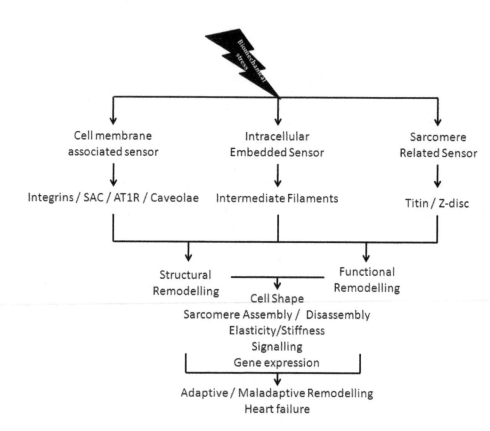

Legend to figure 1: The figure summarizes the most important stress and strain sensors present in cardiac myocytes. All sensors affect cell shape, sarcomere assembly and disassembly, elasticity and stiffness as well as gene expression which will finally decide whether adaptive or maladaptive remodelling will take place (abbreviations: SAC: stretch activated channels, AT1R: angiotensin II type 1 receptor).

Fig. 1. Summary of cardiac myocyte stress and strain sensors

Here we shall introduce the reader into different concepts of cardiac mechanosensation:
1. Receptor / cell membrane mediated mechanosensation (centralized models):
   i. Integrin mediated effects
   ii. Stretch activated channels
   iii. Angiotensin receptor mediated mechanosensation and other receptors
   iv. Caveolae
2. Intracellular stretch sensors:
   i. Intermediate filaments
3. Intrasarcomeric mechanosensors
   i. Z-disc associated mechanosensor complex
   ii. N2A and N2B – titin mechanosensor complex
   iii. Titin kinase mechanosensor complex

These different mechanosensory signalosomes integrate a variety of mechanical stimuli such as mechanical stress, shear stress, torsion and compression as well as the resulting strains into electrochemical and biochemical signals. They are translated into short term effects (i.e. changes in ion concentrations may lead to changes in action potential durations or changes in calcium concentration which may lead to changes in kinase and phosphatase activities) and long term effects via changes in gene expression.

1.1 Integrin mediated effects

Integrins are large heterodimeric transmembrane proteins, consisting of α and β subunits. They act as receptors and are enriched at focal adhesions or costameres, sites where the Z-discs become attached to the cell membrane. The extracellular part of the molecule interacts with fibronectin, laminin or collagen, whereas the intracellular domains interact with signalling proteins such as integrin linked kinase (ILK), focal adhesion kinase (FAK), or cytoskeletal components such as actin, talin and vinculin. As such, integrins link the extracellular matrix (ECM) to the cytoplasm and are able to respond to changes in the composition of the ECM as well as with regard to forces transmitted via the ECM and vice versa (inside out and outside in signalling). They are linked via $G\alpha$ proteins to cAMP and protein kinase A (PKA) mediated effects, they activate via FAK and SH2 phospholipase C (PLC) as well as phosphatidyl inositol 3 kinase (PI3K) and Akt mediated survival pathways (figure 1, 2). Integrins activate as well Src kinase which phosphorylates particularly p130 CAS, which is an important mechanosensory element [3]. Indeed tyrosine kinase activation, such as Src activation, has been observed as early as one minute after stretch and as such is one of the earliest observable effects following mechanical stimuli [4]. It has been postulated, although not yet shown, that orphan tyrosine kinases such as Src might become activated via conformational changes upon membrane stretch. If verified, this could be another mechanism whereby stress is directly translated into enzyme activity (please see also titin kinase chapter). Integrins are also linked via Ras mediated signalling to mitogen activated protein kinases (MAPK) such as ERK and as such to serum response factor (SRF) mediated transcriptional events.

In this regard, it is no surprise that loss of integrins in genetically altered animals is associated with severe heart failure [5] and that human mutations in laminin alpha 4 (LAMA4) and ILK are associated with dilated cardiomyopathy (DCM) [6]. Although integrins are meanwhile well established mechanosensors, other transmembrane protein systems such as the dystrophin associated glycoprotein complex (DAG) are certainly as well important, but they are less well studied with regard to mechanosensation and mechanotransduction.

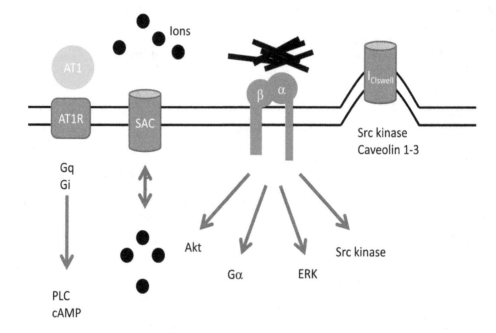

Legend to figure 2: The figure depicts four major membrane associated mechanosensory pathways, namely the angiotensin receptor (AT1R) mediated pathway, stretch activated channels (SAC), integrins and caveolae (abbreviations: Gq, Gi, Gα – Gq, Gi, and Gα mediated effects, PLC – phospholipase C, ERK – extracellular regulated kinase, Akt – Akt kinase, black dots indicate ions such as K+, Na+, Ca++, Cl-, etc.).

Fig. 2. Membrane associated mechanosensory pathways

1.2 Stretch activated channels (SAC)

Stretch activated or stretch gated ion channels respond to strain by opening or closing their pores. They were first found in skeletal muscle [7] and since then have been identified in every living cell of every kingdom, including Archaea, Bacteria, Plant, Fungi and Eukaryote (figure 1, 2). These channels open, or even close, upon membrane stretch and allow ions such as chloride, calcium, potassium, and sodium which are permeable to this channel, to follow the electrochemical gradient and to change the membrane potential. However mechanosensitivity is not restricted to a small subset of ion channels, in fact many proteins and voltage gated channels are mechanosensitive. The difficulty is to identify whether or not the mechanosensitivity of a single protein or channel is biologically relevant [8].

At least two different mechanisms can be made responsible for the opening mechanism:

i.   stretch from the plasma membrane is transferred directly to the channel resulting in a conformational change (lipid bilayer tension or stretch model) and

ii. a spring like tether, connecting ECM, channel and intracellular space, responds to changes by opening the channel (spring like tether model).

Mechanosensitive channels such as the L-type calcium channel are particularly important in cardiac myocytes where they have been made at least partially responsible for post-ischemic arrhythmias. Other effects include their ability to respond to a stretch early in the action potential and to produce a repolarizing tendency whereas if stretched late, the channel causes depolarization, an effect called: "reversal potential" [9-10]. Although it is a general principle in biology to amplify a signal via changes in ion concentrations, which supports a role for SAC in mechanosensation, inhibition of SAC by using Gadolinium is unable to inhibit major stretch induced features such as immediate early gene expression or the increase in protein synthesis [11]. Therefore additional effects must be at play.

1.3 Angiotensin receptor mediated mechanosensation and other receptors

While mechanical activation affects directly transmembrane proteins and causes via direct or indirect effects conformational changes which elicit profound intracellular signaltransduction cascades, another mechanism proposes that mechanical stimulation leads to autocrine angiotensin II release which activates the angiotensin II type 1 (AT1) receptor [12]. As such $G_{q/11}$ and G_i mediated effects, which lead to phospholipase C activation and increased intracellular calcium concentrations and/or a decrease in cAMP via adenylyl cyclase inhibition, may cause long term effects such as cardiac myocyte hypertrophy. However an even more important mechanism has been discovered only recently when it was demonstrated that the AT1 receptor, even without binding to its ligand, can be activated by mechanical stimulation [13]. In addition, beta receptors have also been implicated in mechanosensation, although evidence for their role here is available, but they are less well studied with regard to mechanosensation (please see for a brief overview [14]). Angiotensin converting enzyme (ACE) inhibitors, angiotensin receptor blockers and beta blockers belong to the most powerful therapeutic tools in cardiovascular medicine. Based on the direct involvement of the AT1 receptor in mechanosensation, their actions might at least be partially attributable to their effects here.

1.4 Caveolae

Caveolae are small (50 – 100 nm) invaginations of the plasma membrane found in a variety of different cell types, including cardiac myocytes. They may represent a cellular compartment where ion channels such as the mechanosensitive $I_{Clswell}$, signal transduction components such as Src kinase and caveolins 1-3, among others, can be found enriched (figure 2). $I_{Clswell}$ channels are important for intracellular homeostasis, particularly during hypo-osmotic conditions. Only recently it was shown that caveolae provide significant membrane reserve [15] and that caveolae are important for proper activation of $I_{Clswell}$ channel and as such can be seen as a mechanosensitive structure [16].

2. Intracellular stretch sensors

2.1 Intermediate filaments

Intermediate filaments (IF) are a group of related proteins that share common structural and sequence features, such as amino and carboxy-terminus globular parts which surround the alpha helical rod domain. They were initially named after their diameter which is with ~ 10 nm in the between of actin filaments and myosins and were subdivided into types I - VI. Most types of IFs are cytoplasmic, except for the lamins which are present in the nucleus or in the nuclear membrane. At least 91 different diseases are associated with mutations in these genes and as such a comprehensive discussion of all of them within the context of this chapter is impossible. However desmin is a major IF and present in almost every cell type. In cardiac myocytes desmin connects desmosomes with other organelles such as the Z-disc or the nucleus. Mutations in this gene result in a variety of different cardiac diseases such as desmin related myopathy [17-18], limb girdle muscular dystrophy [19], dilated cardiomyopathy (DCM) [20], arrhythmogenic right ventricular cardiomyopathy (ARVC) [21], cardiomyopathy with advanced AV block and arrhythmia [22], familial restrictive cardiomyopathy [23] and DCM with conduction system defects [24]. IFs interact with a variety of different proteins and because of their elasticity they are able to sense any deformation of cellular structure. As such, IFs have been linked to mechanosensation and might well have a function via "tensegration", i. e. their elasticity may enable them to change their conformation in response to any type of mechanical stimulation.   As such, lamin A/C knockout animals develop severe heart failure most probably due to defects in mechanosensation. In this regard, lamin A/C mutations are one of the major causes of DCM and associated arrhythmia and it is interesting to note, that treatment of animals carrying human LMN A/C mutations with carvedilol an agent with alpha and beta receptor blocking properties improves heart failure significantly [25].

3. Intrasarcomeric mechanosensors

3.1 Z-disc associated mechanosensor complex (MLP/Telethonin)

While all other so far discussed mechanosensors are associated with cell structures found in almost every other cell types, the intrasarcomeric mechanosensors are skeletal and cardiac myocyte specific (figure 3). Any pharmacological intervention at this level might offer the possibility of targeting cross striated myocytes specifically.

Moreover, all other mechanosensors are probably able to sense primarily "external stimuli", whereas the sarcomere associated signalosomes are able to sense force, stress and strain produced primarily within the cell. In addition, all sarcomere associated sensors are directly or indirectly associated with titin, the giant molecular ruler which spans half the sarcomere from the Z-disc to the M-band.

In this regard, the sarcomeric Z-disc which is probably one of the most complex macromolecular structures in biology contains at its periphery a variety of small molecules, namely muscle LIM protein (MLP, CSRP3) and telethonin (TCAP), which interact with the very aminoterminus of titin [26]. Interestingly MLP deficient papillary muscles develop a defect in passive elasticity and isolated cardiac myocytes have a defect in their BNP response following stretch whereas other signal transduction pathways, such as G_q mediated effects are still able to induce this gene. A human mutation in the MLP gene (W4R-MLP), significantly associated with DCM, was also identified and shown to lead to a significant loss of affinity between MLP and telethonin (TCAP). In comparison to the MLP knockout animals, W4R-MLP knock in mice develop a similar phenotype, for example they develop myocardial hypertrophy followed by heart failure, their papillary muscles develop less stiffness when stretched and isolated cardiac myocytes exhibit a similar defect in BNP response [27-28], albeit the effects are smaller and are gene dosage and age dependent. In this regard, MLP was also shown to shuttle into the nucleus and to be necessary for myocardial hypertrophy [29,28].

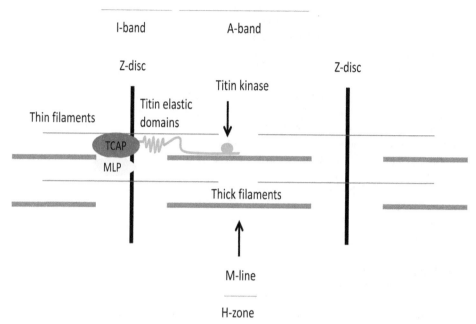

Legend to figure 3: The figure shows a schematic diagram of a sarcomere and depicts major structural elements. Please note the green titin molecule, spanning from the Z-disc to the M-line. At the aminoterminus TCAP (Telethonin) and MLP (muscle LIM protein) are localized. Titin's elastic domains are localized within the I-band and the kinase domain is localized close to the M-line.

Fig. 3. Sarcomere associated mechanosensors

Moreover, it was also shown that MLP interacts with and is necessary for the activation of the serine threonine phosphatase calcineurin (PP2A), which is an important link to myocardial hypertrophy via transcription factors such as nuclear factor of activated T-cells (NFAT) [30]. In addition, MLP interacts with the integrin linked kinase (ILK) and as such provides a molecular link between the sarcomeric Z-disc and integrin mediated signalling (please see also chapter integrins) [6]. However, in addition to MLP mutations, telethonin mutations have also been shown to be associated with types of muscular dystrophy as well as with hypertrophic cardiomyopathy (HCM) and DCM [31-32,27,33-34]. In summary, MLP and telethonin are likely to be involved in Z-disc mediated stress sensation, and mutations in these genes are involved in the pathogenesis of various diseases, but the precise molecular mechanism remains to be defined [35].

3.2 N2A and N2B – Titin mechanosensor complexes (FHL1/MARP)

With a molecular mass of up to 4.2 MDa, titin is the largest molecule in biology and well known for its multiple functions such as serving as a molecular ruler, its importance during embryonic development, and for its role in providing mechanical stability – just to name a few. However the molecule contains at its I-band region several elastic domains, such as the distal and proximal Immunoglobulin (Ig) domains, the N2B and N2BA domains, the N2A domain, which is embedded within the N2BA domain, as well as the PEVK domain. All of these domains unfold upon stretch and release and/or store energy during every cycle of contraction and relaxation (i. e. entropic springs [36]). Differential splicing particularly of the N2B and the more compliant N2BA domains add an additional level of complexity, which is of course species specific, depends on the developmental stage, the environment as well as on different states of disease, where DCM and hypothyroidism lead to increased stiffness [37]. Moreover, PKA and PKG mediated phosphorylation causes the elastic domains to "soften" whereas PKC mediated effects causes them to "stiffen" (figure 3).

The N2B domain binds specifically to four and a half LIM protein 1 (FHL1), which in turn is the core of a signalosome consisting of RAF, MEK1/2, and ERK2, thus connecting growth factor mediated Gq signalling to titin extensibility and finally to changes in gene expression. Interestingly, loss of FHL1 blunts pathologic hypertrophy and as such inhibition of this pathway might be beneficial [38].

Another important pathway is linked to the N2A elastic titin domain, were the muscle ankyrin repeat proteins (MARP) including cardiac ankyrin repeat protein (CARP), ankrd2/Arpp and DARP interact to constitute a signalosome which responds to passive stretch *in vitro* [39].

3.3 Titin kinase mechanosensor complex

While titin's elastic I-band domains may be able to sense strain, titin's amino-terminus, which is anchored within the Z-disc and its carboxy-terminus, anchored within the M-line, may well be able or may at least be involved in the sensation of stress. Interestingly titin's M-line (or better H-band) domain contains a mechanically modulated kinase able to bind and to phosphorylate nbr1 and p62 (SQSTM1) *in vitro*. MURF1 and 2 (and probably MURF3 which has not been analyzed yet) also bind to this complex and will translocate into the nucleus upon mechanical inactivity, where they downregulate and or induce the nuclear export of SRF and as such aggravate the transcriptional atrophy programme [40]. This is supported by the R279W-Titin kinase mutation which is associated with hereditary myopathy with early respiratory failure (HMERF) and which leads to a dramatic loss of affinity to nbr1 [41]. Additional evidence for this model is supported by in vitro experiments whereby stretching of the kinase domain leads to activation of the kinase, thus effectively linking mechanosensation to kinase activity ("mechanozymatics") [42]. Moreover titin's kinase domain is linked via nbr1 and p62 to autophagy, a process of regulated protein and or organelle turnover [43].

4. Summary

Every cell is capable of mechanical stress sensation either via local or decentralized molecular mechanisms and to transform these signals into electrochemical and biochemical mediators. Because of their force generating ability cardiac myocytes developed additional sarcomere titin I-band related strain and Z-disc as well as M-line related stress sensors. It is a general principle in biology to amplify a signal via an increase in local ion concentrations as such SAC play certainly a major role in nerve and muscle cells. Mechanical stimulation also might lead via conformational changes to the direct activation of tyrosine kinases and or the titin kinase - an effect which might be called "mechanozymatics". Direct activation of AT1 receptors via mechanical stimuli has been shown and in this context it might well be possible that other receptors, such as β-receptors, play a role in mechanosensation as well.

Mutations in components of any of the above mentioned systems have been found to cause muscle and or heart failure phenotypes (figure 1, 2) [44-45].

5. Abbreviations

Cardiovascular disease: CVD
Dilated cardiomyopathy: DCM
Extracellular matrix: ECM
Focal adhesion kinase: FAK
Hypertrophic cardiomyopathy: HCM
Immunoglobulin: Ig
Integrin linked kinase: ILK
Muscle Ankyrin Repeat Proteins: MARP
Muscle LIM protein: MLP, CSRP3
Nuclear factor of activated T-cells: NFAT
Protein kinase A, C, G: PKA/C/G
Sarcomere length: SL
Serum response factor: SRF
Telethonin: TCAP

6. References

[1] Kung C (2005) A possible unifying principle for mechanosensation. Nature 436 (7051):647-654. doi:nature03896 [pii] 10.1038/nature03896

[2] Knöll R, Hoshijima M, Chien K (2003) Cardiac mechanotransduction and implications for heart disease. J Mol Med Dec;81(12):750-756.

[3] Sawada Y, Tamada M, Dubin-Thaler BJ, Cherniavskaya O, Sakai R, Tanaka S, Sheetz MP (2006) Force sensing by mechanical extension of the Src family kinase substrate p130Cas. Cell 127 (5):1015-1026. doi:S0092-8674(06)01405-X [pii] 10.1016/j.cell.2006.09.044

[4] Sadoshima J, Izumo S (1997) The cellular and molecular response of cardiac myocytes to mechanical stress. Annu Rev Physiol 59:551-571.

[5] Shai SY, Harpf AE, Babbitt CJ, Jordan MC, Fishbein MC, Chen J, Omura M, Leil TA, Becker KD, Jiang M, Smith DJ, Cherry SR, Loftus JC, Ross RS (2002) Cardiac myocyte-specific excision of the beta1 integrin gene results in myocardial fibrosis and cardiac failure. Circulation research 90 (4):458-464.

[6] Knöll R, Postel R, Wang J, Kratzner R, Hennecke G, Vacaru AM, Vakeel P, Schubert C, Murthy K, Rana BK, Kube D, Knoll G, Schafer K, Hayashi T, Holm T, Kimura A, Schork N, Toliat MR, Nurnberg P, Schultheiss HP, Schaper W, Schaper J, Bos E, Den Hertog J, van Eeden FJ, Peters PJ, Hasenfuss G, Chien KR, Bakkers J (2007) Laminin-alpha4 and integrin-linked kinase mutations cause human cardiomyopathy via simultaneous defects in cardiomyocytes and endothelial cells. Circulation 116 (5):515-525

[7] Guharay F, Sachs F (1984) Stretch-activated single ion channel currents in tissue-cultured embryonic chick skeletal muscle. J Physiol 352:685-701

[8] Sachs F (2010) Stretch-activated ion channels: what are they? Physiology (Bethesda) 25 (1):50-56. doi:25/1/50 [pii] 10.1152/physiol.00042.2009

[9] Lab MJ (1978) Mechanically dependent changes in action potentials recorded from the intact frog ventricle. Circulation research 42 (4):519-528

[10] Zabel M, Koller BS, Sachs F, Franz MR (1996) Stretch-induced voltage changes in the isolated beating heart: importance of the timing of stretch and implications for stretch-activated ion channels. Cardiovasc Res 32 (1):120-130. doi:0008636396000892 [pii]

[11] Sadoshima J, Takahashi T, Jahn L, Izumo S (1992) Roles of mechano-sensitive ion channels, cytoskeleton, and contractile activity in stretch-induced immediate-early gene expression and hypertrophy of cardiac myocytes. Proc Natl Acad Sci U S A 89 (20):9905-9909

[12] Sadoshima J, Xu Y, Slayter HS, Izumo S (1993) Autocrine release of angiotensin II mediates stretch-induced hypertrophy of cardiac myocytes in vitro. Cell 75 (5):977-984

[13] Yasuda N, Akazawa H, Qin Y, Zou Y, Komuro I (2008) A novel mechanism of mechanical stress-induced angiotensin II type 1-receptor activation without the involvement of angiotensin II. Naunyn Schmiedebergs Arch Pharmacol 377 (4-6):393-399. doi:10.1007/s00210-007-0215-1

[14] Lab MJ (2006) Mechanosensitive-mediated interaction, integration, and cardiac control. Ann N Y Acad Sci 1080:282-300. doi:1080/1/282 [pii] 10.1196/annals.1380.022

[15] Kohl P, Cooper PJ, Holloway H (2003) Effects of acute ventricular volume manipulation on in situ cardiomyocyte cell membrane configuration. Prog Biophys Mol Biol 82 (1-3):221-227. doi:S0079610703000245 [pii]

[16] Kozera L, White E, Calaghan S (2009) Caveolae act as membrane reserves which limit mechanosensitive I(Cl,swell) channel activation during swelling in the rat ventricular myocyte. PLoS One 4 (12):e8312. doi:10.1371/journal.pone.0008312

[17] Dalakas MC, Dagvadorj A, Goudeau B, Park KY, Takeda K, Simon-Casteras M, Vasconcelos O, Sambuughin N, Shatunov A, Nagle JW, Sivakumar K, Vicart P, Goldfarb LG (2003) Progressive skeletal myopathy, a phenotypic variant of desmin myopathy associated with desmin mutations. Neuromuscul Disord 13 (3):252-258. doi:S0960896602002717 [pii]

[18] Dalakas MC, Park KY, Semino-Mora C, Lee HS, Sivakumar K, Goldfarb LG (2000) Desmin myopathy, a skeletal myopathy with cardiomyopathy caused by mutations in the desmin gene. N Engl J Med 342 (11):770-780. doi:10.1056/NEJM200003163421104

[19] Walter MC, Reilich P, Huebner A, Fischer D, Schroder R, Vorgerd M, Kress W, Born C, Schoser BG, Krause KH, Klutzny U, Bulst S, Frey JR, Lochmuller H (2007) Scapuloperoneal syndrome type Kaeser and a wide phenotypic spectrum of adult-onset, dominant myopathies are associated with the desmin mutation R350P. Brain 130 (Pt 6):1485-1496. doi:awm039 [pii] 10.1093/brain/awm039

[20] Li D, Tapscoft T, Gonzalez O, Burch P, Quinones M, Zoghbi W, Hill R, Bachinski L, Mann D, Roberts R (1999) Desmin mutation responsible for idiopathic dilated cardiomyopathy. Circulation 100 (5):461-464

[21] Klauke B, Kossmann S, Gaertner A, Brand K, Stork I, Brodehl A, Dieding M, Walhorn V, Anselmetti D, Gerdes D, Bohms B, Schulz U, Zu Knyphausen E, Vorgerd M, Gummert J, Milting H (2010) De novo desmin-mutation N116S is associated with arrhythmogenic right ventricular cardiomyopathy. Hum Mol Genet 19 (23):4595-4607. doi:ddq387 [pii] 10.1093/hmg/ddq387

[22] Otten E, Asimaki A, Maass A, van Langen IM, van der Wal A, de Jonge N, van den Berg MP, Saffitz JE, Wilde AA, Jongbloed JD, van Tintelen JP (2010) Desmin

mutations as a cause of right ventricular heart failure affect the intercalated disks. Heart Rhythm 7 (8):1058-1064. doi:S1547-5271(10)00398-X [pii] 10.1016/j.hrthm.2010.04.023

[23] Pruszczyk P, Kostera-Pruszczyk A, Shatunov A, Goudeau B, Draminska A, Takeda K, Sambuughin N, Vicart P, Strelkov SV, Goldfarb LG, Kaminska A (2007) Restrictive cardiomyopathy with atrioventricular conduction block resulting from a desmin mutation. Int J Cardiol 117 (2):244-253. doi:S0167-5273(06)00565-1 [pii] 10.1016/j.ijcard.2006.05.019

[24] Taylor MR, Slavov D, Ku L, Di Lenarda A, Sinagra G, Carniel E, Haubold K, Boucek MM, Ferguson D, Graw SL, Zhu X, Cavanaugh J, Sucharov CC, Long CS, Bristow MR, Lavori P, Mestroni L (2007) Prevalence of desmin mutations in dilated cardiomyopathy. Circulation 115 (10):1244-1251. doi:CIRCULATIONAHA.106.646778 [pii] 10.1161/CIRCULATIONAHA.106.646778

[25] Chandar S, Yeo LS, Leimena C, Tan JC, Xiao XH, Nikolova-Krstevski V, Yasuoka Y, Gardiner-Garden M, Wu J, Kesteven S, Karlsdotter L, Natarajan S, Carlton A, Rainer S, Feneley MP, Fatkin D (2010) Effects of mechanical stress and carvedilol in lamin A/C-deficient dilated cardiomyopathy. Circulation research 106 (3):573-582. doi:CIRCRESAHA.109.204388 [pii] 10.1161/CIRCRESAHA.109.204388

[26] Zou P, Pinotsis N, Lange S, Song YH, Popov A, Mavridis I, Mayans OM, Gautel M, Wilmanns M (2006) Palindromic assembly of the giant muscle protein titin in the sarcomeric Z-disk. Nature 439 (7073):229-233

[27] Knöll R, Hoshijima M, Hoffman HM, Person V, Lorenzen-Schmidt I, Bang ML, Hayashi T, Shiga N, Yasukawa H, Schaper W, McKenna W, Yokoyama M, Schork NJ, Omens JH, McCulloch AD, Kimura A, Gregorio CC, Poller W, Schaper J, Schultheiss HP, Chien KR (2002) The cardiac mechanical stretch sensor machinery involves a Z disc complex that is defective in a subset of human dilated cardiomyopathy. Cell 111 (7):943-955.

[28] Knöll R, Kostin S, Klede S, Savvatis K, Klinge L, Stehle I, Gunkel S, Kotter S, Babicz K, Sohns M, Miocic S, Didie M, Knoll G, Zimmermann WH, Thelen P, Bickeboller H, Maier LS, Schaper W, Schaper J, Kraft T, Tschope C, Linke WA, Chien KR (2010) A common MLP (muscle LIM protein) variant is associated with cardiomyopathy. Circulation research 106 (4):695-704. doi:CIRCRESAHA.109.206243 [pii] 10.1161/CIRCRESAHA.109.206243

[29] Boateng SY, Senyo SE, Qi L, Goldspink PH, Russell B (2009) Myocyte remodeling in response to hypertrophic stimuli requires nucleocytoplasmic shuttling of muscle LIM protein. J Mol Cell Cardiol 47 (4):426-435. doi:S0022-2828(09)00154-0 [pii] 10.1016/j.yjmcc.2009.04.006

[30] Heineke J, Ruetten H, Willenbockel C, Gross SC, Naguib M, Schaefer A, Kempf T, Hilfiker-Kleiner D, Caroni P, Kraft T, Kaiser RA, Molkentin JD, Drexler H, Wollert KC (2005) Attenuation of cardiac remodeling after myocardial infarction by muscle LIM protein-calcineurin signaling at the sarcomeric Z-disc. Proc Natl Acad Sci U S A 102 (5):1655-1660

[31] Bos JM, Poley RN, Ny M, Tester DJ, Xu X, Vatta M, Towbin JA, Gersh BJ, Ommen SR, Ackerman MJ (2006) Genotype-phenotype relationships involving hypertrophic cardiomyopathy-associated mutations in titin, muscle LIM protein, and telethonin. Mol Genet Metab 88 (1):78-85. doi:S1096-7192(05)00342-2 [pii] 10.1016/j.ymgme.2005.10.008

[32] Hayashi T, Arimura T, Itoh-Satoh M, Ueda K, Hohda S, Inagaki N, Takahashi M, Hori H, Yasunami M, Nishi H, Koga Y, Nakamura H, Matsuzaki M, Choi BY, Bae SW,

You CW, Han KH, Park JE, Knoll R, Hoshijima M, Chien KR, Kimura A (2004) Tcap gene mutations in hypertrophic cardiomyopathy and dilated cardiomyopathy. J Am Coll Cardiol 44 (11):2192-2201. doi:S0735-1097(04)01749-8 [pii] 10.1016/j.jacc.2004.08.058

[33] Moreira ES, Wiltshire TJ, Faulkner G, Nilforoushan A, Vainzof M, Suzuki OT, Valle G, Reeves R, Zatz M, Passos-Bueno MR, Jenne DE (2000) Limb-girdle muscular dystrophy type 2G is caused by mutations in the gene encoding the sarcomeric protein telethonin. Nat Genet 24 (2):163-166

[34] Olive M, Shatunov A, Gonzalez L, Carmona O, Moreno D, Quereda LG, Martinez-Matos JA, Goldfarb LG, Ferrer I (2008) Transcription-terminating mutation in telethonin causing autosomal recessive muscular dystrophy type 2G in a European patient. Neuromuscul Disord 18 (12):929-933. doi:S0960-8966(08)00607-X [pii] 10.1016/j.nmd.2008.07.009

[35] Buyandelger B, Ng KE, Miocic S, Piotrowska I, Gunkel S, Ku CH, Knoll R (2011) MLP (muscle LIM protein) as a stress sensor in the heart. Pflugers Arch. doi:10.1007/s00424-011-0961-2

[36] Linke WA, Grutzner A (2008) Pulling single molecules of titin by AFM--recent advances and physiological implications. Pflugers Arch 456 (1):101-115. doi:10.1007/s00424-007-0389-x

[37] LeWinter MM, Granzier H (2010) Cardiac titin: a multifunctional giant. Circulation 121 (19):2137-2145. doi:121/19/2137 [pii] 10.1161/CIRCULATIONAHA.109.860171

[38] Sheikh F, Raskin A, Chu PH, Lange S, Domenighetti AA, Zheng M, Liang X, Zhang T, Yajima T, Gu Y, Dalton ND, Mahata SK, Dorn GW, 2nd, Heller-Brown J, Peterson KL, Omens JH, McCulloch AD, Chen J (2008) An FHL1-containing complex within the cardiomyocyte sarcomere mediates hypertrophic biomechanical stress responses in mice. J Clin Invest 118 (12):3870-3880

[39] Miller MK, Bang ML, Witt CC, Labeit D, Trombitas C, Watanabe K, Granzier H, McElhinny AS, Gregorio CC, Labeit S (2003) The muscle ankyrin repeat proteins: CARP, ankrd2/Arpp and DARP as a family of titin filament-based stress response molecules. J Mol Biol 333 (5):951-964. doi:S0022283603011380 [pii]

[40] Braun T, Gautel M (2011) Transcriptional mechanisms regulating skeletal muscle differentiation, growth and homeostasis. Nat Rev Mol Cell Biol 12 (6):349-361. doi:nrm3118 [pii] 10.1038/nrm3118

[41] Lange S, Xiang F, Yakovenko A, Vihola A, Hackman P, Rostkova E, Kristensen J, Brandmeier B, Franzen G, Hedberg B, Gunnarsson LG, Hughes SM, Marchand S, Sejersen T, Richard I, Edstrom L, Ehler E, Udd B, Gautel M (2005) The Kinase Domain of Titin Controls Muscle Gene Expression and Protein Turnover. Science

[42] Puchner EM, Alexandrovich A, Kho AL, Hensen U, Schafer LV, Brandmeier B, Grater F, Grubmuller H, Gaub HE, Gautel M (2008) Mechanoenzymatics of titin kinase. Proc Natl Acad Sci U S A 105 (36):13385-13390. doi:0805034105 [pii] 10.1073/pnas.0805034105

[43] Gautel M (2011) Cytoskeletal protein kinases: titin and its relations in mechanosensing. Pflugers Arch. doi:10.1007/s00424-011-0946-1

[44] Buyandelger B, Ng KE, Miocic S, Gunkel S, Piotrowska I, Ku CH, Knoll R (2011) Genetics of Mechanosensation in the Heart. J Cardiovasc Transl Res. doi:10.1007/s12265-011-9262-6

[45] Kimura A (2010) Molecular basis of hereditary cardiomyopathy: abnormalities in calcium sensitivity, stretch response, stress response and beyond. J Hum Genet 55 (2):81-90. doi:jhg2009138 [pii] 10.1038/jhg.2009.138

6

Familial Hypertrophic Cardiomyopathy-Related Troponin Mutations and Sudden Cardiac Death

Laura Dewar, Bo Liang, Yueh Li, Shubhayan Sanatani and Glen F. Tibbits
Simon Fraser University
Canada

1. Introduction

Hypertrophic cardiomyopathy (HCM) is a common structural anomaly of the myocardium that is unexplained by an underlying condition such as hypertension. The main findings in HCM are varying degrees of ventricular and/or septal hypertrophy, myocyte disarray and increased myocardial fibrosis (Maron et al., 1995). There is significant variation in the clinical manifestation among patients, from asymptomatic, to mild dyspnea upon exertion, to substantive heart failure. While many individuals will present with clinical symptoms, including a cardiac murmur related to outflow tract obstruction, in some families, diagnosis is not established until the sudden death of, or incidental finding of hypertrophy within, a family member. Transthoracic echocardiography has traditionally been the clinician's primary tool for determination of asymmetric hypertrophy of the left interventricular septum, with or without left ventricular outflow tract obstruction. Given the heterogeneity in severity of disease and penetrance within HCM-affected families, it is important to rule out other secondary causes of hypertrophy, such as hypertension or aortic stenosis. Diagnosis can be difficult, especially in elite athletes who may present with physiological left ventricular hypertrophy (Maron, 2009). Clinically identifiable HCM has a prevalence of 1:500 in young adults in the general population, making it the most common genetic cardiovascular disease in many countries (Maron et al., 1995).

Although familial hypertrophic cardiomyopathy (FHC) was first described clinically more than half a century ago (Teare, 1958), it was only about 20 years ago that the underlying molecular causes of FHC began to be established, with the finding of a mutation in the beta-myosin heavy chain (*MYH7*) gene (Geisterfer-Lowrance et al., 1990). Since this seminal discovery, there have been more than 900 different mutations identified in over 20 FHC candidate genes (Tester & Ackerman, 2009). Historically, attempts to establish the link between genotype and phenotype were based on studying FHC cohorts with severe, well established disease with cardiac remodelling and in some patients, progression to end-stage cardiac dilatation and failure. It is increasingly apparent that focussing on the end phenotype as a link to genotype is problematic; families are highly heterogeneous in their disease presentation with, in many cases, low penetrance (at least on echocardiography diagnoses) and with novel mutations not seen in other families. There are few large FHC-affected families, leading to linkage analysis difficulties. When a pathogenic FHC mutation is uncovered in the proband, genetic testing of all first degree relatives is highly recommended. When other family members are genotyped, mutation-positive relatives can be closely monitored for disease progression (Colombo et al., 2008).

Up to 60% of patients with a high index of suspicion for FHC are found to have a genetic mutation in one of the FHC-susceptibility genes. A subset of FHC patients do not have identifiable mutations, perhaps because of reduced screening sensitivity that does not incorporate deep intronic sequencing, identify large insertions or deletions in the known candidate genes or include non-hot spot encoding regions. In addition, some patients may have mutations in as-yet unrecognized candidate genes (Rodriguez et al., 2009). The majority of documented FHC mutations occur as single nucleotide substitutions or "missense" mutations, although nucleotide deletions and insertions have also been identified. Insertions and deletions can potentially truncate the gene product by causing a shift in the reading frame leading to a premature stop codon. Mutations that occur at exon/intron boundaries can cause splice anomalies, leading to abnormal and potentially dysfunctional protein products (Wheeler et al., 2009).

Two prominent hypotheses have been developed to explain how sarcomere protein mutations cause the FHC phenotype: first is the "poison polypeptide" hypothesis, in which a single mutant protein disrupts the function of the entire sarcomere unit in a dominant negative manner (Thierfelder et al., 1994). The mutant protein is translated and incorporated into the sarcomere, where it can impair contraction. The second hypothesis is that sarcomeric protein mutations can lead to haploinsufficiency, in which mutations disrupt one copy of the gene, leaving the wild-type gene copy to produce the protein product in inadequate quantities for a balanced sarcomere unit (Thierfelder et al., 1994). In this situation, there is a 50% reduction in peptide concentration due to disruption in translation or trafficking of the mutant. Inadequate levels of incorporated wild-type protein create an imbalance in thin filament stoichiometry.

2. Sudden cardiac death in FHC

FHC is the most common cause of sudden cardiac death (SCD) in young people, affecting approximately 1-2% of children and adolescents, and up to 1% of young adults in HCM community cohorts (Elliott et al., 2000; Maron, 2002). Although SCD is considered rare in competitive athletes (1 in 200,000), HCM is associated with nearly one third of such occurrences (Maron, 2003). Children have the highest SCD rates of FHC patients suggesting that early onset can result from a more severe phenotype that includes lethal arrhythmias (Maron et al., 1999; Ostman-Smith et al., 2008). The highest mortality rates are seen in children aged 9 to 14 years, averaging 7.2%. The SCD risk peaks in girls at 10 to 11 years of age and occurs in boys at 15 to 16 years of age, leading to some researchers to propose that the surge in androgens that occurs prior to puberty may be associated with rapid disease progression and increased SCD risk (Ostman-Smith et al., 2008). There is a male preponderance for FHC-related SCD, especially among athletes (Maron et al., 1996). FHC patients with 2 or more mutations (Hershberger, 2010; Van Driest et al., 2004), and homozygous mutation patients, have more severe disease phenotypes with higher penetrance and greater incidence of SCD over single mutation patients (Ho et al., 2000; Ingles et al., 2005). Modifier gene polymorphisms such as angiotensin I converting enzyme (ACE) D allele, (Marian et al., 1993) and lifestyle/environmental factors such as diet, exercise, body mass and hypertension may also affect the FHC phenotype. With such complexities in disease manifestation, SCD risk assessment has been problematic. Younger age at onset, history of syncope with exertion, history of SCD within close relatives, severity of symptoms and degree of ventricular and septal wall thickness have been used in risk stratification algorithms; however, many risk factor studies involved non-genotyped patients with sometimes conflicting or confusing results and frequently with no single risk factor being identified. Prognosis for genotyped patients varies with the gene and in many cases, specific mutations within a gene; however, the mechanisms by which such mutations have an increased propensity for sudden death in some individuals, while in others appear to be relatively benign, are not well understood. The primary prevention risk factors for SCD in FHC include family history of SCD, unexplained recent syncope, runs of non-sustained ventricular tachycardia on ambulatory 24 hour Holter monitor, hypotensive response to exercise and severe left ventricular wall thickness (over 30 mm) (Maron, 2010). With respect to the latter, mild ventricular hypertrophy, however, does not correlate with low SCD risk, especially with thin filament mutations, as discussed later.

3. The role of the troponin complex in cardiac dynamics

The focus of this chapter is on three genes that encode the troponin complex found within the sarcomere; TNNT2, encoding cardiac troponin T, TNNI3, encoding cardiac troponin I and TNNC1, encoding troponin C. These genes encode the cardiac troponin genes that are unique from their skeletal counterparts and have evolved to help regulate excitation-contraction coupling in the heart. The troponin (Tn) proteins are part of a thin filament regulatory unit of the sarcomere. Cardiac troponin C (cTnC) is the Ca^{2+}-binding subunit that acts as a cytosolic Ca^{2+} sensor, cardiac troponin I (cTnI) is the inhibitory subunit that inhibits contraction when intracellular Ca^{2+} levels are below activation levels and cardiac troponin T (cTnT) is the subunit responsible for attaching the troponin complex to the thin filament via binding with tropomyosin (Tm) and believed responsible for movement of Tm on the thin filament modulating binding of the myosin head to actin. The subunits are arranged in a 1:1:1 stoichiometric ratio along the thin filament with one Tn:Tm complex bound to every seven actin monomers. Actin monomers are arranged in a double helix oriented in parallel to myosin-containing thick filaments. These protein-protein configurations allow for thin filament activation (Figure 1), which in turn facilitates cross-bridge cycling through the action of myosin binding to actin and the production of force (Gordon et al., 2000).

Takeda and collaborators (Takeda et al., 2003) successfully crystallized the globular core of the Tn complex, which revealed that the complex is highly flexible, an inherent feature crucial to its role in heart muscle contraction. The structure consists of two domains: the regulatory head composed of the N-terminus of TnC (residues 3 – 84) and two α-helices of TnI (denoted as H3 and H4, residues 150 - 188), and the highly conserved IT arm composed of the C-terminus of TnC (residues 93-161), two α-helices of TnI (H1 and H2, residues 42-136) and two α-helices of TnT (H3 and H4, residues 203-271). Although crystallography allowed most of the Tn complex structure to be observed, some regions remain unresolved, including the inhibitory region of TnI, and both the N- and C-terminal regions of TnT. These regions are likely highly flexible, allowing them to bind to other thin filament proteins (i.e. actin) to modulate thin filament activation. The primary role of the regulatory domain is as the "Ca^{2+} sensor", while the rigid IT domain appears to be sensitive to myosin binding during contraction (Sun, Bradmeier & Irving, 2006, as cited in Willott et al., 2010).

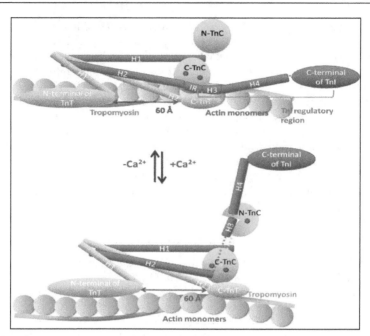

Fig. 1. A schematic representation of cardiac troponin in relation to the thin filament in the absence and presence of Ca²⁺. The inhibitory region of TnI (IR), and the N-terminal and C-terminal domains of TnT are not clearly observed in the crystal structure, likely due to their inherent flexibility (see text). The red dots represent Ca²⁺ ions. The figure is adapted from Takeda, 2003 (Li, 2009).

Most researchers believe that a "3 state model" exists to explain myofilament contraction. Interestingly, it was the study of how various mutations disrupt these interactions that lead to further development and confirmation of the 3 state model (Gordon et al., 2000). During diastole, the ventricles fill with blood to their end-diastolic volumes. The sarcomeres are stretched to longer lengths but without developing significant diastolic pressures. Cross-bridge cycling is physically blocked by the Tm:Tn complex at this stage and is referred to as the "blocked" or "B" state. Recently it has been postulated that perhaps only 50% of the cross-bridges are sterically blocked. The rest may be in a weakly-bound non-force generating state that facilitates the transition of cross-bridge cycling into the systolic state. There are two actin-binding regions on cTnI that play an essential role in diastole. There is an inhibitory region (residues 137-148) and a downstream helix (H3, residues 150-159) that tightly binds to actin, which along with cTnT, anchor Tm into the blocking position (see review by Parmacek & Solaro, 2004).

Calcium initially enters the cell mainly through L-type Ca²⁺ channels and initiates Ca²⁺-induced Ca²⁺ release from the sarcoplasmic reticulum. As cytosolic Ca²⁺ levels rise, the sarcomeres develop tension that increases ventricular isovolumic pressure until the aortic and pulmonary valves open. Blood is expelled from the ventricles by sarcomeres shortening to their end-systolic lengths. At the subcellular level, myofilament activation begins with Ca²⁺ binding to cTnC site II, exposing a hydrophobic region at the N lobe of cTnC and creating a new binding site for cTnI. Cardiac TnI then dissociates from actin and binds ightly to the hydrophobic region of cTnC, causing a cascade of protein-protein interactions that allows Tm to move closer into the thin filament groove. This stage is referred to as the 'closed" or "C" state. This movement exposes myosin binding sites on actin and also appears to alter thin filament structure, allowing more cross-bridges to occur and moving Tm further into the thin filament groove (thus shifting into the "open" or "M" state). Positive feedback may arise from bound cross-bridges causing an increased affinity for Ca^{2+} by cTnC (Pan & Solaro, 1987 as cited in Solaro & Kobayashi, 2011). At basal states of contractility, only 25% of available cTnC regulatory (site II) Ca^{2+} binding sites are occupied due to low cytosolic Ca^{2+} levels, resulting in a substantial cardiac reserve for recruitment of blocked cross-bridges when required.

After the valves close, the sarcomeres are quiescent as the ventricles prepare for refilling. This relaxation phase is highly dependent upon the rate of cytosolic Ca^{2+} removal, the off-loading of Ca^{2+} from cTnC, and the cross-bridges returning to the weakly bound or blocked state. Phosphorylation of the thin filament proteins, in particular the N-terminus of cTnI, plays a crucial role in drawing upon cardiac reserve, cross-bridge cycling rate and hence, relaxation, in a signaling cascade initiated by β-adrenergic stimulation (see review by Tardiff, 2011). These mechanisms are critically important when increased heart rate is required during exercise. Considering that SCD in young FHC patients frequently occurs during exercise (Cha et al., 2007), thin filament mutations may have an inhibitory effect on phosphorylation signalling and cardiac reserve as well as other cross-bridge cycling effects.

4. Mechanisms of Sudden Cardiac Death in FHC troponin mutations

Various mechanisms for SCD due to FHC have been suggested including arrhythmias arising from sinus nodal and atrioventricular nodal conduction abnormalities, and tachycardia due to re-entrant depolarization pathways from myocardial disarray and fibrosis, abnormal Ca^{2+} homeostasis, ventricular diastolic dysfunction or left ventricular outflow tract obstruction (Fatkin & Graham, 2002). With several underlying mechanisms leading to SCD, research is only beginning to define the link between the underlying molecular pathology and arrhythmogenesis in FHC-associated troponin mutations.

One emerging issue is that studying patients with well established disease for the purpose of linking phenotype to genotype has proven extremely difficult. Like all monogenic disorders, there are myriad disease modifiers including genetic, environmental and lifestyle factors that influence disease progression and severity in a manner that is poorly understood. What is also becoming apparent is that ventricular hypertrophy, fibrosis and obstructive disease are likely compensatory FHC features and based on complex signalling cascades arising from pathologies within the sarcomere, as discussed later in this chapter. Perhaps longitudinal studies of patients prior to the onset of structural disease may uncover mutation-specific disease progression that parallels the molecular and biophysical effects observed in *in vitro* experiments, animal models and *in silico* predictions (Tardiff, 2011). There is likely a less complex phenotype in FHC patients in the early disease stages allowing a more discernable link between genotype and phenotype. A study of preclinical FHC patients provides evidence for this hypothesis (Ho et al., 2002). In their study, most FHC cohorts presented with one common phenotype, namely prolonged diastolic relaxation on echocardiography, despite patients having different mutations within different genes. This approach may also benefit treatment outcomes for preclinical FHC cohorts with targeted mutation-specific treatment to attenuate disease progression. It makes sense to treat presymptomatic FHC patients long before gross phenotype becomes established. Diltiazem, a calcium channel blocker, normalized Ca^{2+} regulation and attenuated ventricular hypertrophy in a mouse model (Semsarian et al., 2002) and formed the basis of an ongoing clinical trial, in which preclinical FHC patients receive diltiazem therapy while being monitored for disease progression (http://clinicaltrials.gov/ct2/show/NCT00319982).

Recent approaches to identifying the pathophysiology of FHC mutations includes investigation of the dynamic properties of cross-bridge cycling at the molecular level and how Tn mutations disrupt precise molecular movements. Such high resolution investigations commonly incorporate computational approaches to examine protein flexibility and to predict changes in protein mobility caused by mutations, using molecular dynamics simulation programs such as GROMACS (Van Der Spoel et al., 2005) and CHARMM (Brooks et al., 2009). Another approach is Nuclear Magnetic Resonance (NMR) imaging, allowing investigators to compare recombinant wild-type and mutated Tn complexes in different metal-binding states to measure conformational changes (Lassalle, 2010).

4.1 Troponin T mutations

Since the identification of cTNNT2 in 1993 as the first Tn-based gene associated with FHC (Thierfelder et al., 1993), cTnT mutations have been extensively studied and account for up to 15% of all FHC mutations (Watkins et al., 1995). To date, there are at least 68 cTnT mutations identified associated with FHC (Willott et al., 2010), with a subset that present with a high frequency of SCD and/or ventricular arrhythmia in humans (Table 1). Alternative splicing of exons 4 and 5 of the cTNNT2 gene in the human heart results in four temporally regulated isoforms: one adult isoform (TnT3) and 3 fetal isoforms (TnT1,TnT2 and TnT4). The variable cTnT N-domain contributes to the Ca^{2+} sensitivity of force development and the presence of fetal isoforms in adult myofilaments has been associated with increased myofilament Ca^{2+} sensitivity and diastolic dysfunction (Gomes et al., 2002 as cited in Gomes et al., 2004). Tn complexes with fetal isoforms TnT1 and TnT2 (containing exon 5) have a reduced inhibition of actomyosin ATPase activity compared with the adult TnT3 isoform which suggests that the TnT isoforms have varying ability to modulate cross-bridge cycling and hence, cardiac contraction (Gomes et al., 2002). These findings are noteworthy in that increased myofilament Ca^{2+} sensitivity and diastolic dysfunction occur with many FHC causing Tn mutations; however, studies investigating the expression of cTnT isoforms in diseased hearts and a possible contributory role in altered contractile performance remain unresolved with no as-yet obvious correlation between fetal isoform TnT4 expression and Ca^{2+} sensitivity in diseased hearts (see review by Parmacek & Solaro, 2004).

The majority of cTnT mutations occur within the two structurally poorly resolved regions with a clustering of mutations within residues 69 to 110. There are three "hot spots" occurring at residues 92, 94 and 110, of which R92L and F110I have been associated with high rates of SCD and/or ventricular arrhythmia (Table 1). Another mutational "hotspot" occurs at residues 160 to 163, which is found within a highly charged and a highly conserved sequence from 157 to 166. This region is believed to be a flexible linker between H1 and H2 and whose structure has so far eluded resolution. Closer to the C terminus is a scattering of mutations associated with dilated cardiomyopathy (DCM) as well as several FHC mutations. It is believed that residues in this particular region affect Ca^{2+} sensitivity via allosteric interactions with the cTnC C domain, although actual evidence is lacking (Tardiff, 2011).

Troponin subunit	Mutation(s)	SCD or Ventricular Arrhythmia	References
cTnT	I79N, F87L, R92L, R92W, R94L, A104V, ΔE160*, S179F, Intron 16G1→A[ᵀ]	SCD	(Gimeno et al., 2009; Knollmann & Potter, 2001; Moolman et al., 1997; Thierfelder et al., 1993; Thierfelder et al., 1994)
	F110I	Ventricular arrhythmia	(Watkins et al., 1995)
cTnI	R145G, A157V, R162Q, ΔK183*, R186Q, S199N	SCD	(Ashrafian et al., 2003; Niimura et al., 2002; Van Driest et al., 2003)
	R141Q, G203R	Ventricular arrhythmia	(Alcalai et al., 2008; Ashrafian et al., 2003)
cTnC	Q122AfsX30[¥]	SCD	(Chung et al., 2011)

Table 1. Troponin mutations associated with SCD and ventricular arrhythmia. *Δ denotes deletion of the noted residue causing an in-frame mutation; [ᵀ] denotes a splice donor site mutation that removes 28 residues at the C terminus and replaces them with 7 nonsense codons resulting in a truncated cTnT mutant; [¥] denotes a nucleotide duplication (G) at position 363, causing a frame-shift substitution on residue 122 (Q122A) and a premature stop codon (X) at residue 30 resulting in a truncated cTnC mutant.

4.1.1 In vitro and in vivo approaches, animal models and in silico predictions

Cardiac TnT mutations are predicted to affect the regulatory role of the Tn-Tm complex on sarcomere activation given that TnT functions to attach the Tn complex to Tm and actin (Tobacman, 1996). In vitro studies with different FHC mutations (including cTnT mutants) show faster contraction kinetics and increased Ca^{2+} sensitivity of force generation. Some studies show increased sarcomeric activation at lower Ca^{2+} levels, resulting in myofilament activation and contraction at shorter sarcomere lengths against an increased passive force (Haim et al., 2007; Tardiff et al., 1999). The shorter baseline sarcomere length may be an important factor in why cTnT R92Q transgenic mutant mice have smaller myocytes and negligent or minimal ventricular hypertrophy (Tardiff et al., 1999).

Abnormal Ca^{2+} homeostasis may result from a variety of factors including altered Ca^{2+} availability and altered myofibrillar Ca^{2+} sensitivity. In vitro studies of skinned myocardial fibres reconstituted with mutant cTnT mutations (I79N, R92Q, F110I, ΔE160) show increased myofilament Ca^{2+} sensitivity, which researchers postulate is an important mechanism for the high incidence of SCD even with mild or absent hypertrophy and fibrosis (Gomes & Potter, 2004a; Gomes & Potter, 2004b; Knollmann & Potter, 2001). In silico studies based on results from in vivo transgenic I79N cTnT mouse fibres predict a higher basal contractility, increased rate of force development, delayed relaxation and increased resting tension compared with wild-type fibres (Miller et al., 2001).

In intact transgenic mouse hearts and in isolated voltage-clamped cardiomyocytes, Knollmann et al. produced compelling evidence that ventricular arrhythmias may arise from action potential remodelling related to altered Ca^{2+} regulation in mice carrying the human cTnT I79N mutation (Knollmann et al., 2003). A more recent study elegantly demonstrated that the degree of myofilament sensitivity may be correlated positively with the risk of developing ventricular tachycardia (Baudenbacher et al., 2008). Given that the transgenic mice had no evidence of hypertrophy, fibrosis or myocyte disarray, this study provided further evidence that altered myofilament function is the underlying pathophysiological mechanism of FHC and may be the causal link of FHC to SCD. Many of the most "deleterious" cTnT mutations are located within the H1 domain of the N-terminus. Previous studies have demonstrated that the N-terminus plays an important role in the inhibition of myofilament activation (reviewed in Tardiff, 2011). It stands to reason that disruption of this inhibitory N-terminal function by mutations in this region may allow Tm movement (and hence, cross-bridge cycling) under conditions of low Ca^{2+}, exhibiting an apparent increased Ca^{2+} sensitivity of myofilament activation (Tardiff, 2011).

4.1.2 Human cardiac TnT mutation studies

FHC patients harbouring the I79N cTnT mutation commonly present with minimal or absent hypertrophy on echocardiography and are frequently asymptomatic (i.e. no syncope, dyspnea or chest pain at rest or with exertion), yet have the highest incidence of SCD among young cTnT mutation carriers (Watkins et al., 1995) and is one of the most investigated of all FHC mutations (see review by Gomes et al., 2004). The F87L mutation also presents with mild hypertrophy (less than 16 mm ventricular wall thickness) but with a high incidence of SCD, including sub-adult patients, in a study of one multigenerational family (Gimeno et al., 2009). Of great significance, the youngest mutation carriers were completely asymptomatic. The R94L was also studied within a single family and found to have marked myocyte disarray and frequent SCD in the absence of ventricular hypertrophy (Varnava et al., 1999 as cited in Gomes et al., 2004). FHC patients with the A104V cTnT mutation also have a high incidence of SCD with only moderate left ventricular hypertrophy (Szczesna et al., 2000 as cited in Gomes & Potter, 2004; Gomes et al., 2004). A longitudinal study involving R92W cTnT FHC patients revealed that clinically identifiable hypertrophy did not occur in this cohort until after 35 years of age and yet the highest occurrence of SCD was prior to cardiac remodelling, particularly in young males (Revera et al., 2007, as cited in Revera et al., 2008). Another study by the same group (Revera et al., 2008) reported that phenotype-negative R92W patients had higher basal contractility and delayed relaxation compared to their genotype-negative relatives. Given the mild phenotype of many cTnT mutation patients, there is likely a reporting and referral bias in these patients and are therefore likely under-recognized in FHC clinics where the majority of patients have substantial hypertrophy and outflow obstruction that are relatively easy to diagnose non-invasively by echocardiography (Tardiff, 2011).

A study comparing FHC cTnT mutation patients with other FHC patients who died suddenly revealed that the cTnT mutation patients were younger, had less hypertrophy and fibrosis, but more myocardial disarray than other patients (Varnava, Elliott, Baboonian et al., 2001). Such findings suggest that the pathological mechanism is essentially myocellular as opposed to being related to the sequelae of ventricular hypertrophy and that ventricular wall thickness may not be an appropriate risk factor for SCD in cTnT patients.

4.2 Troponin I mutations

The first report of FHC-causing mutations in the *TNNI3* gene was in 1997 (Kimura et al., 1997), in which 5 missense mutations were discovered that co-segregated with FHC. Since then, approximately 35 mutations have been reported linked to FHC, of which several missense and deletion mutations are associated with SCD and/or ventricular arrhythmia (Table 1). There are 3 genes encoding 3 TnI protein isoforms, of which two are expressed in the human heart on a temporal basis. The slow skeletal TnI (ssTnI from the *TNNI1* gene) is the predominant isoform expressed within the fetal heart. This isoform declines rapidly after birth and is generally replaced by the cardiac isoform (cTnI from the *TNNI3* gene) by approximately 9 months of age in humans (Bhavsar et al., 1991, Hunkeler, Kullman and Murphy, 1991 and Sasse et al., 1993 in Parmacek & Solaro, 2004). The 31 residue N-terminus in cTnI is entirely absent in ssTnI and contains two serine residues at positions 23 and 24, that are substrates for phosphorylation by protein kinase A (PKA). Given that PKA phosphorylation of these serine residues reduces myofilament Ca^{2+} sensitivity and accelerates cross-bridge cycling during high heart rates (see below), it is not surprising that fetal myofilaments have an increased Ca^{2+} sensitivity and reduced length dependence of Ca^{2+} activation (Arteaga et al., 2000, Fentzke et al., 1999 and Wolksa et al., 2001 as cited in Parmacek & Solaro, 2004). However, increased ssTnI expression is not observed in hearts with severe FHC phenotype (Sasse et al., 1993 as cited in Parmacek & Solaro, 2004), suggesting that other factors, such as myocellular modifications due to FHC mutations, are at play.

The clustering of FHC mutations within the highly flexible inhibitory domain and the mobile region of cTnI with its actin-Tm binding site are of extreme interest to researchers. Perhaps this clustering represents a "tolerance" to alterations of the highly mobile regions of the thin filament, providing evidence that Tn mutations frequently modulate, but do not obliterate, thin filament movements. Some researchers have proposed that under sub-maximal cardiac loads, many of the discussed mutations are relatively benign. However, increased cardiac loads can create the arrhythmogenic substrate leading to SCD in a subset of FHC patients, which is in keeping with the observed high frequency of SCD occurring during or following physical activity (Maron, 2003).

PKA phosphorylation of cTnI affects the cross-bridge cycling rate in response to β-adrenergic activation and represents a post-translational mechanism through which mutations can cause adverse effects to cardiac output and response to increased cardiac demands. Phosphorylation of cTnI at S23 and S24 causes a decrease in Ca^{2+} sensitivity of force generation, increase in off-rates of Ca^{2+} from TnC site II, increase in cross-bridge cycling rate and increase in relaxation rate (Metzger & Westfall, 2004 in Tardiff, 2011). Functional studies with the FHC cTnI R145G mutation provide evidence of an interaction between the N-terminus and the inhibitory domain of cTnI, as the expected desensitization after PKA-mediated phosphorylation was not observed with this mutant. Perhaps the loss of a basic residue (arginine to glycine) depresses inhibition in the inhibitory domain and alters electrostatic interactions with the N-terminal of cTnI (Deng, Y. et al., 2001 as cited in Tardiff, 2011).

4.2.1 *In vitro* and *in vivo* approaches

Similar to other FHC mutations, cTnI mutations demonstrate increased myofilament Ca^{2+} sensitivity which is believed to contribute to pathological hypertrophy and SCD (Parmacek

& Solaro, 2004). Elliot et al. (2000) reported that R145G and R162G mutations demonstrated significantly increased Ca^{2+} sensitivity of ATPase regulation (i.e. force generation) and reduced inhibition of actomyosin ATPase activity *in vitro*. Skinned reconstituted rabbit fibres incorporating R145G, R162G and ΔK183 mutants provide further evidence with increased Ca^{2+} sensitivity consistent with myofilament activation at lower Ca^{2+} levels and predicting an impairment in cardiac relaxation (Takahashi-Yanaga et al., 2001). An *in vivo* study with a cTnI R145G transgenic mouse model also confirmed these results (James et al., 2000). Other animal models recapitulate human FHC findings of myocellular dysfunction preceding structural phenotype; young transgenic cTnI G203S mice display abnormal Ca^{2+} cycling with prolonged decay rates of Ca^{2+} transients long before phenotypic expression of hypertrophy, fibrosis and myocyte disarray (Tsoutsman et al., 2006). Transgenic rabbits expressing low protein levels of R145G cTnI displayed apical myocyte disarray, interstitial fibrosis, but with only mild ventricular hypertrophy at later ages (1.5 to 2 years of age) (Sanbe et al., 2005). Rabbit models more closely resemble human cardiac physiology in that myocellular Ca^{2+} handling and alterations in Ca^{2+} flux during heart failure is much more similar to humans than mouse models (Bers, 2002, as cited in Sanbe et al., 2005). Another limitation for mouse models is their heart rate is roughly 10 times faster than humans, which in turn influences the refractory period associated with arrhythmia incidence (Boyett and Jewell, 1978 as cited in Sanbe et al., 2005).

4.2.2 Human cardiac TnI mutation studies

As with cTnT mutations, studies into patients with cTnI mutations are confounded by small family sizes and referral biases. Nonetheless, characterization of the ΔK183 mutation in several families lead to striking discoveries of high penetrance, age-independent SCD and highly variable ventricular remodeling with some patients, particularly in patients over 40 years, progressing to left ventricular dilatation (referred to as "burned out" hypertrophic cardiomyopathy) within single, multigenerational families (Kokado et al., 2000). A landmark study (Mogensen et al., 2004) reported the phenotype with 748 families ranging from severe restrictive cardiomyopathy, biventricular hypertrophy, or apical hypertrophy in some relatives to no disease features in others, complicating treatment options and risk stratification within families and suggesting that other genetic and/or environmental factors play a role in disease manifestation (Parmacek & Solaro, 2004). Unlike cTnT mutations, however, there have been no reported cases of SCD with mild disease presentation (Mogensen et al., 2004). Interestingly, most of the 13 cTnI mutations within this large cohort are found with the relatively narrow range of exons 7 and 8 encompassing the inhibitory and mobile domains of the C terminal domain.

4.3 Troponin C mutations

Cardiac TnC has only recently joined the list of FHC-causing genes and so far, 6 mutations have been identified (Chung et al., 2011; Chung et al., 2011; Hoffmann et al., 2001; Landstrom et al., 2008; Willott et al., 2010). Cardiac TnC is a highly conserved protein found in all striated muscle among vertebrate species. In mammals, there are two paralogs of TnC: the fast skeletal TnC (sTnC) and the cardiac/slow skeletal TnC (cTnC), consisting of N- and C-terminal domains connected by a long central α-helix. Each domain contains a pair of EF-hand (helix-loop-helix) motifs that bind Ca^{2+} (Kretsinger & Nockolds, 1973, as cited in Li, 2009) and are numbered I to IV (Potter & Gergely, 1975; Zot & Potter, 1982 as cited in Li,

!009). Site III and site IV in the C-terminal domain have high Ca^{2+} binding affinity and are generally occupied by Mg^{2+} and Ca^{2+} ions under physiological conditions. Thus, the C-terminal domain almost always adopts a more open conformation, making it a "structural" domain that maintains the integrity of the Tn complex (Potter & Gergely, 1975; Zot & Potter, 982 as cited in Li, 2009). The N-terminal domain exhibits a lower Ca^{2+} binding affinity of $.0^6$ M^{-1} (more than one order of magnitude lower affinity than sites III and IV) and is herefore sensitive to changes in cytosolic Ca^{2+} concentration, making it the "regulatory domain" (Potter & Gergely, 1975; Zot & Potter, 1982 as cited in Li, 2009). It was proposed hat the N-terminal domain changes from a "closed" state to an "open" state upon Ca^{2+} binding. A reorientation of helices exposes the hydrophobic residues of the central helix, where the inhibitory domain of TnI binds and triggers the overall conformational change of he Tn complex. As cTnC does not have a functional Ca^{2+} binding site I, it tends to have a more closed conformation compared to sTnC even when site II is coordinating Ca^{2+} Herzberg, Moult & James, 1986 in Li, 2009).

4.3.1 *In vitro* analyses and human cardiac TnC mutation studies

What makes cTnC mutations unique is that they are dispersed relatively evenly throughout he gene. As with other Tn mutations, investigations into cTnC mutations are confounded by small family sizes and in some cases, are limited to a single patient. Commercial and research laboratories have only recently added cTnC to their molecular genetic testing platforms (and some continue to omit cTnC from their screenings), leading one to propose perhaps some purportedly genotype-negative FHC patients could potentially harbour cTnC mutations.

The first observed FHC related cTnC mutation, L29Q, was discovered in a 59 year old man who presented with dyspnea upon exertion (Hoffmann et al., 2001). An ECG revealed an abnormal QRS complex suggestive of ventricular hypertrophy and confirmed by echocardiography. There has yet to be any follow-up study with this patient who would now be approximately 70 years of age, which limits knowledge of disease progression with this mutation.

Leucine 29 of cTnC is located in the dysfunctional Ca^{2+} binding site I of the N-domain. Although it is not Ca^{2+} binding, it is important in maintaining the structural integrity of the first helix of cTnC (Sia et al., as cited in Li, 2009). It is located at the cTnI binding site (Schmidtmann et al., 2005). Replacement of a non-polar leucine with a polar glutamine is predicted to have an impact on overall function of the Tn complex with Tm. However, several studies show that in the absence of phosphorylated cTnI, the L29Q mutation can decrease, increase, or have no affect on Ca^{2+} sensitivity (Baryshnikova et al., 2008; Liang et al., 2008; Schmidtmann et al., 2005) leading to scepticism of its status as a pathogenic FHC mutation. For example, *in vitro* assays conducted on L29Q show that the Ca^{2+} sensitivity of ATPase in reconstituted thin filaments is not affected by PKA-dependent phosphorylation of cTnI (Schmidtmann et al., 2005). This finding implies that L29Q may decrease the Ca^{2+} sensitivity and disrupt the signal from the phosphorylated cTnI to cTnC. However, this finding contradicts other reports of FHC mutations generally having higher myofilament Ca^{2+} sensitivities (Chang et al., 2005; Gomes & Potter, 2004; Karibe et al., 2001). Recent NMR and ultraviolet/visual spectrum titration studies showed that L29Q essentially has the same Ca^{2+} affinity as that of wild-type cTnC (Baryshnikova et al., 2008) although this technique presents challenges for measuring Ca^{2+} affinity (see below).

Conversely, our research group demonstrated that L29Q significantly increases the Ca^{2+} sensitivity of force generation using single skinned cardiac myocytes, but in a manner that was extremely sarcomere length dependent (Liang et al., 2008). Cardiac TnC F27W was used as a fluorescence reporter to monitor the *in vitro* Ca^{2+} binding and exchange with binding site II of cTnC. Our results showed that L29Q has a significantly increased Ca^{2+} binding affinity compared to the wild-type, and its response to sarcomere length change was significantly reduced. The increased Ca^{2+} sensitivity suggests that L29Q mutants bind Ca^{2+} more tightly and cause Ca^{2+} to dissociate more slowly from cTnC site II. Reduced length dependence of myofilament Ca^{2+} sensitivity likely influences the heart's ability to regulate ventricular output in response to changes in ventricular filling (Liang et al., 2008). Overall, the heart is maintained in systole longer, resulting in diastolic dysfunction (Wen et al., 2008 in Pinto et al., 2009). Changes in Ca^{2+} affinity is hypothesized to disrupt myocellular homeostasis, triggering Ca^{2+}-regulated pathways leading to SCD (Baudenbacher et al., 2008) and/or hypertrophy (Heineke & Molkentin, 2006) as discussed later in this chapter.

Choice of experimental techniques may account for the conflicting results. Compared to studies using single cardiac myocytes, ATPase and *in* vitro motility assays are excellent techniques for defining molecular interactions, but lack the geometric and mechanical constraints from other proteins within the sarcomere (Liang et al., 2008). Additionally, NMR techniques are limited in terms of accurate Ca^{2+} measurement as Ca^{2+} chelators, such as EGTA, cannot be utilized in NMR studies (Liang et al., 2008). The reduced length dependence of Ca^{2+} sensitivity is likely why other researchers, who had no or only marginal sarcomeric length control in their experimental techniques, have observed such variable results. Our experimental technique using single cardiac myocytes held at a constant sarcomere length may be more precise and closer to physiological conditions. Further to this, our work on cTnC and the L29Q mutation precedes the discovery of a human L29Q cTnC FHC patient. Salmonid cTnC has a greater than two-fold Ca^{2+} affinity over mammalian cTnC (Gillis et al., 2003) with four sequence differences between the mammalian and salmonid homologues responsible for the high Ca^{2+} affinity: D2N, V28I, L29Q, and G30D (NIQD). When the mammalian residues were mutated to the salmonid-equivalent, including L29 to Q29, the Ca^{2+}-binding affinities of the mammalian cTnC mutants increased to the level of the salmonid cTnC (Gillis et al., 2005).

Seven years after the initial FHC cTnC report, a large study cohort of 1025 unrelated patients was screened for FHC mutations and four novel cTnC mutations were reported: A8V, C84Y, E134D and D145E (Landstrom et al., 2008). All four patients were symptomatic for FHC, with findings of syncope upon exertion (C84Y) and dyspnea and chest pain in the other three patients. They were all positive for varying degrees of ventricular hypertrophy. All were young or relatively young (17, 22, 37 and 58 years old) when diagnosed, but SCD was not reported in any patients or relatives. Functional analysis of the four variants using skinned porcine papillary fibres revealed increased Ca^{2+} sensitivity of force development for A8V, C84Y and D145E mutations, and A8V and D145E also showed increases in maximal force consistent with other *in vitro* studies of FHC-associated mutants (Landstrom et al., 2008). Actomyosin ATPase activity in reconstituted thin filaments and spectroscopic properties of the four mutants confirmed increased myofilament Ca^{2+} sensitivity, except for E134D which was not significantly different from wild-type (Pinto et al., 2009). Isolated cTnC, Tn complex and thin filament assays, however, did not recapitulate the Ca^{2+} sensitivity findings observed in the reconstituted fibre assays, suggesting that the entire reconstituted myofilament (that included the S1 myosin head) is required to recreate the increased Ca^{2+} sensitivity changes observed in skinned fibre assays. This research group also proposed that the D145E mutation influences regulation of contraction by disrupting Ca^{2+} binding to site IV of cTnC and demonstrated that this mutation reduced the cTnC α helicity in the metal-bound state as determined by circular dichroism (Pinto et al., 2009). Another report investigated the effects of IAANS-labeled cTnC mutants on Ca^{2+} off-rate kinetics and concluded that both A8V and D145E mutations had significantly slower off-rate kinetics over the wild-type, suggesting that both mutations alter muscle relaxation properties by reducing ventricular filling time which correlates with the diastolic dysfunction seen in FHC patients (Pinto et al., 2011).

Only one cTnC mutation so far has been directly linked to the SCD of a previously undiagnosed and asymptomatic 19 year old man who had a witnessed collapse while working at his computer (Chung et al., 2011). Autopsy revealed ventricular hypertrophy. Genetic testing of his family revealed a novel cTnC duplication at nucleotide 363, leading to a frameshift mutation at Q122A and causing a premature stop codon at position 30 in the new reading frame (Q122AfsX30) in 4 out of 7 relatives. The primary concern was for his 16 year old genotype-positive, phenotype-negative sister, who can be monitored for disease manifestation (Chung et al., 2011). To date, no functional analysis has been done on this mutation finding. The premature stop codon created by this frameshift mutation is close to the C terminus, leading to speculation that the mutant protein is successfully translated, incorporated into the thin filament and creates adverse effects on Ca^{2+} sensitivity of force production similar to other cTnC mutations. One could also propose that the protein undergoes nonsense-mediated decay, leading to haploinsufficiency of cTnC within the cardiac myocytes. Future investigations will hopefully provide further insight to the pathogenic mechanisms of this newest cTnC mutation finding.

5. Arrhythmogenic mechanisms in FHC

Many studies comparing FHC phenotype with suspected underlying mechanisms are plagued by the lack of genotyping of cardiomyopathy patients, perhaps related to the high cost and time-consuming work of genetic testing. To address this issue, Colombo et al. (Colombo et al., 2008) argue that some genotype-phenotype correlations can provide important information to target DNA analyses in specific FHC candidate genes. Genetic testing may also clarify diagnosis and assist with optimal treatment strategies for more malignant phenotypes. In addition, genetic screening of first-degree relatives can assist in early identification and diagnosis of individuals at greatest risk for developing cardiomyopathy, allowing physicians to focus clinical resources on high-risk family members. Determining the underlying mechanism of SCD resulting from FHC remains elusive, though recent studies have begun to focus on the three cardinal manifestations of FHC separately (i.e. cardiac hypertrophy, myocyte disarray and fibrosis), as researchers are postulating that they may arise from distinct and independent mechanisms (Varnava, Elliott, Baboonian et al., 2001; Varnava, Elliott, Mahon et al., 2001; Wolf et al., 2005). Myocyte hypertrophy is postulated by some to increase arrhythmia vulnerability through intrinsic automaticity changes, as some studies demonstrate that hypertrophied myocytes exhibit pacemaker current up-regulation (re-expression) and action potential prolongation by down-regulation of the potassium transient outward I_{to} current (Sanguinetti, 2002 as cited in Wolf et al., 2005).

Triggered arrhythmias can occur as delayed after-depolarizations (DADs), early after-depolarizations (EADs) or increased automaticity in non-ischemic FHC and are likely related to myocellular Ca^{2+} signalling and transport (Bers, 2008). DADs are commonly believed to be caused by spontaneous Ca^{2+} release from the SR that occurs as a consequence of high SR Ca^{2+} levels. This SR Ca^{2+} release causes a transient inward current (I_{ti}) that can cause a threshold depolarization leading to an action potential. Several studies suggest that the Na^+/ Ca^{2+} exchanger current (I_{NCX}) is responsible for I_{ti} in human ventricular myocytes (Pogwizd et al., 2001). Further to this, Ter Keurs' research group has been investigating myofilament arrhythmogenic Ca^{2+} release to determine if non-uniform excitation-contraction coupling plays a role in the initiation of extra-systoles that create arrhythmias ((Ter Keurs et al., 2006). Ter Keurs developed a model of non-uniform excitation-contraction using rat trabeculae and exposed a small muscle segment to BDM, a cross-bridge inhibitor (Backx et al., 1995 as cited in Ter Keurs et al., 2006), to recapitulate non-contracting myocardium as found in diseased hearts. Triggered propagating contractions were observed in the border zone of myocardium between non-contractile and contractile tissue when the trabeculae were stimulated to contract. The triggered contractions may be due to a quick release-induced Ca^{2+} dissociation from cTnC site II, leading to a local Ca^{2+} surge that is above the threshold for inducing Ca^{2+}-induced Ca^{2+} release. This mechanism, referred to as "reverse excitation contraction coupling" (RECC), occurs when Ca^{2+} reuptake mechanisms have sufficiently recovered from the previous contraction during diastole (Boyden & ter Keurs, 2001). In FHC, the myocardium may have focal regions of non-uniformity due to structural anomalies, such as fibrosis or myocardial disarray, or perhaps due to electrical remodelling or gene dosage effects from Tn mutations. Increased Ca^{2+} binding to cTnC leading to a high Ca^{2+} buffering capacity may cause a large Ca^{2+} surge during rapid myofilament shortening during RECC. Hence, RECC may be an underlying pathological mechanism of arrhythmogenesis seen in FHC patients and warrants further investigation.

Electrical alternans, in which there is alternating long and short action potential duration (APD), increases the risk of ventricular tachycardia that can degrade to ventricular fibrillation and SCD. The underlying mechanism may to be related to Ca^{2+} transient amplitude alternans. At high pacing frequencies, slow ryanodine receptor and/or Ca^{2+} current recovery may result in alternating SR Ca^{2+} release, due to alternating availability of ryanodine receptors (RyR). Prolonged Ca^{2+} transient decay rates, as seen in some transgenic FHC animal models may play a role here (see below). Spatially discordant alternans is thought to be a prerequisite to dangerous arrhythmias, as there is a non-synchronous electrical substrate within the heart (Bers, 2008). Animal models support this hypothesis; increased myofilament Ca^{2+} sensitivity was associated with an arrhythmogenic substrate in transgenic cTnT mice, despite the absence of structural heart disease (Baudenbacher et al., 2008). Addition of a myofilament Ca^{2+} sensitizing agent, EMD, resulted in repolarization alternans at high pacing rates, beat to beat variation in APD, shorter effective refractory periods and increased spatial conduction velocity dispersion in wild-type cat and mouse hearts, paralleling the findings as observed in mutant cTnT I79N transgenic mice. Several mechanisms were proposed for the induction of ventricular tachyarrhythmias: increased Ca^{2+} binding to cTnC resulting in reduced Ca^{2+} transients with slower decay rates responsible for the shorter APD seen in transgenic I79N cTnT mice, and dysfunctional myocardial relaxation as seen in transgenic mice and in human patients also causing APD shortening. However, transgenic mice have differing ion channel and Ca^{2+}-handling protein expression from human hearts (Wetzel & Klitzner, 1996). The high heart rates of mice, roughly 10 times faster than humans, can influence the refractory period associated with the incidence of arrhythmias, as mentioned previously. Additionally, studies of human HCM patients suggested that T-wave alternans (surface ECG recording associated with action potential alternans) may not be a useful SCD prediction tool (Fuchs & Torjman, 2009).

5.1 Clinical findings in FHC patients

It has proven difficult to elucidate the exact mechanisms linking FHC pathology and arrhythmogenicity in humans with limited access to fresh cardiac tissue from FHC patients. Studies currently utilize tissue from myectomy samples and explanted hearts in which there is profound disease phenotype. Thus, explorations of disease progression in pre-clinical patients are normally limited to non-invasive imaging techniques and electrophysiology. In addition, there is inherent patient referral bias for research studies as most FHC patients seen in surgical referral centres already have profound disease manifestation (Tardiff, 2011).

Stored electrograms from implantable cardiac defibrillators indicate that SCD largely results from sustained ventricular tachycardia and/or ventricular fibrillation (B.J. Maron, 2010). One suggested trigger for SCD is sympathetic excitation, given that the initiating rhythm in many cases is sinus tachycardia, which may underlie the high SCD rate in athletes and sub-adult FHC populations (Cha et al., 2007). Several studies of HCM patients wearing Holter monitors identified a higher rate of SCD for younger patients (age 30 and under) with non-sustained ventricular tachycardia (NSVT) detected at least once during the 48 hour monitoring period. While NSVT is usually asymptomatic and frequently occurs during periods of increased parasympathetic (vagal) tone, it is associated with an increased SCD risk, especially in children and young adults (Elliott et al., 2000; Monserrat et al., 2003). However, most SCDs occur in patients without ambulatory ECG episodes of NSVT; clearly other contributory factors leading to risk of SCD are at play. A more recent study identified an increased SCD risk with ventricular arrhythmias triggered by exercise (Gimeno, Tome-Esteban et al., 2009), which is more in keeping findings of triggered arrhythmias during sinus tachycardia, implicating sympathetic excitation during physical activity (Cha et al., 2007). This is also in keeping with the *in vitro* experimental evidence of a blunted response to β-adrenergic stimulation through phosphorylation of cTnI (i.e. reduced inhibitory response of phosphorylated cTnI on Ca^{2+} sensitivity for cTnC) and the resultant diastolic dysfunction as discussed previously.

Cardiac magnetic resonance (CMR) imaging has allowed clinicians to precisely determine myocyte fibrosis and scarring in non-ischemic FHC, including phenotype-negative FHC patients who have experienced life-threatening arrhythmias (Makhoul et al., 2011; Strijack et al., 2008). Detection of fibrosis by late gadolinium enhancement in CMR is associated with increased propensity for VT on ambulatory ECG monitoring (Adabag et al., 2008) and is being considered as a clinical SCD risk marker (Maron, 2010). Fibrosis and scarring may promote localized zones of slowed conduction resulting in re-entrant arrhythmias (Cha et al., 2007). NMR imaging can detect focal or diffuse regions of fibrosis and hypertrophy morphologies that are missed by traditional echocardiography (M. S. Maron, 2009) and will likely continue to improve in resolution leading to improved risk stratification for FHC patients.

Myocyte disarray is another common feature in FHC patients and a recent study of myectomy samples from a small pediatric HCM cohort suggests that myocyte disarray has a significantly higher correlation with diastolic dysfunction than either hypertrophy or fibrosis (Menon et al., 2009). Extensive myocyte disarray has been linked to SCD in younger FHC patients (Varnava, Elliott, Mahon et al., 2001), especially those with cTnT mutations (Varnava, Elliott, Baboonian et al., 2001) in the absence of, or with minimal hypertrophy.

6. Future considerations

Of interest to investigators is the potential role of Ca^{2+} dysregulation in ER stress pathways. The SR in myocardial cells has long been thought to be the cardiac equivalent to ER with its main role as the intracellular regulator of Ca^{2+} fluxes and hence, excitation-contraction coupling in the heart. Some researchers propose that the SR contains a functional ER "compartment" with physiological roles such as protein synthesis, translocation and integration into membranes, folding and post-translational modifications including glycosylation and Ca^{2+} homeostasis (Mesaeli et al., 2001), although studies are lacking. ER stress occurs in response to environmental or genetic factors causing ER metabolic disturbances, accumulation of misfolded proteins, oxidative stress and/or depletion of ER Ca^{2+} stores. The "unfolded protein response" (UPR) is one mechanism by which the ER attempts to reestablish homeostasis by reducing protein expression, by increasing production of chaperones to handle accumulation of misfolded protein, promoting ER-associated degradation to remove misfolded proteins (Schroder & Kaufman, 2005). This initial response of protein synthesis, suppression and upregulation of ER resident chaperones is designed to resolve the ER stress and enhance survival, but if the ER stress is severe or prolonged, the UPR may stimulate apoptosis (cell death). Do FHC mutations play a role in ER stress pathways, such as through Ca^{2+} dysregulation? Activation of the "fetal gene program" is a response to elevated Ca^{2+} to increase cardiac efficiency in the stressed heart. This response, unfortunately, also commonly results in detrimental cardiac hypertrophy (Eizirik et al., 2008; Wang et al., 2000). Elevated Ca^{2+} activates calcineurin A that dephosphorylates the transcription factor NFAT which translocates to the nucleus to stimulate cardiac remodelling and hypertrophy associated with the fetal gene program (Heineke & Molkentin, 2006). Other factors, such as MEF2, GATA and CamKII are also activated which initiate transcription programs associated with hypertrophy, remodelling and heart failure with increased risk of cardiac death (Molkentin et al., 1998). GATA-4 may play a significant role in FHC pathogenesis due to its ability to stimulate transcription of the cardiac-specific Tn genes (Liang et al., 2001; Molkentin & Olson, 1997; Molkentin et al., 1998). Therefore, ER stress may turn on the fetal gene program in response to pathological insult. MicroRNAs (miRs) likely play a role in these regulatory processes with miRNA coding sequences often located within the newly transcribed genes (Eizirik et al., 2008; Wang et al., 2000). The hypothesis of elevated Ca^{2+} causing transcriptional activation of hypertrophy and perhaps pathological arrhythmia substrates (see below) is provocative and will likely continue to be an area of active investigation.

Research into miRs that play a role in regulation of cardiac function and the recent findings that miR expression is deranged in cardiac disease may help to uncover the pathways to FHC disease progression and arrhythmogenesis. MiRs are short, non-coding RNA sequences that regulate expression of genes involved in orchestrating growth, development, function and stress responses in a spatio-temporal manner. MiRs target specific mRNA equences generally to inhibit protein expression, either by degradation of the bound nRNA target or by directly inhibiting translation of the mRNA sequence (Bartel, 2004). To late, there are at least 4 miRs shown to be involved in cardiac development, apoptosis and hypertrophy, namely: miR-1, miR-133, miR-208 and miR-499 (van Rooij et al., 2006). Several mportant target genes for miRs related to cardiac electrophysiology have been identified, ncluding connexin 43 and inwardly-rectifying potassium channel Kir2.1 (Zhao et al., 2007) and miR-1 expression changes have been associated with arrhythmogenesis due to up-regulation or down-regulation of these gene products (Girmatsion et al., 2009; Yang et al., 2007). Recent studies are beginning to elucidate the link between miRs and SCD due to arrhythmias by identifying the effects of altered expression levels of miRs in the heart on cardiac conduction and excitability (Callis et al., 2009; Matkovich et al., 2010; Zhao et al., 2007). A database has been developed online (http://www.mir2disease.org/) for miRs involved in human disease, including FHC.

Sudden Infant Death Syndrome (SIDS) refers to the sudden death of an infant under 1 year of age which remains unexplained after a thorough medicolegal investigation (Willinger et al., 1991). Researchers are now considering inherited cardiac arrhythmia syndromes in its etiology. Recent research has revealed that up to 20% of SIDS cases may be associated with inheritable arrhythmia syndromes, such as long QT syndrome (Klaver et al., 2011). Given that FHC is the most common cause of SCD in young individuals, it stands to reason that some infants may die from SCD attributed to FHC. Further to this, as discussed earlier, some Tn mutants, particularly the cTnT mutants, have negligible or mild hypertrophy that may not be observed grossly during the post mortem exam. To date, only one study has screened SIDS cases for FHC mutations (Brion et al., 2009). Their findings of 14 cases with 7 genetic variants from 4 different FHC genes, including cTnT and cTnI, from 140 SIDS tissues suggests that some SIDS cases may be associated with FHC-causing mutations. The relatively recent emergence of FHC-associated Tn (in particular, cTnC) gene mutations make these candidate genes previously unrecognized and perhaps under-represented factors to be considered in future SIDS investigations. Besides SIDS cases, how many FHC mutation positive cases have gone unrecognized in post mortem investigations following the sudden, unexpected death of children and young adults?

7. Conclusions

Sudden cardiac death affects approximately 1-2% of children and adolescents, and up to 1% of young adults in FHC-affected populations. *In vitro* analysis of single molecule mechanics and reconstituted skinned myocytes have identified intracellular Ca^{2+} dysregulation, altered myofibrillar Ca^{2+} sensitivity and altered energy metabolism as potential mechanisms at the sarcomere and cellular level. Animal models incorporating specific FHC mutations have broadened our understanding of the pathogenesis of FHC, including structural and electrophysiological remodelling associated with the arrhythmogenic substrate. There are, however, caveats to using in vitro and animal model analyses, given that some may not necessarily recapitulate the physiological substrate in human FHC patients. Most models, however, share a consistent molecular phenotype, namely increased myofilament Ca^{2+} sensitivity and increased energetic cost of force development, that underlies the complex and heterogeneous phenotype that exists at the human patient level. Other genetic, environmental and biological factors such as age, lifestyle and other health issues are also likely disease-modifying factors. Research into molecular approaches and post-translational mechanisms associated with FHC, including effects of phosphorylation and a potential role in ER stress mechanisms, will likely continue to elucidate the link between genotype and phenotype.

8. Acknowledgements

GFT is a Canada Research Chair and the authors acknowledge the generous support of the Heart and Stroke Foundation of BC and Yukon.

9. References

Adabag, A. S., Maron, B. J., Appelbaum, E., Harrigan, C. J., Buros, J. L., Gibson, C. M., Maron, M. S. (2008). Occurrence and frequency of arrhythmias in hypertrophic cardiomyopathy in relation to delayed enhancement on cardiovascular magnetic resonance. *Journal of the American College of Cardiology, 51*(14), 1369-1374. doi:10.1016/j.jacc.2007.11.071

Alcalai, R., Seidman, J. G., & Seidman, C. E. (2008). Genetic basis of hypertrophic cardiomyopathy: From bench to the clinics. *Journal of Cardiovascular Electrophysiology, 19*(1), 104-110. doi:10.1111/j.1540-8167.2007.00965.x

Ashrafian, H., Redwood, C., Blair, E., & Watkins, H. (2003). Hypertrophic cardiomyopathy:A paradigm for myocardial energy depletion. *Trends in Genetics : TIG, 19*(5), 263-268.

Bartel, D. P. (2004). MicroRNAs: Genomics, biogenesis, mechanism, and function. *Cell, 116*(2), 281-297.

Baryshnikova, O. K., Li, M. X., & Sykes, B. D. (2008). Modulation of cardiac troponin C function by the cardiac-specific N-terminus of troponin I: Influence of PKA phosphorylation and involvement in cardiomyopathies. *Journal of Molecular Biology, 375*(3), 735-751. doi:10.1016/j.jmb.2007.10.062

Baudenbacher, F., Schober, T., Pinto, J. R., Sidorov, V. Y., Hilliard, F., Solaro, R. J., Knollmann, B. C. (2008). Myofilament Ca2+ sensitization causes susceptibility to cardiac arrhythmia in mice. *The Journal of Clinical Investigation, 118*(12), 3893-3903. doi:10.1172/JCI36642

Bers, D. M. (2008). Calcium cycling and signaling in cardiac myocytes. *Annual Review of Physiology, 70*, 23-49. doi:10.1146/annurev.physiol.70.113006.100455

Boyden, P. A., & ter Keurs, H. E. (2001). Reverse excitation-contraction coupling: Ca2+ ions as initiators of arrhythmias. *Journal of Cardiovascular Electrophysiology, 12*(3), 382-385.

Brion, M., Allegue, C., Gil, R., Torres, M., Santori, M., Poster, S., .. Carracedo, A. (2009). Involvement of hypertrophic cardiomyopathy genes in sudden infant death syndrome (SIDS). *Forensic Science International: Genetics Supplement Series, 2*(1), 495-496. doi:DOI: 10.1016/j.fsigss.2009.09.040

Brooks, B. R., Brooks, C. L.,3rd, Mackerell, A. D.,Jr, Nilsson, L., Petrella, R. J., Roux, B., Karplus, M. (2009). CHARMM: The biomolecular simulation program. *Journal of Computational Chemistry, 30*(10), 1545-1614. doi:10.1002/jcc.21287

Callis, T. E., Pandya, K., Seok, H. Y., Tang, R. H., Tatsuguchi, M., Huang, Z. P., .. Wang, D. Z. (2009). MicroRNA-208a is a regulator of cardiac hypertrophy and conduction in mice. *The Journal of Clinical Investigation, 119*(9), 2772-2786. doi:10.1172/JCI36154; 10.1172/JCI36154

Cha, Y. M., Gersh, B. J., Maron, B. J., Boriani, G., Spirito, P., Hodge, D. O., .. Shen, W. K. (2007). Electrophysiologic manifestations of ventricular tachyarrhythmias provoking appropriate defibrillator interventions in high-risk patients with hypertrophic cardiomyopathy. *Journal of Cardiovascular Electrophysiology, 18*(5), 483-487. doi:10.1111/j.1540-8167.2007.00780.x

Chang, A. N., Harada, K., Ackerman, M. J., & Potter, J. D. (2005). Functional consequences of hypertrophic and dilated cardiomyopathy-causing mutations in alpha-tropomyosin. *The Journal of Biological Chemistry, 280*(40), 34343-34349. doi:10.1074/jbc.M505014200

Chung, W. K., Kitner, C., & Maron, (2011). Novel frameshift mutation in troponin C (TNNC1) associated with hypertrophic cardiomyopathy and sudden death. *Cardiology in the Young, , 1-4.* doi:10.1017/S1047951110001927

Colombo, M. G., Botto, N., Vittorini, S., Paradossi, U., & Andreassi, M. G. (2008). Clinical utility of genetic tests for inherited hypertrophic and dilated cardiomyopathies. *Cardiovascular Ultrasound, 6,* 62. doi:10.1186/1476-7120-6-62

Elliott, P. M., Poloniecki, J., Dickie, S., Sharma, S., Monserrat, L., Varnava, A., .. McKenna, W. J. (2000). Sudden death in hypertrophic cardiomyopathy: Identification of high risk patients. *Journal of the American College of Cardiology, 36*(7), 2212-2218.

Eizirik, D. L., Cardozo, A. K., & Cnop, M. (2008). The role for endoplasmic reticulum stress in diabetes mellitus. *Endocrine Reviews, 29*(1), 42-61. doi:10.1210/er.2007-0015

Fatkin, D., & Graham, R. M. (2002). Molecular mechanisms of inherited cardiomyopathies. *Physiological Reviews, 82*(4), 945-980. doi:10.1152/physrev.00012.2002

Fuchs, T., & Torjman, A. (2009). The usefulness of microvolt T-wave alternans in the risk stratification of patients with hypertrophic cardiomyopathy. *The Israel Medical Association Journal : IMAJ, 11*(10), 606-610.

Geisterfer-Lowrance, A. A., Kass, S., Tanigawa, G., Vosberg, H. P., McKenna, W., Seidman, C. E., & Seidman, J. G. (1990). A molecular basis for familial hypertrophic cardiomyopathy: A beta cardiac myosin heavy chain gene missense mutation. *Cell, 62*(5), 999-1006.

Gillis, T. E., Liang, B., Chung, F., & Tibbits, G. F. (2005). Increasing mammalian cardiomyocyte contractility with residues identified in trout troponin C. *Physiological Genomics, 22*(1), 1-7. doi:10.1152/physiolgenomics.00007.2005

Gillis, T. E., Moyes, C. D., & Tibbits, G. F. (2003). Sequence mutations in teleost cardiac troponin C that are permissive of high Ca2+ affinity of site II. *American Journal of Physiology.Cell Physiology, 284*(5), C1176-84. doi:10.1152/ajpcell.00339.2002

Gimeno, J. R., Monserrat, L., Perez-Sanchez, I., Marin, F., Caballero, L., Hermida-Prieto, M., Valdes, M. (2009). Hypertrophic cardiomyopathy. A study of the troponin-T gene in 127 spanish families. *Revista Espanola De Cardiologia, 62*(12), 1473-1477.

Gimeno, J. R., Tome-Esteban, M., Lofiego, C., Hurtado, J., Pantazis, A., Mist, B., .. Elliott, P. M. (2009). Exercise-induced ventricular arrhythmias and risk of sudden cardiac death in patients with hypertrophic cardiomyopathy. *European Heart Journal, 30*(21), 2599-2605. doi:10.1093/eurheartj/ehp327

Girmatsion, Z., Biliczki, P., Bonauer, A., Wimmer-Greinecker, G., Scherer, M., Moritz, A., Ehrlich, J. R. (2009). Changes in microRNA-1 expression and IK1 up-regulation in human atrial fibrillation. *Heart Rhythm : The Official Journal of the Heart Rhythm Society, 6*(12), 1802-1809. doi:10.1016/j.hrthm.2009.08.035

Gomes, A. V., Guzman, G., Zhao, J., & Potter, J. D. (2002). Cardiac troponin T isoforms affect the Ca2+ sensitivity and inhibition of force development. insights into the role of troponin T isoforms in the heart. *The Journal of Biological Chemistry, 277*(38), 35341-35349. doi:10.1074/jbc.M204118200

Gomes, A. V., Barnes, J. A., Harada, K., & Potter, J. D. (2004). Role of troponin T in disease. *Molecular and Cellular Biochemistry, 263*(1-2), 115-129.

Gomes, A. V., & Potter, J. D. (2004). Molecular and cellular aspects of troponin cardiomyopathies. *Annals of the New York Academy of Sciences, 1015*, 214-224. doi:10.1196/annals.1302.018

Gordon, A. M., Homsher, E., & Regnier, M. (2000). Regulation of contraction in striated muscle. *Physiological Reviews, 80*(2), 853-924.

Haim, T. E., Dowell, C., Diamanti, T., Scheuer, J., & Tardiff, J. C. (2007). Independent FHC-related cardiac troponin T mutations exhibit specific alterations in myocellular contractility and calcium kinetics. *Journal of Molecular and Cellular Cardiology, 42*(6), 1098-1110. doi:10.1016/j.yjmcc.2007.03.906

Heineke, J., & Molkentin, J. D. (2006). Regulation of cardiac hypertrophy by intracellular signalling pathways. *Nature Reviews.Molecular Cell Biology, 7*(8), 589-600. doi:10.1038/nrm1983

Hershberger, R. E. (2010). A glimpse into multigene rare variant genetics: Triple mutations in hypertrophic cardiomyopathy. *Journal of the American College of Cardiology, 55*(14), 1454-1455. doi:10.1016/j.jacc.2009.12.025

Ho, C. Y., Lever, H. M., DeSanctis, R., Farver, C. F., Seidman, J. G., & Seidman, C. E. (2000). Homozygous mutation in cardiac troponin T: Implications for hypertrophic cardiomyopathy. *Circulation, 102*(16), 1950-1955.

Ho, C. Y., Sweitzer, N. K., McDonough, B., Maron, B. J., Casey, S. A., Seidman, J. G., .. Solomon, S. D. (2002). Assessment of diastolic function with doppler tissue imaging to predict genotype in preclinical hypertrophic cardiomyopathy. *Circulation, 105*(25), 2992-2997.

Hoffmann, B., Schmidt-Traub, H., Perrot, A., Osterziel, K. J., & Gessner, R. (2001). First mutation in cardiac troponin C, L29Q, in a patient with hypertrophic cardiomyopathy. *Human Mutation, 17*(6), 524. doi:10.1002/humu.1143

Ingles, J., Doolan, A., Chiu, C., Seidman, J., Seidman, C., & Semsarian, C. (2005). Compound and double mutations in patients with hypertrophic cardiomyopathy: Implications for genetic testing and counselling. *Journal of Medical Genetics, 42*(10), e59. doi:10.1136/jmg.2005.033886

James, J., Zhang, Y., Osinska, H., Sanbe, A., Klevitsky, R., Hewett, T. E., & Robbins, J. (2000). Transgenic modeling of a cardiac troponin I mutation linked to familial hypertrophic cardiomyopathy. *Circulation Research, 87*(9), 805-811.

Karibe, A., Tobacman, L. S., Strand, J., Butters, C., Back, N., Bachinski, L. L., .. Fananapazir, L. (2001). Hypertrophic cardiomyopathy caused by a novel alpha-tropomyosin mutation (V95A) is associated with mild cardiac phenotype, abnormal calcium binding to troponin, abnormal myosin cycling, and poor prognosis. *Circulation, 103*(1), 65-71.

Kimura, A., Harada, H., Park, J. E., Nishi, H., Satoh, M., Takahashi, M., .. Sasazuki, T. (1997). Mutations in the cardiac troponin I gene associated with hypertrophic cardiomyopathy. *Nature Genetics, 16*(4), 379-382. doi:10.1038/ng0897-379

Klaver, E. C., Versluijs, G. M., & Wilders, R. (2011). Cardiac ion channel mutations in the sudden infant death syndrome. *International Journal of Cardiology,* doi:10.1016/j.ijcard.2010.12.051

Knollmann, B. C., Kirchhof, P., Sirenko, S. G., Degen, H., Greene, A. E., Schober, T., .. Morad, M. (2003). Familial hypertrophic cardiomyopathy-linked mutant troponin T causes stress-induced ventricular tachycardia and Ca2+-dependent action potential remodeling. *Circulation Research,* 92(4), 428-436. doi:10.1161/01.RES.0000059562.91384.1A

Knollmann, B. C., & Potter, J. D. (2001). Altered regulation of cardiac muscle contraction by troponin T mutations that cause familial hypertrophic cardiomyopathy. *Trends in Cardiovascular Medicine,* 11(5), 206-212.

Kokado, H., Shimizu, M., Yoshio, H., Ino, H., Okeie, K., Emoto, Y., .. Mabuchi, H. (2000). Clinical features of hypertrophic cardiomyopathy caused by a Lys183 deletion mutation in the cardiac troponin I gene. *Circulation,* 102(6), 663-669.

Landstrom, A. P., Parvatiyar, M. S., Pinto, J. R., Marquardt, M. L., Bos, J. M., Tester, D. J., .. Ackerman, M. J. (2008). Molecular and functional characterization of novel hypertrophic cardiomyopathy susceptibility mutations in TNNC1-encoded troponin C. *Journal of Molecular and Cellular Cardiology,* 45(2), 281-288. doi:DOI: 10.1016/j.yjmcc.2008.05.003

Lassalle, M. W. (2010). Defective dynamic properties of human cardiac troponin mutations. *Bioscience, Biotechnology, and Biochemistry,* 74(1), 82-91.

Li, Y. A. (2009). *Crystallographic analysis of the regulatory domain of human cardiac troponin C.* (Master of Science, Simon Fraser University).

Liang, B., Chung, F., Qu, Y., Pavlov, D., Gillis, T. E., Tikunova, S. B., .. Tibbits, G. F. (2008). Familial hypertrophic cardiomyopathy-related cardiac troponin C mutation L29Q affects Ca2+ binding and myofilament contractility. *Physiological Genomics,* 33(2), 257-266. doi:10.1152/physiolgenomics.00154.2007

Liang, Q., De Windt, L. J., Witt, S. A., Kimball, T. R., Markham, B. E., & Molkentin, J. D. (2001). The transcription factors GATA4 and GATA6 regulate cardiomyocyte hypertrophy in vitro and in vivo. *The Journal of Biological Chemistry,* 276(32), 30245-30253. doi:10.1074/jbc.M102174200

Makhoul, M., Ackerman, M. J., Atkins, D. L., & Law, I. H. (2011). Clinical spectrum in a family with tropomyosin-mediated hypertrophic cardiomyopathy and sudden death in childhood. *Pediatric Cardiology,* 32(2), 215-220. doi:10.1007/s00246-010-9843-1

Marian, A. J., Yu, Q. T., Workman, R., Greve, G., & Roberts, R. (1993). Angiotensin-converting enzyme polymorphism in hypertrophic cardiomyopathy and sudden cardiac death. *Lancet,* 342(8879), 1085-1086.

Maron, (2002). Hypertrophic cardiomyopathy: A systematic review. *JAMA : The Journal of the American Medical Association,* 287(10), 1308-1320.

Maron, (2003). Sudden death in young athletes. *The New England Journal of Medicine,* 349(11), 1064-1075. doi:10.1056/NEJMra022783

Maron, (2009). Distinguishing hypertrophic cardiomyopathy from athlete's heart physiological remodelling: Clinical significance, diagnostic strategies and implications for preparticipation screening. *British Journal of Sports Medicine,* 43(9), 649-656. doi:10.1136/bjsm.2008.054726

Maron, (2010). Contemporary insights and strategies for risk stratification and prevention of sudden death in hypertrophic cardiomyopathy. *Circulation, 121*(3), 445-456. doi:10.1161/CIRCULATIONAHA.109.878579

Maron, B. J., Casey, S. A., Poliac, L. C., Gohman, T. E., Almquist, A. K., & Aeppli, D. M. (1999). Clinical course of hypertrophic cardiomyopathy in a regional united states cohort. *JAMA : The Journal of the American Medical Association, 281*(7), 650-655.

Maron, B. J., Gardin, J. M., Flack, J. M., Gidding, S. S., Kurosaki, T. T., & Bild, D. E. (1995). Prevalence of hypertrophic cardiomyopathy in a general population of young adults. echocardiographic analysis of 4111 subjects in the CARDIA study. coronary artery risk development in (young) adults. *Circulation, 92*(4), 785-789.

Maron, B. J., Shirani, J., Poliac, L. C., Mathenge, R., Roberts, W. C., & Mueller, F. O. (1996). Sudden death in young competitive athletes. clinical, demographic, and pathological profiles. *JAMA : The Journal of the American Medical Association, 276*(3), 199-204.

Maron, M. S. (2009). The current and emerging role of cardiovascular magnetic resonance imaging in hypertrophic cardiomyopathy. *Journal of Cardiovascular Translational Research, 2*(4), 415-425. doi:10.1007/s12265-009-9136-3

Matkovich, S. J., Wang, W., Tu, Y., Eschenbacher, W. H., Dorn, L. E., Condorelli, G., .. Dorn, G. W.,2nd. (2010). MicroRNA-133a protects against myocardial fibrosis and modulates electrical repolarization without affecting hypertrophy in pressure-overloaded adult hearts. *Circulation Research, 106*(1), 166-175. doi:10.1161/CIRCRESAHA.109.202176

Menon, S. C., Eidem, B. W., Dearani, J. A., Ommen, S. R., Ackerman, M. J., & Miller, D. (2009). Diastolic dysfunction and its histopathological correlation in obstructive hypertrophic cardiomyopathy in children and adolescents. *Journal of the American Society of Echocardiography : Official Publication of the American Society of Echocardiography, 22*(12), 1327-1334. doi:10.1016/j.echo.2009.08.014

Mesaeli, N., Nakamura, K., Opas, M., & Michalak, M. (2001). Endoplasmic reticulum in the heart, a forgotten organelle? *Molecular and Cellular Biochemistry, 225*(1-), 1-6.

Miller, T., Szczesna, D., Housmans, P. R., Zhao, J., de Freitas, F., Gomes, A. V., .. Potter, J. D. (2001). Abnormal contractile function in transgenic mice expressing a familial hypertrophic cardiomyopathy-linked troponin T (I79N) mutation. *The Journal of Biological Chemistry, 276*(6), 3743-3755. doi:10.1074/jbc.M006746200

Mogensen, J., Murphy, R. T., Kubo, T., Bahl, A., Moon, J. C., Klausen, I. C., .. McKenna, W. J. (2004). Frequency and clinical expression of cardiac troponin I mutations in 748 consecutive families with hypertrophic cardiomyopathy. *Journal of the American College of Cardiology, 44*(12), 2315-2325. doi:10.1016/j.jacc.2004.05.088

Molkentin, J. D., Lu, J. R., Antos, C. L., Markham, B., Richardson, J., Robbins, J., .. Olson, E. N. (1998). A calcineurin-dependent transcriptional pathway for cardiac hypertrophy. *Cell, 93*(2), 215-228.

Molkentin, J. D., & Olson, E. N. (1997). GATA4: A novel transcriptional regulator of cardiac hypertrophy? *Circulation, 96*(11), 3833-3835.

Monserrat, L., Elliott, P. M., Gimeno, J. R., Sharma, S., Penas-Lado, M., & McKenna, W. J. (2003). Non-sustained ventricular tachycardia in hypertrophic cardiomyopathy: An independent marker of sudden death risk in young patients. *Journal of the American College of Cardiology, 42*(5), 873-879.

Moolman, J. C., Corfield, V. A., Posen, B., Ngumbela, K., Seidman, C., Brink, P. A., & Watkins, H. (1997). Sudden death due to troponin T mutations. *Journal of the American College of Cardiology, 29*(3), 549-555.

Niimura, H., Patton, K. K., McKenna, W. J., Soults, J., Maron, B. J., Seidman, J. G., & Seidman, C. E. (2002). Sarcomere protein gene mutations in hypertrophic cardiomyopathy of the elderly. *Circulation, 105*(4), 446-451.

Ostman-Smith, I., Wettrell, G., Keeton, B., Holmgren, D., Ergander, U., Gould, S., .. Verdicchio, M. (2008). Age- and gender-specific mortality rates in childhood hypertrophic cardiomyopathy. *European Heart Journal, 29*(9), 1160-1167. doi:10.1093/eurheartj/ehn122

Parmacek, M. S., & Solaro, R. J. (2004). Biology of the troponin complex in cardiac myocytes. *Progress in Cardiovascular Diseases, 47*(3), 159-176.

Pinto, J. R., Parvatiyar, M. S., Jones, M. A., Liang, J., Ackerman, M. J., & Potter, J. D. (2009). A functional and structural study of troponin C mutations related to hypertrophic cardiomyopathy. *The Journal of Biological Chemistry, 284*(28), 19090-19100. doi:10.1074/jbc.M109.007021

Pinto, J. R., Reynaldo, D. P., Parvatiyar, M. S., Dweck, D., Liang, J., Jones, M. A., .. Potter, J. D. (2011). Strong cross-bridges potentiate the ca(2+) affinity changes produced by hypertrophic cardiomyopathy cardiac troponin C mutants in myofilaments: A fast kinetic approach. *The Journal of Biological Chemistry, 286*(2), 1005-1013. doi:10.1074/jbc.M110.168583

Pogwizd, S. M., Schlotthauer, K., Li, L., Yuan, W., & Bers, D. M. (2001). Arrhythmogenesis and contractile dysfunction in heart failure: Roles of sodium-calcium exchange, inward rectifier potassium current, and residual beta-adrenergic responsiveness. *Circulation Research, 88*(11), 1159-1167.

Revera, M., van der Merwe, L., Heradien, M., Goosen, A., Corfield, V. A., Brink, P. A., & Moolman-Smook, J. C. (2008). Troponin T and beta-myosin mutations have distinct cardiac functional effects in hypertrophic cardiomyopathy patients without hypertrophy. *Cardiovascular Research, 77*(4), 687-694. doi:10.1093/cvr/cvm075

Rodriguez, J. E., McCudden, C. R., & Willis, M. S. (2009). Familial hypertrophic cardiomyopathy: Basic concepts and future molecular diagnostics. *Clinical Biochemistry*, doi:10.1016/j.clinbiochem.2009.01.020

Sanbe, A., James, J., Tuzcu, V., Nas, S., Martin, L., Gulick, J., .. Robbins, J. (2005). Transgenic rabbit model for human troponin I-based hypertrophic cardiomyopathy. *Circulation, 111*(18), 2330-2338. doi:10.1161/01.CIR.0000164234.24957.75

Schmidtmann, A., Lindow, C., Villard, S., Heuser, A., Mugge, A., Gessner, R., .. Jaquet, K. (2005). Cardiac troponin C-L29Q, related to hypertrophic cardiomyopathy, hinders the transduction of the protein kinase A dependent phosphorylation signal from cardiac troponin I to C. *The FEBS Journal, 272*(23), 6087-6097. doi:10.1111/j.1742-4658.2005.05001.x

Schroder, M., & Kaufman, R. J. (2005). The mammalian unfolded protein response. *Annual Review of Biochemistry, 74*, 739-789. doi:10.1146/annurev.biochem.73.011303.074134

Semsarian, C., Ahmad, I., Giewat, M., Georgakopoulos, D., Schmitt, J. P., McConnell, B. K., .. Seidman, J. G. (2002). The L-type calcium channel inhibitor diltiazem prevents cardiomyopathy in a mouse model. *The Journal of Clinical Investigation, 109*(8), 1013-1020. doi:10.1172/JCI14677

Solaro, R. J., & Kobayashi, T. (2011). Protein phosphorylation and signal transduction in cardiac thin filaments. *The Journal of Biological Chemistry* doi:10.1074/jbc.R110.197731

Strijack, B., Ariyarajah, V., Soni, R., Jassal, D. S., Greenberg, C. R., McGregor, R., & Morris A. (2008). Late gadolinium enhancement cardiovascular magnetic resonance in genotyped hypertrophic cardiomyopathy with normal phenotype. *Journal of Cardiovascular Magnetic Resonance : Official Journal of the Society for Cardiovascular Magnetic Resonance, 10,* 58. doi:10.1186/1532-429X-10-58

Takahashi-Yanaga, F., Morimoto, S., Harada, K., Minakami, R., Shiraishi, F., Ohta, M., . Ohtsuki, I. (2001). Functional consequences of the mutations in human cardiac troponin I gene found in familial hypertrophic cardiomyopathy. *Journal of Molecular and Cellular Cardiology, 33*(12), 2095-2107. doi:10.1006/jmcc.2001.1473

Takeda, S., Yamashita, A., Maeda, K., & Maeda, Y. (2003). Structure of the core domain of human cardiac troponin in the ca(2+)-saturated form. *Nature, 424*(6944), 35-41 doi:10.1038/nature01780

Tardiff, J. C. (2011). Thin filament mutations: Developing an integrative approach to a complex disorder. *Circulation Research, 108*(6), 765-782 doi:10.1161/CIRCRESAHA.110.224170

Tardiff, J. C., Hewett, T. E., Palmer, B. M., Olsson, C., Factor, S. M., Moore, R. L., . Leinwand, L. A. (1999). Cardiac troponin T mutations result in allele-specific phenotypes in a mouse model for hypertrophic cardiomyopathy. *The Journal of Clinical Investigation, 104*(4), 469-481. doi:10.1172/JCI6067

Teare, D. (1958). Asymmetrical hypertrophy of the heart in young adults. *British Heart Journal, 20*(1), 1-8.

Ter Keurs, H. E., Wakayama, Y., Miura, M., Shinozaki, T., Stuyvers, B. D., Boyden, P. A., & Landesberg, A. (2006). Arrhythmogenic ca(2+) release from cardiac myofilaments *Progress in Biophysics and Molecular Biology, 90*(1-3), 151-171 doi:10.1016/j.pbiomolbio.2005.07.002

Tester, D. J., & Ackerman, M. (2009). Cardiomyopathic and channelopathic causes of sudden, unexpected death in infants and children. *Annual Review of Medicine,* doi:10.1146/annurev.med.60.052907.103838

Thierfelder, L., MacRae, C., Watkins, H., Tomfohrde, J., Williams, M., McKenna, W., . Bowcock, A. (1993). A familial hypertrophic cardiomyopathy locus maps to chromosome 15q2. *Proceedings of the National Academy of Sciences of the United States of America, 90*(13), 6270-6274.

Thierfelder, L., Watkins, H., MacRae, C., Lamas, R., McKenna, W., Vosberg, H. P., .. Seidman, C. E. (1994). Alpha-tropomyosin and cardiac troponin T mutations cause familial hypertrophic cardiomyopathy: A disease of the sarcomere. *Cell, 77*(5), 701- 712.

Tobacman, L. S. (1996). Thin filament-mediated regulation of cardiac contraction. *Annual Review of Physiology, 58,* 447-481. doi:10.1146/annurev.ph.58.030196.002311

Tsoutsman, T., Chung, J., Doolan, A., Nguyen, L., Williams, I. A., Tu, E., .. Semsarian, C. (2006). Molecular insights from a novel cardiac troponin I mouse model of familial hypertrophic cardiomyopathy. *Journal of Molecular and Cellular Cardiology, 41*(4), 623-632. doi:10.1016/j.yjmcc.2006.07.016

Van Der Spoel, D., Lindahl, E., Hess, B., Groenhof, G., Mark, A. E., & Berendsen, H. J. (2005). GROMACS: Fast, flexible, and free. *Journal of Computational Chemistry, 26*(16), 1701-1718. doi:10.1002/jcc.20291

Van Driest, S. L., Ellsworth, E. G., Ommen, S. R., Tajik, A. J., Gersh, B. J., & Ackerman, M. J. (2003). Prevalence and spectrum of thin filament mutations in an outpatient referral population with hypertrophic cardiomyopathy. *Circulation, 108*(4), 445-451. doi:10.1161/01.CIR.0000080896.52003.DF

Van Driest, S. L., Vasile, V. C., Ommen, S. R., Will, M. L., Tajik, A. J., Gersh, B. J., & Ackerman, M. J. (2004). Myosin binding protein C mutations and compound heterozygosity in hypertrophic cardiomyopathy. *Journal of the American College of Cardiology, 44*(9), 1903-1910. doi:10.1016/j.jacc.2004.07.045

van Rooij, E., Sutherland, L. B., Liu, N., Williams, A. H., McAnally, J., Gerard, R. D., .Olson, E. N. (2006). A signature pattern of stress-responsive microRNAs that can evoke cardiac hypertrophy and heart failure. *Proceedings of the National Academy of Sciences of the United States of America, 103*(48), 18255-18260. doi:10.1073/pnas. 0608791103

Varnava, A. M., Elliott, P. M., Baboonian, C., Davison, F., Davies, M. J., & McKenna, W. J. (2001). Hypertrophic cardiomyopathy: Histopathological features of sudden death in cardiac troponin T disease. *Circulation, 104*(12), 1380-1384.

Varnava, A. M., Elliott, P. M., Mahon, N., Davies, M. J., & McKenna, W. J. (2001). Relation between myocyte disarray and outcome in hypertrophic cardiomyopathy. *The American Journal of Cardiology, 88*(3), 275-279.

Wang, Y., Shen, J., Arenzana, N., Tirasophon, W., Kaufman, R. J., & Prywes, R. (2000). Activation of ATF6 and an ATF6 DNA binding site by the endoplasmic reticulum stress response. *The Journal of Biological Chemistry, 275*(35), 27013-27020. doi:10.1074/jbc.M003322200

Watkins, H., McKenna, W. J., Thierfelder, L., Suk, H. J., Anan, R., O'Donoghue, A., Seidman, J. G. (1995). Mutations in the genes for cardiac troponin T and alpha-tropomyosin in hypertrophic cardiomyopathy. *The New England Journal of Medicine, 332*(16), 1058-1064. doi:10.1056/NEJM199504203321603

Wetzel, G. T., & Klitzner, T. S. (1996). Developmental cardiac electrophysiology recent advances in cellular physiology. *Cardiovascular Research, 31 Spec No*, E52-60.

Wheeler, M., Pavlovic, A., DeGoma, E., Salisbury, H., Brown, C., & Ashley, E. A. (2009). A new era in clinical genetic testing for hypertrophic cardiomyopathy. *Journal of Cardiovascular Translational Research, 2*(4), 381-391. doi:10.1007/s12265-009-9139-0

Willinger, M., James, L. S., & Catz, C. (1991). Defining the sudden infant death syndrome (SIDS): Deliberations of an expert panel convened by the national institute of child health and human development. *Pediatric Pathology / Affiliated with the International Paediatric Pathology Association, 11*(5), 677-684. doi:10.3109/15513819109065465

Willott, R. H., Gomes, A. V., Chang, A. N., Parvatiyar, M. S., Pinto, J. R., & Potter, J. D. (2010). Mutations in troponin that cause HCM, DCM AND RCM: What can we learn about thin filament function? *Journal of Molecular and Cellular Cardiology, 48*(5), 882-892. doi:10.1016/j.yjmcc.2009.10.031

Wolf, C. M., Moskowitz, I. P., Arno, S., Branco, D. M., Semsarian, C., Bernstein, S. A., Seidman, J. G. (2005). Somatic events modify hypertrophic cardiomyopathy pathology and link hypertrophy to arrhythmia. *Proceedings of the National Academy of Sciences of the United States of America, 102*(50), 18123-18128. doi:10.1073/pnas.0509145102

Yang, B., Lin, H., Xiao, J., Lu, Y., Luo, X., Li, B., Wang, Z. (2007). The muscle-specific microRNA miR-1 regulates cardiac arrhythmogenic potential by targeting GJA1 and KCNJ2. *Nature Medicine, 13*(4), 486-491. doi:10.1038/nm1569

Zhao, Y., Ransom, J. F., Li, A., Vedpantham, V., von Drehle, M., Muth, A. N., Srivastava, D. (2007). Dysregulation of cardiogenesis, cardiac conduction, and cell cycle in mice lacking miRNA-1-2. *Cell, 129*(2), 303-317. doi:10.1016/j.cell.2007.03.030

7

Consequences of Mutations in Genes Encoding Cardiac Troponin C, T and I – Molecular Insights

Kornelia Jaquet and Andreas Mügge

Molecular Cardiology & Clinic of Cardiology, St. Josef-Hospital & Bergmannsheil,
University Hospitals of the Ruhr-University of Bochum,
Germany

1. Introduction

Cardiac troponin is the main regulatory protein of the thin filament and mediates the Ca^{2+}-sensitivity of the actin-myosin interaction. Troponin forms a heterotrimeric complex composed of the tropomyosin binding subunit (cTnT), the inhibitory subunit (cTnI) and the Ca^{2+}-binding subunit (cTnC). A complex interplay between the cardiac troponin subunits and other thin filament proteins, as tropomyosin (Tm) and actin, is essential to regulate muscle contraction, which can be described by cross bridge cycling on the molecular level. Troponin is located on both sides of the thin filament with a stagger of about 27 Angstroms between two adjacent troponin molecules (Ebashi, 1972; Paul et al., 2009). In the thin filament each troponin binds to one tropomyosin, which covers 7 actin monomers. It is no surprise that mutations in genes encoding proteins, which participate in crossbridge cycling and its regulation, derange interactions and lead to contractile dysfunction and disease. In all three cardiac troponin subunits, changes in amino acid sequence have been identified in families with hypertrophic (HCM), restrictive (RCM) and dilated cardiomyopathy (DCM). Therefore knowledge of structure, function and interactions of the proteins is a prerequisite to understand dysfunction in disease.

1.1 Cardiac troponin T (cTnT)

One of the main tasks of cardiac troponin T (30-35kDa) is to fix the troponin complex to the thin filament. Furthermore cTnT participates in conferring calcium sensitivity to actin/myosin (Tobacman, 1988). Tobacman also showed that the N-terminal half of cTnT, TnT1 (amino acids 1-158, skeletal muscle numbering), was able to keep the thin filament in the blocked state without TnI. In the blocked state of the thin filament no interaction between actin and myosin is possible, i.e. no force production occurs. Thus cTnT plays an active role in inhibition of actin/myosin interaction in the resting state. It further promotes tropomyosin polymerization and binding of tropomyosin to actin.

Structural information on cTnT is poor. According to EM analysis of thin filaments and low resolution co-crystallization of Tm in complex with cTnT, cTnT is highly asymmetric. It is a 180-202 nm long comma –shaped molecule, with the N-terminal rod like part arranged along the thin filament and a C-terminal more globular domain (Ohtsuki, 1979, Flicker et al., 1982, White et al., 1987). The high resolution crystal structure available for the core troponin complex contains only the less flexible C-terminal part of cTnT, which binds the other two troponin subunits, cTnI and cTnC (Takeda et al., 2003). There is strong evidence from latest single particle reconstruction studies of the thin filament by Paul et al., (2009), that the N-terminal tail of cTnT points to the M-band of the sarcomere, whereas the core domain of the troponin complex is oriented versus the Z-band.

The N-terminal tail fraction of cTnT contains a hypervariable N-terminal part and a highly conserved region, which is located in the central region of the cTnT molecule (Fig. 1). This conserved region contains the main interaction site for tropomyosin (Biesiadecki et al., 2007, Perry, 1998) comprising 39 amino acids (residues 98-136 (human cardiac sequence)) (Jin & Chong, 2010). The Tm interaction site forms a helix according to Murakami et al., (2008) and binds to the overlapping region of two tropomyosin molecules (Jin & Chong, 2010). Crystal structure of the tropomyosin overlap region and the Tm binding helix reveals the formation of a four helix bundle between tropomyosin ends and cTnT (Murakami et al., 2008). The hypervariable region of the cTnT tail fraction does not bind to tropomyosin and can be truncated without losing binding ability of the rest of the molecule (Zhang et al., 2006). Phylogenetically the hypervariable region might be added to the conserved core region of cTnT (Conserved tail region and C-terminal domain) (Jin & Samanez, 2001; Biesiadecki et al., 2007). Its function is not completely elucidated, but the hypervariable region may play a role as modulator of the core molecule thus subtly affecting binding affinities of Tm and cTnT (Biesiadecki et al, 2007; Feng et al., 2008).

A second interaction site for tropomyosin is located at the beginning of the C-terminal half of cTnT and has lately been analysed by Jin & Chong (2010) using antibodies. They showed that highly conserved amino acid sequences are involved comprising amino acid residues 197-236 (human sequence). This interaction site binds to the middle part of tropomyosin near Cys190. Earlier studies (Pearlstone et al., 1983; Morris & Lehrer, 1984) propose the second interaction with tropomyosin at the very C-terminus of cTnT involving residues 272-288. Whichever amino acids are included in the cTnT/Tm interactions, in the presence of cTnC binding of the TnT-C-Terminus to tropomyosin near Cys190 is Ca^{2+} dependent (Chong & Hodges, 1982). Ca^{2+} weakens its binding to tropomyosin though the molecular mechanism, i.e. conformational changes which lead to alteration in Tm/TnT -binding, is not known yet. The TnT-C-Terminus also contains the binding site for the other two troponin subunits, TnI and TnC. According to the 3 D structure of the core cardiac troponin complex, the helix in the C-terminal region of cTnT (residues 226-271), which is highly conserved (Jin et al., 2008) forms a rigid coiled coil with a cTnI-helix (residues 90-136) and is part of a rigid structure within the troponin complex, called the IT-arm (Takeda et al., 2003). At the C-terminal end of the coiled coil the interaction site for cTnC is located and comprises amino acid residues 256- 270. The organisation of cTnT is summarized in Fig.1.

In cardiac muscle the mammalian cTnT- gene (TNNT2) is composed of 17 exons. Exon 5 is absent in adult cTnT (Cooper & Ordahl, 1985). Exon 5 encodes a 10 amino acid long region within the hypervariable N-terminus of cTnT. This sequence contains several acidic residues and contributes to a more negatively charged cTnT. Such a charge difference may modulate function. Indeed fetal cTnT, which contains exon 5, exhibits a higher Ca^{2+}-sensitivity compared to adult cTnT and shows a higher tolerance towards acidic pH (Gomes et al., 2002). Mainly 4 variants of human cTnT ($cTnT_{1-4}$) have been described due to alternative splicing of exons 4 and 5, whereby TnT_1 and TnT_3 are the major isoforms present in fetal and in the adult human cardiac muscle, respectively (Townsend et al., 1995; Anderson et al., 1991). The expression pattern of cTnT isoforms seems to be altered in heart failure and correlates with changes in Ca^{2+}- sensitivity. The modification in Ca^{2+}- sensitivity however, seems not to be caused by an lteration in the isoform expression pattern. Differences in the phosphorylation status of arcomeric proteins, especially of myosin light chain 2 (MLC-2) may be decisive (van der /elden et al., 2003). Also cTnT itself is a phospho protein (Fig. 1) which is constitutively •hosphorylated at Ser1 in several species inclusive men due to the action of casein kinase- 2 Gusev et al., 1980; Risnik & Gusev, 1984, Swiderek et al., 1990). The function of this •hosphorylation is not known up to date. It might prevent degradation and/or interaction of he hypervariable region. At least one further reversible phosphorylation site for PKC is ocated in the C-terminal region of cTnT near the second Ca^{2+}- dependent interaction site for ˉm and thus may affect Ca^{2+}- sensitivity of the actin/myosin interaction. Indeed, according to •umandea et al., reversible phosphorylation of Thr206 (mouse sequence) is critical for function Sumandea et al., 2003). In vitro experiments showed that phosphorylation by PKCα decreases naximal tension, myofilament Ca^{2+} -sensitivity, actomyosin ATPase activity and cooperativity Sumandea et al., 2003). Other protein kinases than PKC, as for example ROCKII (Vahebi et al., !005), phosphorylate cTnT in vitro. The physiological role of cTnT phosphorylation by lifferent protein kinases is not yet clarified. cTnT, however, is not a target of cAMP dependent ›rotein kinase (PKA), which is activated upon ß-adrenergic stimulation. But as recently lescribed by Sumandea et al., (2011) cTnT forms an AKAP for PKA with either regulatory •ubunit I or II (PKA-RI, PKA-RII) and thus provides a platform for sarcomeric protein ›hosphorylation upon ß-adrenergic stimulation. Binding of PKA might occur within the ımino acid region 202-226 which forms an amphiphilic helix needed for the docking of PKA ₹I and − II (Feliciello et al., 2001). The interaction site for PKA-R would then be located just ˥ear the second interaction site with tropomyosin described by (Jin & Chong, 2010) and the ʾKC phosphorylation site. This implies that PKA-R binding might be affected by PKC ›hosphorylation and vice versa.

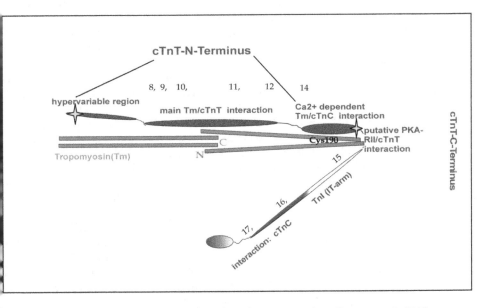

Fig. 1. Organisation , interaction and phosphorylation sites of cardiac troponin T. Exons ⟨nown to contain cardiomyopathy mutations are indicated by numbers

1.2 Cardiac troponin C (cTnC)

cTnC is the calcium binding subunit of the cardiac troponin complex. Structurally the protein belongs to the EF-hand calcium binding protein super family together with parvalbumin, the first described protein of this family, Calmodulin, skeletal muscle troponin C etc. cTnC is composed of two lobes connected by a flexible linker (Sia et al., 1997) (Fig.2).

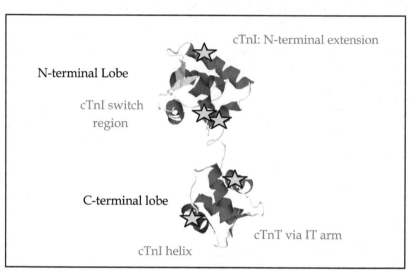

Fig. 2. Interaction sites and cardiomyopathy inducing single amino acid exchanges in cTnC

The structure was taken from PDP 1AJ4 based on the work of (Sia et al., 1997). The 3 D structure of cTnC in calcium (green points) saturated from is shown. Helices are given as magenta ribbons. The position of cardiomyopathy mutations is indicated by stars. Interacting proteins are given in blue.

Each lobe contains two parallel EF hands, each of which forms the helix-loop-helix divalent metal binding domain. Helices in a protein have been labeled by capital letters, with A assigned to the most N-terminally located helix. Thus E and F are the loop flanking helices in parvalbumin forming the metal binding motif. The name EF-hand for the helix loop helix metal binding motif is based on this nomenclature. The short helices of about 10-12 residues are arranged perpendicular. The loop is composed of 12 residues essential for calcium coordination in a pentagonal bipyramidal configuration. The residues 1, 3, 5, 7, 9 and 12 (X, Y, Z, -Y, -X, -Z) are involved in Ca^{2+}-coordination. In position 12 there is a conserved glutamate or aspartate residue providing two oxygens for calcium binding (Structure Reference: PDB: 2PMY). The calcium binding residues preferentially have an acidic side chain, but also the protein backbone is involved. In cTnC the two EF hands (III, IV) in the C-terminal lobe are the high affinity Ca^{2+}-, Mg^{2+}-binding sites, which contain metal ions also at low (relaxing) intracellular Ca^{2+}-concentration. This C-terminal domain of cTnC provides the platform for binding of cTnI and of cTnT and therefore is pivotal for the integrity of the troponin complex. Helices of the metal bound C-terminal domain exhibit a hydrophobic pocket, where cTnI is bound (Gasmi-Seabrook et al., 1999). cTnT binds to Calcium sites III and IV at the end of the rigid coiled coil. Besides the structural role of the C-terminal lobe, there is now strong evidence that it plays an active part in thin filament activation (Fuchs &

Grabarek, 2011). Alteration in Ca^{2+}-/Mg^{2+}-binding to sites III and IV might alter the interaction with cTnT and the coiled coil structure. Also the identification of cardiomyopathy causing alterations in this part of cTnC points to the involvement in regulation.

The N-terminal EF-hand I is not able to bind Ca^{2+} due to an insertion of Val and the replacement of two Asp residues involved in Ca^{2+}-coordination by Ala and Leu residues. Therefore there is only one functional active Ca^{2+}-binding site (site II) in the N-terminal domain of cTnC, which is a high affinity Ca^{2+}-specific binding site. Binding and release kinetics of Ca^{2+} to cTnC within the thin filament are such that Ca^{2+}-binding and release occurs within one contraction cycle (Davis & Tikunova, 2008). Saturation of cTnC with Ca^{2+} is obtained upon increase in intracellular Ca^{2+}-concentration after influx from sarcoplasmatic Ca^{2+}-store upon membrane depolarization. Therefore site II is named the regulatory Ca^{2+}-binding site. Due to the non functional site I there is no conformational switch from closed to open solely upon Ca^{2+}-binding as is observed for skeletal muscle TnC and the C-terminal lobe of cTnC (Sia et al., 1997). For the stabilization of the open conformation of the N-terminal lobe cTnI binding is required (Dong et al., 1999; Li et al., 1999). There exist multiple interaction sites for cTnI throughout the complete cTnC molecule. The amphiphilic part of helix 1 in cTnI (residues 43-65) binds via several polar and van der Waals interaction to the C-terminal cTnC lobe and around residue 10 of the N-terminal helix of cTnC. Furthermore residues 93-161 in the C-terminal lobe of cTnC interact with the IT-arm (Takeda et al., 2003), The N-terminal lobe of cTnC forms the Ca^{2+}-dependent binding site for the cTnI switch region (Takeda et al., 2003) and a phosphorylation dependent binding site near the nonfunctional Ca^{2+}-binding loop with the flexible heart specific N-terminal cTnI extension (see below) (Schmidtmann et al., 2005).

1.3 Cardiac troponin I (cTnI)

cTnI, the inhibitory subunit of the troponin complex is a very flexible molecule consisting of helices and random coils. In solution cTnI exhibits no tertiary structure. A specific spatial orientation is only obtained within the ternary troponin complex. cTnI is build up in a modular fashion (Fig. 3).

1.3.1 The N-terminal extension

The N-terminal extension of about 31 amino acids (length is dependent on species) is heart specific and resembles the hypervaraible region of cTnT. It contains conserved amino acid stretches; thus at the very N-terminus there is a acidic region (Sadayappan et al., 2008) followed by a proline rich sequence, which forms a polyprolin helix and functions as a rigid spacer to keep the N-terminus extended (Howarth et al., 2007). Then the phosphorylation region follows, which contains two adjacent located serine residues at position 22 and 23 (numbered without starter methionine). Both residues are substrates for PKA (Swiderek et al., 1990; Mittmann et al., 1990). In its dephosphorylated state the N-terminal cTnI arm interacts between residues 10-30 with cTnC around amino acid residue 29 (Fig. 2) (Finley et al., 1999; Gaponenko et al., 1999; Abbott et al., 2000; Ward et al.,2003, 2004; Schmidtmann et al., 2002, 2005). This interaction also seems to stabilize the open conformation of the cTnC-N-terminal lobe (Abbott et al., 2000, 2001; Ward et al., 2004). Bisphosphorylation of the two serine residues 22 and 23 by PKA upon ß- adrenergic stimulation releases the interaction with cTnC. According to Howarth et al, (2007) the bisphosphorylated arm contains a helix comprising amino acids 21-30 being stabilized by salt bridges between phosphate and preceeding arginine residues (Jaquet et al. 1998). The release of the extension from cTnC takes place due to the insertion of negative charges followed by conformational changes. This allows a different interaction, which is directed by the acidic part of the N-terminal cTnI arm and therefore needs a positively charged partner (Sadayappan et al., 2008). Clusters of basic amino acid residues are provided by the regulatory C-terminal domain of cTnI itself, but also an additional interaction with actin cannot be excluded. The release of the N-terminal arm from cTnC leads to a reduction of the Ca^{2+} -affinity of cTnC, in myofilament Ca^{2+}-sensitivity (Zhang et al 1995; Reiffert et al., 1996) and to enhanced cross bridge cycling (Kentish et al.,2001; Turnbull et al., 2002). There is evidence that the main action occurs via interaction with cTnI, which stabilizes cTnI binding to the thin filament (Sakthivel et al., 2005).

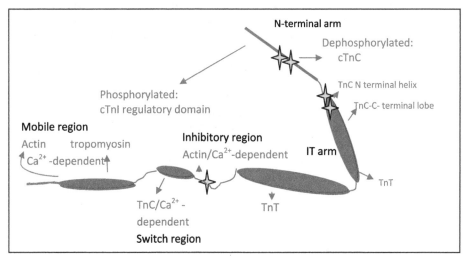

Fig. 3. Organization of cTnI, its interactions (blue) and phosphorylation sites (indicated by ✦)

1.3.2 Constitutive cTnC and cTnT binding sites

The cTnC binding site is located subsequent to the N-terminal extension. It forms a helix (helix 1 according to the nomenclature of Takeda et al., 2003) which contacts the N-terminal cTnC helix and reaches to the C-terminal lobe of cTnC. It strongly binds to the hydrophobic pocket of the C-terminal cTnC lobe. The C-terminal part of helix 1 also interacts with cTnT via several hydrogen bonds and hydrophobic interactions. This helix is followed by another helical binding site for cTnT (helix 2). Helix 2 forms a coiled coil with a helix located in the C-terminal half of cTnT. The two helices are part of the IT arm (Takeda et al., 2003). Both these binding sites in cTnI are independent on reversible Ca^{2+} -binding to the regulatory Ca^{2+} binding loop in cTnC. In helix 1 there are two serine residues (Ser43/45) which are phosphorylated by PKC upon alpha adrenergic stimulation. Ser43/45 are positioned near residue 10 of the N-terminal helix in cTnC-N-terminal lobe as well as near the C-terminal lobe. Thus, phosphorylation might alter these interactions. In mice phosphorylation of these sites by PKC upon α-adrenergic stimulation is responsible for the negative inotropic effect and might be influenced by the cTnT phosphorylation state. The physiological effect of PKA dependent phosphorylation at Ser22/23 seems not to be impaired by Ser43/45 phosphorylation (Montgomery et al., 2002).

1.3.3 Regulatory C-terminal region

The C-terminal region of cTnI can functionally be subdivided into the inhibitory region comprising amino acids 137-148, the helical switch region (amino acids 150-159) and the C-terminal mobile region. The inhibitory region binds to actin/tropomyosin in the relaxed state, i.e. when the regulatory Ca^{2+} binding loop of cTnC contains no Ca^{2+}. Within this region there is another heart specific PKC phosphorylation site at Thr 144. The physiological role of this phosphorylation site is not quite clear (Solaro & Kobayashi, 2011), though investigations by Tachampa et al., (2007) imply that Thr144 is involved in length dependent activation of tension development in thin filament bundles. Phosphorylation might modulate this function probably by loosening the interaction of cTnI inhibitory region with actin. Upon Ca^{2+}- saturation of cTnC the inhibitory region is released from actin and the switch region binds to the cTnC-N-terminal lobe inducing the formation of the hydrophic pocket. Strength of interaction is sensible to small conformational changes in the cTnC-N-lobe also affecting Ca^{2+}-binding affinity. The C-terminal mobile region following the switch region is a very important cTnI region for regulation of muscle contraction, though not much is known about this region. It provides a second actin binding site and a tropomyosin binding site. Under relaxing conditions, this mobile region is fixed to tropomyosin (Pirani et al., 2005; Galinska et al., et al., 2008) and actin, and is released from actin/tropomyosin upon Ca^{2+}-saturation of cTnC. Thus the C-Terminus stabilizes the blocked state of the thin filament (Galinska et al., 2010). Probably this effect is intensified by the interaction of cTnT binding to tropomyosin actin. Thus cTnT- N-terminus and cTnI-C-terminus both support the inhibitory region of cTnI in keeping tropomyosin in the blocking position. Hereby troponin complexes on opposite sites cooperate, one complex providing cTnT/tropomyosin interaction the other cTnI/tropomyosin/actin interaction (Paul et al., 2009; Solaro & Kobayashi, 2011). But cardiac TnI is not only involved in regulation of inhibition, but also of activation. Evidence came from investigations of Galinska et al., (2010) using truncated cTnI and normal length cTnI. They showed that the C-terminus is also involved in stabilization of tropomyosin in the active state (Ca^{2+} - saturated cTnC). Truncation may occur *in vivo* due to proteolysis in myocardial stunning (reversible ischemia/reperfusion injury) (Foster et al., 2003) and due to cardiomyopathy mutations.

2. Cardiomyopathy inducing troponin mutations

A large number of mutations have been detected in genes encoding for the three cTn subunits in patients suffering of cardiomyopathies (tables 1-6). Resulting phenotypes are highly variable, even within a family carrying the same mutation (see below), indicating that modifiers, environment or polymorphisms are involved in disease development. Wang et al., (2005) was the first group who detected a polymorphism in the MYBPC3 (cardiac myosin binding protein C gene) that might be able to modify the expression of hypertrophy. Also combinations of more than one mutation determine the disease development. Therefore it is still impossible to correlate phenotype and genotype, though an immense progress has been made in the understanding of molecular pathogenesis. The goal to understand phenotype development remains. Since the disease is primarily caused by mutations, it is crucial to improve knowledge on the dysfunctions on molecular level in detail of as many mutants as possible. Thus one might be able to detect common features and mechanisms which might allow detection of a link to phenotype development. Though the molecular effects of only a couple of mutations have been thoroughly investigated a first common rule, namely an enhancement in Ca^{2+}- sensitivity of the myofilament for HCM/RCM-mutants and a decrease in Ca^{2+}- sensitivity for DCM mutants has been stated by Robinson et al., (2007). However it seems to be too simple and does not explain the development of HCM or RCM or the often very low degree of hypertrophy despite large Ca2+ sensitivity changes and susceptibility to malignant arrhythmia. Furthermore, the rule does not apply to all mutations investigated. One problem is that analysis of Ca^{2+} - sensitivity resulted in many opposing statements. Thus for example Nakaura et al., 1999 did not observe enhanced Ca^{2+} -sensitivity of force in skinned fibres with cTnT-F110I, whereas Hernandez et al., 2005 described enhanced Ca^{2+} -sensitivity of force development as well as of actomyosin ATPase activity. One main reason lies in the complexity of the systems used, as reconstituted proteins, skinned fibers, myofibrils, isolated cardiomyocytes (adult or neonatal), transgenic animals. In general results obtained with higher organised system sseem to be more reliable. But additionally species differences might account for differing results. For example according to Rust et al., (1999) overexpression of cTnT-I79N in rat cardiomyocytes resulted in suppressed contractile performance, whereas others using mice myofibrils suggested hypercontractility.

2.1 Mutations in TNNT2, the gene encoding cTnT

Most mutations in TNNT2 detected in patients lead to familial hypertrophic cardiomyopathy (HCM), only a few to restricted cardiomyopathy (RCM) or dilated hypertrophic cardiomyopathy (DCM) (Table 1). Families with DCM mutations in TNNT2 mostly exhibit a severe disease progression with poor prognosis.

2.1.1 HCM inducing mutations

HCM-mutations in TNNT2 are found in about 10% of the HCM cases, and thus TNNT2 belongs to the more abundant troponin disease genes. There is no known HCM mutation which is located within the hypervariable N-terminal region of cTnT. All mutations identified in patients suffering from HCM are located either near or within the N-terminal main interaction site for tropomyosin (amino acids 79-182) or within the C-terminal half (amino acids 203-288) which contains multiple interaction and putative phosphorylation sites (Table 1; Fig. 1). This distribution of mutations implies that they affect the interaction either with tropomyosin (Tm) and/ or the other troponin subunits and might influence phosphorylation dependent effects. The majority of gene loci, where mutations have been identified in patients encode the N-terminal region of cTnT interacting with the overlap of Tm (Table 1; Fig. 1). Mutations in the Tm binding region of cTnT (amino acids 92-183) destabilize Tm binding to actin filaments (Palm et al., 2001). Mutations within the main Tm binding site further weaken the end-to-end Tm interaction, which is responsible for the cooperativity (Palm et al., 2001). Also a lowered affinity of troponin to actin/Tm could be expected. Indeed cTnT-F110I, located at the C-terminal end of the main Tm binding region, impairs binding of troponin to actin/Tm by altering the dynamic properties of the tail region (Hinkle & Tobacman, 2002). It reduces its flexibility. Flexibility of the cTnT-tail is an important feature for its interaction with Tm overlap region (Hinkle & Tobacman, 2002).

Mutation	Disease	Exon/Intron	Reference
Phe70Leu (F70L)	HCM	8	Richard et al., (2003) Circ. 107: 2227-32
Pro77Leu (P77L)	HCM	8	Varnava et al., (2001) Circ. 104: 1380-4
Ile79Asn (I79N)	HCM , RCM, DCM	8	Thierfelder et al., (1994) Cell 77:701-12; Watkins et al., (1995) NEJM. 332: 1058-64; Rust et al., (1999) JCI. 104: 1459-67; Yanaga et al., JBC. (1999) 74:8806-12; Varnava et al., (2001) Circ. 104: 1380-4 ; Palm et al., (2001) Biophys J. 81: 827-37 ; Westermann et al., (2006) Eur J Heart Fail. 8:115-21 ; Menon et al., (2008) Clin Genet, 74(5): 445-54 ; Baudenbacher et al.,(2008) JCI. 118 :3893-903 ; Midde et al., (2011) JMCC [Epub ahead of print]
Glu83Lys (E83K)	HCM	8	Mogensen et al., (2003) J Med Genet 40: e59
Val85Leu (V85L)	HCM	8	Konno et al., (2005) J Intern Med. 258: 216-24.
Asp86Ala (D86A)	HCM	8	Van Driest et al., (2003) Circ. 108: 445-51
Arg92Trp (R92W)	HCM	9	Moolman et al., (1997) JACC. 29: 549-55; Moolman-Smook et al., (1999) Am J Hum Genet. 65:1308-20; Fujino et al., (2001) Clin Cardiol. 24: 397-402; Varnava et al., (2001) Circ. 104:1380-4; Palm et al., (2001) Biophys J. 81:2827-37; Waldmuller et al., Hum Mutat (2002) 19:560-9; Ackerman et al., (2002) JACC. 39: 2042-8; Van Driest et al., (2003) Circ. 108: 445-51; Shimizu et al., (2003) Clin Cardiol 26: 536-9; Konno et al., (2005) J Intern Med. 258:216-24
Arg92Leu (R92L)	HCM	9	Forissier et al., (1996) Circ. 94: 3069-73 ; Varnava et al., (2001) Circ. 104: 1380-4 ; Palm et al., (2001) Biophys J. 81:2827-37 ; Richard et al., (2003) Circ. 107: 2227-32
Arg92Gln (R92Q)	HCM	9	Thierfelder et al., (1994) Cell 77:701-12; Watkins et al., (1995) NEJM. 332:1058-64; Yanaga et al., (1999) JBC. 274: 8806-12; Palm et al., (2001) Biophys J. 81:2827-37 ; Cuda et al., (2002) Hum Mutat 19:309-10; Robinson et al., (2002) JBC. 277: 40710-6; Hinkle & Tobacman (2003)JBC. 278: 506-13; Javadpour et al., (2003) JCI. 112: 768-75; Torricelli et al., (2003) Am J Cardiol 92:1358-62; Van Driest et al., (2004) JACC. 44: 1903-10
Arg94Leu (R94L)	HCM	9	Varnava et al., (1999) Heart 82: 621-4; Varnava et al., (2001) Circ. 104:1380-4 ; Palm et al., (2001) Biophys J. 81:2827-37
Arg94Cys (R94C)	HCM	9	Mogensen et al., (2003) J Med Genet. 40: e59
Lys97Asn (K97N)	HCM	9	Barr, Seidman et al., (2001) originally posted on URL: http://www.cardiogenomics.org
Ala104Val (A104V)	HCM	9	Nakajima-Taniguchi et al., (1997) JMCC. 29: 839-43; Palm et al., (2001) Biophys J. 81: 2827-37 ; Hinkle & Tobacman (2003) JBC. 278: 506-13.

Mutation	Disease	Exon/Intron	Reference
Phe110Ile (F110I)	HCM	9	Watkins et al., (1995) NEJM. 332: 1058-64; Anan et al., (1998) Circ. 98: 391-7; Yanaga et al., (1999) JBC. 274: 8806-12; Lin et al., (2000) Cardiol. 93:155-62 ; Palm et al., (2001) Biophys J. 81: 2827-37 ; Hinkle & Tobacman (2003) JBC. 278: 506-13; Konno et al., (2005) J Intern Med. 258: 216-24; Hernandez et al., (2005) JBC. 280: 37183-94
Phe110Leu (F110L)	HCM	9	Torricelli et al., (2003) Am J Cardiol. 92: 1358-62
Phe110Val (F110V)	HCM	9	Richard et al., (2003) Circ. 107: 2227-32 ; Torricelli F et al., (2003) Am J Cardiol. 92: 1358-62
Lys124Asn (K124N)	HCM	9	An et al., (2004) Zhonghua Xue Za Zhi 84:1 340-3
Arg130Cys (R130C)	HCM	10	Torricelli et al., (2003) Am J Cardiol. 92: 1358-62 ; Song et al., (2005) Clin Chim Acta 351: 209-16
Glu163Lys (E163K)	HCM	11	Watkins et al., (1995) NEJM. 332: 1058-64; Palm et al., (2001) Biophys J. 81: 2827-37
Glu160del (ΔE160)	HCM	11	Watkins et al., (1995) NEJM. 332: 1058-64; Palm et al., (2001)Biophys J. 81: 2827-37 ; Richard et al., (2003) Circ. 107: 2227-32 ; Mogensen et al., (2003) J Med Genet. 40:e59; Torricelli et al., (2003) Am J Cardiol. 92:1358-62; Capek & Skvor (2006) Meth Inf Med. 45: 169-72
Ser179Phe (S179F)	HCM	11	Ho et al., (2000) Circ. 102:1950-5
Glu244Asp (E244D)	HCM	14	Watkins et al., (1995) NEJM. 332: 1058-64; Yanaga et al., (1999) JBC. 274: 8806-12; Moore, Seidman et al., (2004) URL: http://www.cardiogenomics.org
Lys247Arg (K247R)	HCM	14	Garcia-Castro et al., (2003) Clin Chem. 49: 1279-85
Asn271Ile (N271I)	HCM	15	Richard (2003) Circ. 107:2227-32
Lys273Glu (K273E)	HCM	15	Fujino et al., (2002) Am J Cardiol. 89:29-33; Venkatraman et al., (2003) JBC 278: 41670-6; Konno et al., (2005) J Intern Med. 258: 216-24
IVS15+1G>A	HCM	15	Thierfelder et al., (1994) Cell 77: 701-12; Watkins et al., (1995) NEJM. 332: 1058-64; Watkins et al., (1996) JCI. 98: 2456-61. ; Mukherjea et al., (1999) Biochem. 38: 13296-301; Redwood et al., (2000) Circ Res. 86: 1146-52; Varnava et al., (2001) Circ. 104: 1380-4

Mutation	Disease	Exon/Intron	Reference
Arg278Cys (R278C)	HCM	16	Watkins et al., (1995) NEJM. 332:1058-64; Yanaga et al., (1999) JBC. 274:806-12; Elliott et al., (1999) NEJM. 341: 1855-6; Barr, Seidman et al., 2002 and Moore, Seidman et al., (2003, 2004) URL:http://www. cardiogenomics.org; Van Driest et al., (2003) Circ. 108: 445-51; Garcia-Castro et al., (2003) Clin Chem 49: 1279-85; Garcia-Castro et al., (2003) Rev Esp Cardiol. 56: 1022-5; Torricelli (2003) Am J Cardiol 92: 1358-62; Theopistou et al., (2004) Am J Cardiol 94: 246-9; Miliou et al., (2005) Heart 91: 966-7; Hernandez et al., (2005) JBC. 280:371 83-94; Ingles et al., . (2005) J Med Genet. 42:e59, Sirenko et al., (2006) J Physiol. 5755.1: 201-13
Arg278Pro (R278P)	HCM	16	Erdmann et al., 1998. (on-line); Van Driest et al., (2003) Circ. 108: 445-51; Miliou et al., (2005) Heart 91: 966-7
Arg286Cys (R286C)	HCM	16	Richard et al., (2003) Circ. 107: 2227-32 ; Miliou et al., (2005) Heart 91: 966-7
Arg286His (R286H)	HCM	16	Van Driest et al., (2003) Circ. 108: 445-51 ; Van Driest et al., (2004) JACC. 44: 1903-10
Trp287ter (W287ter)	HCM	16	Richard et al., (2003) Circ. 107: 2227-32.
Arg113Trp (R113W)	DCM	9	Mogensen et al., (2004) JACC. 44: 2033-40 ; Mirza et al., (2005) JBC. 280 :28498-506
Arg141Trp (R141W)	DCM	10	Li et al., (2001) Circ. 104:2188-93 ; Venkatraman et al., (2003) JBC. 278: 41670-6 ; Villard et al., (2005) EHJ. 26: 794-803 ; Mirza et al., (2005) JBC. 280 :28498-506
Ala172Ser (A172S)	DCM	11	Stefanelli et al., (2004) Mol Genet Metab. 83: 188-96
Arg205Leu (R205L)	DCM	13	Mogensen et al., (2004) JACC 44: 2033-40; Mirza et al., (2005) JBC. 280 :28498-506
Lys210del (ΔK210)	DCM	13	Kamisago et al., (2000) NEJM. 343: 1688-96; Hanson et al., (2002) J Card Fail. 8 : 28-32 ; Venkatraman et al., (2003) JBC 278: 41670-6 ; Mogensen et al., (2004) JACC 44: 2033-40.
Asp270Asn (D270N)	DCM	15	Mirza et al., (2005) JBC. 280 :28498-506
Glu96del (ΔE96)	RCM	9	Peddy et al., (2006) Pediatrics 117:1830-3; Pinto et al., (2008) JBC. 283:2156-66
Asn100del/Glu101 Del (ΔN100/ΔE101)	RCM	9	Pinto et al., (2011)JBC 286:20901-12 (double mutation)
Glu136Lys (E136K)	RCM	10	Kaski et al., (2008) Heart 94:1478-84

Updated from: Genomics of Cardiovascular Development, Adaptation, and Remodeling. NHLBI Program for Genomic Applications, Harvard Medical School. [june, 2011 accessed] and OMIM database. er designates termination of sequence resulting in a truncated protein, del and Δ are synonyms for a deleted amino acid. The one letter code is given in brackets.

Table 1. Mutations in TNNT2

Since the cTnT- N-terminus contributes to the inhibition of the actin/myosin interaction (Tobacman, 1988), one might assume that also inhibition is affected by mutations. Indeed inhibition of is reduced due to cTnT-F110I (Knollmann & Potter, 2001; Gomes et al., 2004). A similar decrease in inhibition has been described for I79N (Yanaga et al., 1999), though this amino acid exchange is positioned N-terminally of the main Tm interaction site. Nevertheless I79N and F110I exhibit several similarities. Thus, Midde et al., 2011 showed that rigor crossbridges in I79N or F110I containing filaments were disordered, indicating that disruption in thin filament structure may lead to severe contractile dysfunction. I79N, as most investigated HCM mutants, enhances the Ca^{2+}- sensitivity of force development and actomyosin ATPase activity, which might contribute to enhanced contractility and higher energy consumption (Lin et al., 1996; Sweeney et al., 1998; Chandra et al., 2005). Furthermore, mouse hearts with I79N or R92Q could not increase cardiac performance upon ß-adrenergic stimulation (Knollmann et al., 2001; Javadpour et al., 2003), performance of I79N transgenic even worsened upon isoproterenol treatment (Sirenko et al., 2006). Such an effect as well as Ca^{2+} –sensitivity increase has not been observed with a R278C, a mutation located in the cTnT-C-terminus. These findings suggest that the region around amino acids 79 and 92 is important for Ca^{2+} -signal transmission and affects Ca^{2+}-regulation. Furthermore dysfunction is especially prominent under ß-adrenergic stimulation, which might explain the high risc for cardiac sudden death of these mutations. Causality between enhanced Ca^{2+}-sensitivity and the potential for the development of malignant arrhythmias has been shown by Baudenbacher et al., (2008) for I79N. They described altered action potential duration due to the mutation.

Mutations in TNNT2 gene encoding the C-terminal half of cTnT might affect the interaction with tropomyosin at the second Ca^{2+} -dependent binding site, as well as binding to cTnI and cTnC. Most mutations in this part lead either to single amino acid exchanges, deletions of single amino acids or to C-terminally truncated cTnT molecules due to splice site mutations. IVS15+1G>A is a splicing donor mutant which might result in two truncated proteins. In one mutant exon 16 is skipped encoding the C-terminal 14 amino acids, in the other mutants seven amino acids replace the C-terminal 28 amino acids encoded by exon 15 and 16 (Thierfelder et al., 1994). Both mutants are able to form a heterotrimeric troponin complex, however their affinity towards cTnI is drastically reduced (Mukherjea et al., 1999). The impaired interaction with cTnI may be the cause for reduced inhibitory capacity of troponin at low Ca^{2+}-concentrations described by Redwood et al., (2000) and accelerated cross bridge kinetics (Stelzer et al., 2004). Furthermore a reduced binding of troponin to the thin filament has been reported dependent on its regulatory states (Knollmann & Potter, 2001; Burhop et al., 2001), indicating that the C-terminal part of cTnT stabilizes binding of cTn to the thin filament and affects Ca^{2+} -regulation. Increased Ca^{2+}-sensitivity and cooperativity (Nakaura et al., 1999)) and impaired switching off myosin cycling at low Ca^{2+}-concentrations is observed (Burhop et al., 2001). Up to date nearly nothing is known on how cardiomyopathy inducing mutations in TNNT2 influence phosphorylation dependent effects of PKC dependent cTnT or PKA dependent cTnI phosphorylation. According to a study of Nakaura et al., (1999) effects of truncated cTnT were independent on PKA dependent cTnI phosphorylation.

2.1.2 RCM inducing mutations

There are only few RCM mutations detected in TNNT2 (Table 1). Most RCM mutations in genes encoding for cardiac troponin subunits are found in TNNI3 (see below). However,

nterestingly I79N, originally listed as HCM mutation, might also cause RCM or DCM even
n members of the same family. This indicates that other factors besides the mutation, as for
example polymorphisms etc. (see below) are determinant for the development of the specific
disease. Also in mice RCM might be evolved by I79N (Table 1). The other two RCM
mutations (Table 1), a deletion of an acidic residue (E96del) and replacement of a glutamic
acid residue by a basic lysine (E136K) have been detected in children developing RCM with
very poor prognosis. E96del poorly inhibited actomyosin activity at low Ca^{2+} -
concentrations (Pinto et al., 2008) confirming that the cTnT N-terminus is important for the
inhibitory capacity of the cardiac troponin complex. A first double deletion (Table 1) leads to
the deletion of two amino acids, located adjacently within the main Tm binding site. In
filaments with adult, not fetal cTnT an increase in Ca^{2+}-sensitivity and decrease in
cooperativity has been observed so far (Pinto et al., 2011).

2.1.3 DCM inducing mutations

Patients with DCM mutations in cTNNT2 exhibit a malignant prognosis as do also most of
the FHC mutations in cTNNT2. Investigations on molecular level are largely missing to
date. All patients showed decreased cardiac function (Kamisago et al., 2000) in contrast to
enhanced contractility often observed in patients and transgenic animals carrying HCM
mutations. In accordance *in vitro* analysis of DCM-mutations revealed a decreased Ca^{2+}-
sensitivity (Mirza et al., 2005). Venkatraman et al., 2005 showed that ΔK210, the most
prominent example for DCM causing cTnT-variation, decreases Ca^{2+}-sensitivity of force and
actomyosin ATPase activity as well as maximal force and ATPase activity not only with
adult, but also with fetal cTnT. The deletion of K210 occurs in the second Ca^{2+} -sensitive
tropomyosin binding region near the PKC phosphorylation site and possibly near the
binding site for PKA regulatory subunit II. This implies that Ca^{2+} -regulation as well as PKC
dependent phosphorylation of cTnT and/or PKA dependent phosphorylation of other
sarcomeric proteins might be affected. Detailed information is missing.

2.2 Mutations in TNNC1, the gene encoding cTnC

Mutations in the TNNC1 gene occur seldom. Far less than 1% of the genetic disorders
leading to familial cardiomyopathies in patients are due to mutations in TNNC1. Up to date
only six HCM and one DCM inducing mutations, all single amino acid exchanges, have
been identified (Fig.2; Table 2). A8V, L29Q and C84Y are located in the N-terminal and
N122fs, E134D, D145E and G159D in the C-terminal domain of cTnC (Fig. 2). L29Q was the
first mutation detected in the cTnC gene (Hoffmann et al., 2001). Since there was only one
family showing this mutation, it is not clear if this mutation causes HCM. However,
according to Schmidtmann et al., 2005 and Liang et al., 2008 this amino acid replacement has
the potential to cause a cardiomyopathy. Replacement of leucine by glutamine destabilizes
the interaction of the N-terminal cTnI arm with cTnC (Schmidtmann et al., 2005;
Baryshnikova et al., 2008). The release of the N-terminal cTnI arm occurs also upon
bisphosphorylation of cTnI after ß-adrenergic stimulation and contributes to a reduction in
Ca^{2+}-sensitivity of the actomyosin ATPase activity (see below). Consistent with this effect for
L29Q a small reduction of Ca^{2+}- sensitivity has been described (Schmidtmann et al., 2005).
However, in the phosphorylated state of cTnI, an enhanced Ca^{2+}-sensitivity of the
actomyosin ATPase activity was observed, indicating an altered ß-adrenergic
responsiveness. Divergent results might be obtained in systems differing in complexity

mutation	disease	exon	reference
Leu29Gln (L29Q)	HCM	3	Hoffmann et al., (2001). Hum. Mutat. 17: 524; Dweck et al., (2008). J Biol Chem. 283: 33119-28; Liang et al., (2008). Physiol. Gen. 33:257-66; Schmidtmann et al., (2005). *FEBS J.* 272(23):6087-97.
Ala8Val (A8V)	HCM	1	Landstrom et al., (2008). JMCC 45: 281-288 ; Pinto et al., (2009) JBC. 284(28):19090-100; Pinto et al., (2011).JBC. 286(2):1005-13.
Cys84Tyr (C84Y)	HCM	4	Landstrom et al., (2008). JMCC 45: 281-288. Pinto et al., (2009) JBC. 284(28):19090-100
Gln122Alafsx30 (Q122fs)	HCM	4	Chung et al., (2011) Cardiol. Young [Ehead of print]
Glu134Asp (E134D)	HCM		Pinto et al., (2009) JBC. 284(28):19090-100
Asp145Glu (D145E)	HCM	5	Landstrom et al., (2008). JMCC 45: 281-288. Pinto et al., (2009) JBC. 284(28):19090-100; Pinto et al., (2011).JBC. 286(2):1005-13.
Gly159Asp (G159D)	DCM	6	Mogensen et al., (2004). JACC 44: 2033-2040; Mirza et al., (2005). JBC 280: 28498- 506.

Modified from: OMIM database (http://omim.org); the one letter code is given in brackets; fs designates frameshift.

Table 2. Mutations in TNNC1

(Dweck et al., 2008). Thus, in a higher organized system, namely mouse cardiomyocytes, Liang et al. (2008) described an enhanced Ca^{2+}-sensitivity of force generation dependent on sarcomere length. They showed that also Ca^{2+}- binding affinity to site II was higher in cTnC-L29Q than in cTnC wild type, whereas Ca^{2+}-dissociation rate was not affected. This is in agreement with former findings of Gillis et al., 2005, that residues 2, 28-30 affect Ca^{2+}-binding properties of the regulatory Ca^{2+}-binding site. Replacement of these residues might increase cardiomyocyte contractility. Also the other FHC mutation in TNNC1, leading to A8V, C84Y and D145E replacements in cTnC, enhance Ca^{2+} -sensitivity of force development (Landstrom et al., 2008). For E134D no influence on Ca^{2+}-sensitivity could be observed. It remains unclear how this mutation leads to contractile dysfunction. Since E134 is located near contact sites of cTnI around Ser43/45 effects of PKC dependent phosphorylation might be influenced. Also A8V in the N-terminal helix of cTnC- N-lobe is located near a contact site with cTnI- Ser43 in H1 of cTnI (Li et al., 2004, Takeda et al., 2003). No data on the impact of these mutations on PKC phosphorylation are available up to date.

The proximity of A8 and E134 to the same cTnI region underlines findings of Smth et al. (1999) that the cTnC-N-terminal helix is spatially near the C-lobe. Latest kinetical investigations by Pinto et al, (2011a) showed that Ca^{2+} off rates are delayed for A8V and D145E, both stabilizing cross bridges. Thus structural disturbances at the cTnC-N-terminus not only alter structure of the N- but also of the C-terminal lobe and vice versa and may impair cTnC-cTnI interaction. C84Y is located at the end of the EF hand helix flanking regulatory Ca^{2+}- binding loop at the transition to the central linker region. This residue probably is involved in forming the binding platform for the cTnI switch region and thus might destabilize binding of cTnI in Ca^{2+} -saturated state of cTnC (Fig. 2). D145E is located in Ca^{2+} -binding loop IV, in +Z position (see above) indicating that divalent cation binding might be affected (Pinto et al., 2009). Another amino acid exchange in the C-terminal lobe, G159D, is linked to DCM. Consistent with all other investigated DCM causing mutations G159D reduces Ca^{2+}-sensitivity of the actin-myosin interaction and decreases contractility (Mirza et al., 2005). The hydrophobic residues at position 156,157 and 160 make contact to cTnI (Gasmi-Seabrook et al., 1999). Thus the G156D exchange may considerably disturb the hydrophobic interaction with cTnI and also might affect interaction with cTnT. In the troponin complex G159D reduced the opening (Ca2+ binding) and closing rates (Ca2+ dissociation) of the N-terminal domain of cTnC. Alteration in opening rate was also observed for L29Q, indicating that both mutants alter structural transition kinetics (Dong et al., 2008). PKA dependent phosphorylation of cTnI also affects kinetics in that it enhances the closing rate. This effect was abolished by L29Q and G159D implying that phosphorylation signal transduction is impaired as was earlier proposed for L29Q by Schmidtmann et al. (2005).

2.3 Mutations in TNNI3, the gene encoding cTnI

Most mutations in the gene encoding cTnI, are located in exon 7 and 8, which encode the regulatory C-terminal region of cTnI a few are located in the N-terminal heart specific extension. In patients they mostly induce either HCM or RCM. There are only three mutations identified up to date in TNNI3, which are linked to DCM.

2.3.1 Mutations in TNNI3 linked to HCM

Only one mutation has been identified in exon 3 encoding part of the heart specific N-terminal cTnI arm (Table 3). This mutation results in an R20C (numbering without starter methionine) amino acid exchange, which is located within the consensus sequence for PKA (Fig. 3). The consensus sequence is present in cTnI in a dublicated form (Mittmann et al., 1992) enabling phosphorylation of two adjacent located serine residues (Ser22, 23) by PKA (Fig. 4). The exchange of the middle arginine in a series of three arginine residues (position 20 or 21 dependent on the inclusion of the starter methionine) impairs phosphorylation of the two serine residues and reduces the phosphorylation effect *in vitro* as shown by Gomes et al. (2005). Since both phosphorylation sites are affected, susceptibility towards proteolysis is enhanced. Phosphorylation protects to a certain extent towards proteolysis (Barta et al., 2003). But also the amino acid exchange itself might enhance susceptibility towards protein degradationas proposed by Gomes et al. 2005). Thus probably impairment of PKA dependent phosphorylation as well as enhanced protein digestion might be the main effect of this mutant protein for disease development.

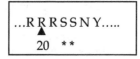

...R R R S S N Y.....
▲
20   **

*Designates phosphorylation sites, arg 20 is indicated

Fig. 4. Consensus sequence in cTnI for PKA.

The first 6 mutations in TNNI3 causing HCM were described by Kimura et al. (1997) (Table 3). R145G, for example, is located within the inhibitor region of cTnI, which binds to actin/tropomyosin at low intracellular Ca^{2+} -concentrations (relaxed state) and blocks actin/myosin interaction (Fig. 3). Mutations located in the inhibitory region most probably affect inhibitory capacity of cTnI by altering actin/cTnI interaction in the relaxed state. Indeed R145G in fibers resulting from transgenic mice reduce inhibition (James et al., 2000, Wen et al., 2008) and binding affinity towards actin. Ca^{2+} -sensitivity of force development in skinned papillary muscles from these mice was enhanced with maximal force being decreased (Krüger et al., 2005; Wen et al ., 2008). These findings are in accordance with enhanced Ca^{2+}-sensitivity and reduced maximal actomyosin ATPase activity described by Deng et al. (2001). Also energy consumption in transgenic mice was increased as shown by Wen et al., 2008, indicating hypercontractility. In isolated rat cardiomyocytes as in myofibrils from transgenic mice contractile parameters were reduced (James et al., 2000, Kruger et al., 2005; Reis et al., 2008) and Ca^{2+} -regulation and ß -adrenergic response was impaired (Lang et al., 2002; Reis et al., 2008). The dynamic properties of contraction were severely suppressed upon ß- adrenergic stimulation (Reis et al., 2008). This again supports the idea that impairment of ß- adrenergic signaling might be important for disease development. Furthermore, R145G might also affect PKC dependent phosphorylation at Thr144, which has not been investigated thoroughly yet. Kobayashi et al. (2004) showed that effects of exchange of all PKC sites Thr144/ Ser43/45 by a glutamic acid residue, which is thought to mimic phosphorylation, are reduced due to the mutation. Pseudophosphorylated PKC sites reduce the Ca^{2+} -dependent opening of the N-terminal lobe of cTnC (Kobayashi et al., 2004). However, a more differentiated analysis is needed.

Mutations in the switch region (Table 3, Fig. 3), which binds to the N-terminal lobe of cTnC upon Ca^{2+}-saturation, are thought to impair binding to N-terminal lobe of cTnC under Ca^{2+}-saturating conditions. Thus, they probably affect Ca^{2+}- dissociation from cTnC and the conformational switch of cardiac troponin I needed for transmission of the Ca^{2+}- signal. An example for such a mutation is Ala157Val.

Mutations located in the mobile C terminal cTnI region may alter cTnI Tm/actin interaction. This may affect inhibition as well as activation. The mobile C-terminus together with N-terminal part of cTnT of the opposing troponin complex stabilizes the tropomyosin position in the blocked state. Indeed for C-terminally truncated cTnI impaired relaxation kinetics, enhanced Ca^{2+} sensitivity and disturbed cooperativity has been observed (Narolska et al., 2006, Tachampa et al., 2009). A small decrease in inhibitory capacity has been described for R162W and K185del (Redwood et al., 1998). Mutations located at the very C-terminus of cTnI as G203S or K206Q do not exhibit an effect on inhibition (Deng et al., 2003, Köhler et al, 2003). Again there are conflicting results concerning Ca^{2+}-sensitivity alterations. Transgenic mice with cTnI-G203S exhibit altered Ca^{2+} -regulation and show prominent altered expression of cytosketetal, contractile proteins and of proteins involved in energy production (Tsoutsman et al., 2006; Lam et al., 2007). Not much is known about other mutations at the same position, G203R (replacement of glycin by the positively charged larger and less flexible amino acid arginine) and a frameshift (fs) mutation (table 3). One would expect that dysfunction due to these sequence alterations are more prominent than for G203S. Also K206Q is not well characterized. It enhances maximal actomyosin ATPase activity and alters dynamics of the actin myosin interaction (Deng et al., 2003). According to our own latest investigations (abstract, Saes et al., DGK, Mannheim April 2011) this part of cTnI interacts with actin; the replacement of lysine in position 206 by glutamine abolishes cTnI-C-terminus/actin interaction indicating a stabilization of the activated state. Furthermore, K206Q as well as G203S impair transduction of the PKA dependent phosphorylation signal *in vitro* (Deng et al., 2003). This implies that PKA dependent phosphorylation at the cTnI-N-terminus modulates not onlyfunction of inhibitory and switch region, but also of the mobile domain.

2.3.2 Mutations in TNNI3 linked to RCM

Mutations linked to RCM occur mostly in the regulatory domain as do HCM inducing mutations and may share even the same locus (Table 3). Thus for example R145G induces FHC and R145W, RCM. Indeed RCM and HCM have some clinical as well as molecular characteristics in common. Both diseases show diastolic dysfunction and all RCM mutations investigated lead to enhanced Ca^{2+}- sensitivity as do most of the HCM inducing mutations. Many of them reduce maximal tension a well as maximal actomyosin ATPase activity and impair inhibition (Gomes et al., 2005; Davis et al., 2008; Kobayashi & Solaro, 2006; for review see Parvatayar et al., 2010). Thus it is unclear how the RCM phenotype develops. But it indicates that the type of exchange (for example R145G HCM and R145W RCM) might be important for the disease development. A glycine exhibits a much smaller van der Waals volume, higher flexibility and higher hydrophilicity than a tryptophan at the same position and thus may alter interactions and dynamic properties very differently. Ca^{2+}-regulation is accompanied by allosteric transitions which are dependent on dynamic properties of the proteins involved. Thus alteration in dynamic properties affects Ca^{2+} regulation and might determine the type of dysfunction (Lassalle, 2010).

2.3.3 Mutations in TNNI3 linked to DCM

The first mutation identified (autosomal recessive) is located at the very N-terminal end of the heart specific N-terminal arm of cTnI and leads to a conservative replacement of the amino acid alanine by valine, which both are hydrophobic (Table 3). However, in contrast to alanine, valine is branched, takes double of the van der Waals volume and has a higher hydropathy index. These altered physicochemical properties might produce local structure disturbances and therefore modify interactions. According to Murphy et al., 2004 this amino acid exchange affects cTnI/cTnT interaction, though no direct interaction of the N-terminal arm with cTnT has been described so far. There are several contacts of the non phosphorylated N-terminus with cTnC- N-terminal lobe and of the phosphorylated N-terminus with the regulatory C-terminal region of cTnI. The mechanism how this mutation may alter cTnI/cTnI interaction is not clear. Further investigations are needed. Lately Carballo et al. (2009) described two new DCM mutations in cTNNI3 with an autosomal dominant trait leading to a severe onset of the disease. K36Q is located near constitutive cTnC interaction site and in the putative hinge region important for phosphorylation dependent movement of the cTnI-N-terminal arm. Therefor this mutation possibly might affect structural integrity of the troponin complex and ß-adrenergic responsiveness. N185K is located within the mobile cTnI C-terminal region. *In vitro* both amino acid replacements reduce Ca^{2+} -sensitivity of the actomyosin ATPase and decreased maximal ATPase activity (Carballo et al., 2009) considered as typical for DCM.

mutation	disease	exon	reference
Arg21Cys (R21C /R20C)	HCM	3	Barr, Seidman et al. (2001) first posted on URL: http: //www. cardiogenomics.org; Arad et al., (2005) Circ. 112:2805-1 ; Gomes et al.,(2005) JMCC 39 :754-65
Arg141Gln (R141Q)	HCM	7	Richard et al., (2003) Circ. 107:2227-32 ; Van Driest et al., (2003) Circ. 108 : 445-51
Leu144Pro (L144P)	HCM	7	Merk, Seidman et al., (2005) first posted on URL:http://www. cardiogenomics.org
Arg145Gly (R145G/R146G)	HCM	7	Kimura et al., (1997) Nat Genet. 16:379-82. Takahashi-Yanaga, et al., (2000) J Biochem (Tokyo) 127:355-7, Elliott et al. (2000) JBC 275:22069-74 ; Deng et al., (2001) Biochem. 40:14593-602; Takahashi-Yanaga et al., (2001)JMCC 33:2095-107 ; Lang et al., (2002) JBC 277(4):11670-8 ; Burton et al., (2002) Biochem J 362:443-51 ; Lindhout et al., (2002) Biochem 41:7267-74 and (2005) Biochem 44:14750-9; Kruger et al., (2005) J Physiol 564: 347-57, Wen et al.,(2008) JBC 283: 20484-94; Reis et al., (2008) *Pflugers Arch.* 457:17-24
Arg145Gln (R145Q)	HCM	7	Kimura et al., (1997) Nat Genet 16:379-82 ; Taka-hashi-Yanaga et al., (2001) JMCC 33: 2095-107; Mogensen et al., (2004) JACC 44: 2315-25.
Ala157Val (A157V)	HCM	7	Richard et al., (2003) Circ. 107: 2227-32 ; Mogensen et al., (2004) JACC 44:2315-25; Brito & Madeira (2005)Rev Port Cardiol. 24:1137-46 ; Meder et al., (2009) J Cardiol 15: 274-8
Arg162Trp (R162W)	HCM	7	Kimura et al., (1997) Nat Genet 16: 379-82; Elliott et al., (2000) JBC 275: 22069-74; Takahashi-Yanaga et al., (2001) JMCC 33: 2095-107
Arg162Gln (R162Q)	HCM	7	Van Driest et al., (2003) Circ.108: 445-51; Mogensen et al., (2004) JACC 44: 2315-25 ; Doolan et al., (2005) JMCC 2005 38: 387-93; Cheng et al., (2005) JACC 46:180-1; Ingles et al., (2005) J Med Genet. 42 :e59.
Arg162Pro (R162P)	HCM	7	Richard et al., (2003)Circ. 2003 107: 2227-32; Doolan et al., (2005) JMCC 38: 387-93; Ingles et al., (2005) J Med Genet. 42: e59
Ser166Phe (S166F)	HCM	7	Van Driest et al., (2003) Circ. 108: 445-51; Van Driest et al., (2004) JACC 44: 1903-10; Mogensen et al., (2004) JACC 44: 2315-25
Lys178del (ΔK178)	HCM	7	Richard et al., (2003) Circ. 107: 2227-32
Lys183Glu (K183E)	HCM	7	Mogensen et al., (2004) JACC 44: 2315-25

mutation	disease	exon	reference
Lys183del (ΔK183)	HCM	7	Kimura et al., (1997) Nat Genet. 16: 379-82; Kokado et al., (2000) Circ. 102: 663-9; Takahashi-Yanaga et al., (2001) JMCC 33: 2095-107; Kohler et al., (2003) Physiol Gen. 14: 117-28 ; Konno et al., (2005) J Int Med. 258: 216-24.
Arg186Gln (R186Q)	HCM	8	Richard et al., (2003) Circ. 107:2227-32; Mogensen et al., (2004) JACC 44: 2315-25
Ile195Met (I195M)	HCM	8	Barr, Seidman et al., (2001) first posted on URL: http://www. cardiogenomics.org
Asp196Asn (D196N)	HCM	8	Richard et al., (2003) Circ. 107: 2227-32; Mogensen et al., (2004) JACC 44: 2315-25; Nimura et al., (2002) Circ. 105 : 446-51
Leu198Val (L198V)	HCM	8	Merk, Seidman et al., (2005) first posted on URL:http://www. cardiogenomics.org
Leu198Pro (L198P)	HCM	8	Doolan et al., (2005) JMCC 38: 387-93
Ser199Gly (S199G)	HCM	8	Mogensen et al., (2004) JACC 44: 2315-25
Ser199Asn (S199N)	HCM	8	Mogensen et al., (2004) JACC 44: 2315-25; Brito & Madeira (2005) Rev Port Cardiol. 24: 1137-46
Glu202Gly (E202G)	HCM	8	Mogensen et al., (2004) JACC 44: 2315-25
Gly203Arg (G203R)	HCM	8	Mogensen et al., (2004) JACC 44: 2315-25
Gly203Ser (G203S)	HCM/ Wolff Parkinson syndrom	8	Kimura et al., (1997) Nat Genet. 16:379-82; Kokado et al., (2000) Circ. 102: 663-9 ; Takahashi-Yanaga et al., (2001) JMCC 33: 2095-107 ; Burton D et al., (2002) Biochem J 362: 443-51; Kohler et al., (2003) Physiol Gen. 14: 117-28, Deng et al., (2003) JMCC 35: 1365-74; Tsoutsman et al., (2006) JMCC 41: 623-32; Nguyen et al., (2007) Int J Cardiol. 119: 245-8; Lam et al., (2010) JMCC 48: 1014-22
Gly203fs (G203fs)	HCM	8	Morner et al., (2000) JMCC 32: 521-5 and (2003) 35: 841-9; Richard et al., (2003) Circ. 107: 2227-32
Arg204Cys (R204C)	HCM	8	Barr, Seidman et al., (2002) first posted on URL: http://www. cardiogenomics.org
Arg204His (R204H)	HCM	8	Doolan et al., (2005) JMCC 38: 387-93; Ingles et al., (2005) J Med Genet. 42: e59
Lys206Gln (K206Q)	HCM	8	Kimura et al., (1997) Nat Genet. 16:379-82; Taka-hashi-Yanaga et al., (2001) JMCC 33: 2095-107; Kohler et al., (2003) Physiol Gen. 14: 117-28; Deng et al., (2003) JMCC 35: 1365-74
Ala2Val (A2V)	DCM, recessive	1	Murphy et al., (2004) Lancet 363: 371-2
Lys36Gln (K36Q)	DCM, dominant	3	Carballo et al., (2009) Circ. 105 : 375-82
Asn135Lys (N135K)	DCM dominant	7	Carballo et al., (2009) Circ. 105 : 375-82
Leu144Gln (L144Q)	RCM	7	Mogensen et al., (2003) JCI 111:209-16; Gomes et al., (2005) JBC 280: 30909-15
Arg145Trp (R145W)	RCM	7	Mogensen et al., (2003) JCI 111: 209-16; Mogensen et al., (2004) JACC 44: 2315-25; Gomes et al., (2005) JBC 280: 30909-15; Cheng (2005) J Am Coll Cardiol 46: 180-1

mutation	disease	exon	reference
Ala171Thr (A171T)	R CM	7	Mogensen et al., (2003) JCI 111: 209-16; Gomes et al., (2005) JBC 280: 30909-15
Lys178Glu (K178E)	RCM	7	Mogensen et al., (2003) JCI 111: 209-16; Gomes et al., (2005) JBC 280: 30909-15
Asp190His (R190H)	RCM	8	Mogensen et al., (2003) JCI 111: 209-16; Gomes et al., (2005) JBC 280: 30909-15
Asp190Gly (D190G)	RCM	8	Davis et al., (2008) JMCC 44: 891-904
Arg192His (R192H)	RCM	8	Mogensen et al., (2003) JCI 111: 209-16; Gomes et al., (2005) JBC 280: 30909-15

In brackets the one letter code and positions due to species specifities are given; fs designates frameshift.

Table 3. Mutations in TNNI3

In summary, there seem to be three major factors on the molecular level which help to understand phenotype development and might be directive for future investigations. 1) Mutations might severely affect affinity to other thin filament proteins and/or enhance susceptibility to proteolysis. In both cases structural integrity of the thin filament would be disturbed, which would in turn affect contractile function. It might even affect sarcomeric structure. 2) Mutations alter dynamical properties of the protein. Changes in dynamics might affect inter- and intramolecular interactions, Ca^{2+}-regulation, ß –adrenergic responsiveness and PKC mediated phosphorylation and thereby may induce contractile dysfunction in various degrees. 3) Combinations of mutations might lead to additive or compensatory effects.

3. Clinical presentation

3.1 Diagnosis of HCM
In 1989 (Jarcho et al., 1989) and 1990 (Geisterfer-Lowrance et al., 1990), the first "disease genes" have been identified in family members with inherited hypertrophic cardiomyopathy (HCM). This identification of disease genes has raised many expectations, among others in the better understanding of the molecular mechanisms of disease development, in a more reliable identification of patients at risk, and in new concepts of treatment (Keren et al.; 2008, Lippi et al., 2009; Marian, 2010; Ho, 2010a; Watkins et al, 1995; 2011). The following paragraphs will focus on the clinical presentation of patients with mutations in the genes encoding troponin C, T and I (TNNC1, TNNT2, and TNNI3) in the context of HCM. For clinical presentation of HCM patients in general the reader is referred to an excellent book chapter from Fatkin et al., (2007).
HCM is clinically suggested in patients by the presence of unexplained left ventricular hypertrophy (LVH, usually defined as ventricular wall thickness ≥ 15 mm or ≥ 13 mm in relatives of a HCM patient; Elliott et al., 2008) and a non-dilated left ventricle with preserved or even enhanced global systolic function (Fig.5). Diagnosis relies on the electrographic and echocardiographic demonstration of hypertrophy. LVH may be diffuse or more segmentally distributed (proximal and/or midportion of the interventricular septum, apex, anterior or lateral wall), but no single morphologic expression appears to be specific (Klues et al., 1995). In fact, differentiation of LVH secondary to HCM may be difficult from other diseases affecting the ventricles, e.g. hypertrophy secondary to infiltrative diseases (e.g. amyloidosis),

abry's disease (Monserrat et al., 2007), glycogen storage disorders (Arad et al., 2005a), or ystemic arterial hypertension. These diagnostic difficulties may rise with advanced age.

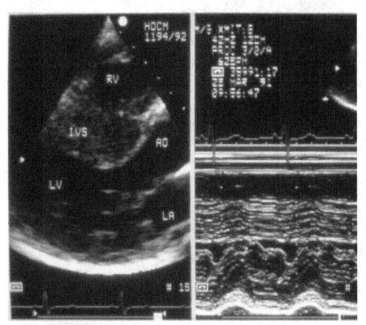

(VS=septum, LV/RV=left/right ventricles, Ao=aorta ascendens, LA=left atrium)

ig. 5. 2D and M-mode echocardiogram demonstrating severe hypertrophy (> 25 mm) of the eptum

esides LVH, left ventricular outflow obstruction is one of the most suspicious features of his disease. Braunwald & Ebert (1962) noted first the dynamic component of this bstruction. Later on the systolic anterior motion ("SAM") of the anterior leaflet of the mitral alve was recognized as the major contributor of left ventricular outflow obstruction and the nore or less significant accompanying mitral regurgitation (Marian 2010). In a series of 320 onsecutive HCM patients, this obstructive pathology at resting conditions (defined as a gradient ≥ 50 mmHg at rest) was found in 37% of patients (Maron et al., 2006). In the emaining patients, 52% developed dynamic outflow gradients during exercise or naneuvers which decrease afterload or increase contractility. These high numbers, however, hould be cautiously extrapolated for the general HCM population because of referral bias nd patients selection criteria.

Abnormal diastolic function (prolonged LV relaxation and increased LV chamber tiffness) is an almost universal feature of HCM. It appears that diastolic dysfunction is a ery early manifestation of HCM, even before morphological evidence of hypertrophy occurs (Nagueh et al., 2001; Ho et al., 2009). Today, diastolic dysfunction is suggested if he ratio between early diastolic peak filling velocity (the E wave in transmitral Doppler) and early diastolic peak velocity of the mitral annulus (the E' derived from tissue Doppler) exceeds the value 15 in the presence of normal systolic function (Fig. 6; Ommen t al., 2000; Paulus et al., 2007).

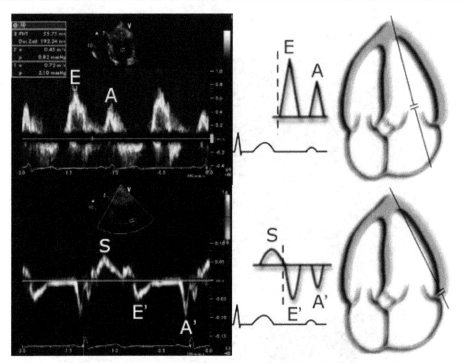

Fig. 6. Transmitral Doppler (top) and tissue Doppler (bottom) allowing quantification of the early diastolic peak filling velocity (E) and early diastolic peak velocity of the mitral annulus (E'). The ratio E/E' is used to determine diastolic dysfunction.

The clinical presentation of HCM patients shows a remarkable diversity: some individuals experience none or minor symptoms, others may develop dyspnoe at exercise or at rest, angina pectoris, palpitations, atrial fibrillation, dizziness, presyncope and syncope, fatigue or finally end stage heart failure requiring cardiac transplantation (Ho, 2010a).

The changes on ECG are very variable and include left axis deviation, occurrence of Q waves, a positive Sokolow index for hypertrophy, conduction abnormalities, ST-T depression or other abnormalities, negative T waves and giant T waves (particularly observed in Japanese patients with apical type of HCM (Sakamoto et al., 1976). The ECG abnormalities may not parallel hypertrophy in all cases. In fact, ECG abnormalities are more frequently found in HCM patients as echocardiographic abnormalities. Konno et al. (2005) observed ECG abnormalities (in particular ST-T abnormalities) in about 54% of genetically affected, but nonhypertrophic patients at echocardiography. However, almost all of ECG abnormalities (perhaps except giant T waves) are unspecific, and do also occur in patients with advanced age for various other reasons.

The underlying histopathology is characterized by gross cardiac hypertrophy, myocyte hypertrophy, disarray of cardiac cells, interstitial fibrosis, hyperplasia of the media of coronary arteries. The cardiac myocyte disarray (Fig. 7) appears to be a hallmark of HCM, not infrequently involving up to 20% of the ventricles (Maron & Roberts, 1979; Elliot & McKenna, 2004).

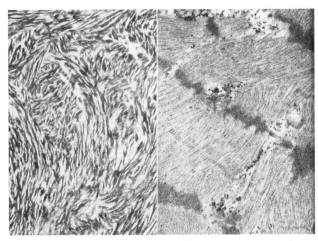

Fig. 7. Histology of the heart of a patient with HCM demonstrating typical disarray of the myocytes and myofibrils.

3.2 Complications and general prognosis in HCM

A major concern in the management of patients with HCM is prognosis. Sudden cardiac death (which may account for 50% of the disease-related death), atrial fibrillation with the risk of stroke, and congestive heart failure (CHF) are the leading contributors to the morbidity and mortality associated with HCM (Keren et al., 2008; Marian 2010). Overall, HCM is a "benign" disease with an annual mortality rate of 0.5-1% in unselected HCM-affected subjects (Cannan et al. 1995). However, sudden death may the first clinical manifestation of this disease, particularly in young otherwise healthy appearing subjects (Maron et al., 1996). In a meta-analysis by Liberthson (1996), HCM was the most frequent single cause of sudden death in children and young adults. This was supported by a large series of Maron (2003) who analyzed 387 young athletes who died suddenly, and found that HCM was the cause in 26.4%. The overall risk of sudden death appears to be similar in males and females (Olivotto et al., 2005), by contrast, 90% of 134 athletes with sudden cardiac death were males (Maron et al., 1996).

The risk for sudden cardiac death can be effectively reduced by the prophylactic implantation of an internal automated defibrillator (ICD), the main problem is, however, to identify those who will profit from this device. So far, no single risk factor (except surviving cardiac arrest) has been identified which may clearly justify prophylactic ICD implantation. Nowadays, a more comprehensive approach is used combining informations/findings (family history of sudden death, severe cardiac hypertrophy, history of presynope or syncope, non-sustained or sustained ventricular tachycardia) (Kofflard et al., 2003; Marian 2003; Frenneaux 2004; Marian 2010). It is a new challenge to integrate genotype testing in this risk assessment algorithm, although the power of genetic testing appears to be up to now more the identification of non-carriers in HCM families obviating the need for clinical screening and follow-up examinations (Keren et al., 2008; Pinto et al., 2011). The ethical, legal and societal implications of genetic testing for cardiac diseases in clinical practice has been discussed elsewhere (Tester & Ackerman, 2011). Furthermore, the pro and contra of genotyping in predicting prognosis in HCM has been recently discussed in Circulation (Ho, 2010b; Landstrom & Ackerman, 2010).

The true penetrance of all clinical presentations is not known and may be underestimated because the clinical diagnosis of HCM is not robust. Furthermore, clinical findings may either vary over time or the disease-related abnormalities may have a variable onset during life. For example, progressive increase in LV wall thickness has been observed in adolescents and young adults with HCM, whereas wall thickness remains to be more stable in the elderly (Maron et al., 1986; Semsarian et al., 1997). This may, however, not be true for all mutations. Revera et al. (2007) re-evaluated 22 carriers with an Arg92Trp (TNNT2 gene) mutation after an average of 11 years. With age, left ventricular hypertrophy increased (≥ 5 mm wall thickness, as assessed by echocardiography) in 50% of individuals. These later points are of particular importance since most clinical studies have a cross-sectional design, and prospective longitudinal studies are scarce.

All groups are in agreement that the phenotypic heterogeneity in HCM patients/families cannot be explained by the genetic defect alone. Other factors must be involved including sex, additional disease such as arterial hypertension, and environmental factors. This heterogeneity is particularly striking in families with one genetic defect, but demonstrating phenotypes of different cardiomyopathies. For example, Menon et al. (2008) identified a large family with a mutation in the TNNT2 gene (Ile79Asn). This mutation affected 9 family members. Mutation carries showed clinically a restrictive cardiomyopathy in 2, a non-obstructive HCM in 3, dilated cardiomyopathy in 2, a mixed cardiomyopathy in 1, and mild concentric hypertrophy in 1 family member. Genetic factors others than the causal sarcomere mutation may affect the penetrance and severity of cardiac abnormalities, referred as the modifier genes. In this regard, variants of the angiotensin-1 converting enzyme (ACE-1) gene are discussed as potential modifiers, increasing the risk for sudden cardiac death (Marian et al., 1993) and the severity of LVH (Lechin et al., 1995). Beside modifier genes, others factors must also determine the phenotype, as pressure or volume load, since manifestations of HCM are predominantly restricted to the LV, although the mutant sarcomeric protein is expressed in both ventricles. Finally, homozygous mutations (as it has been described for a child with a Ser179Phe mutation in the TNNT2 gene who died suddenly at the age of 17 (Ho et al., 2000)), or multiple mutations within the sarcomere protein encoding genes may cause a more severe type of HCM. For example, Girolami et al. (2010) identified in a cohort of 488 unrelated index HCM patients 4 patients (0.8%) who harbored triple mutations of the sarcomere proteins. The triple sarcomere defects were associated with an adverse outcome.

Mutations in the troponin genes (TNNC1, TNNT2, TNNI3) are accounting for less than 10% of patients with HCM. In a large series of 197 index patients living in France, Richard et al. (2003) detected disease-casing mutations in 63%, whereby mutations within the TNNT2 and TNNI3 gene accounted for 4% each.

3.3 TNNT2

In MEDLINE, reports on approx. 194 HCM patients from various living areas with a mutation of the TNNT2 gene have been published so far (Thierfelder et al., 1994; Watkins et al., 1995; Forissier et al., 1996; Moolman et al., 1997; Anan et al., 1998; Elliott et al., 1999; Ho et al., 2000; Varnava et al., 2001; Richard et al., 2003; Van Driest et al, 2003; Garcia-Castro et al., 2003; Torricelli et al., 2003; An et al., 2004; Theopistou et al., 2004; Miliou et al., 2005; Konno et al., 2005; Capek & Skvor, 2006; Menon et al., 2008; Xu et al., 2008; Gimeno et al., 2009). Table 4 summarizes those reports (86 families, 188 genetically affected subjects) which provided at least prognostic informations and/or some data on the phenotype. The median age (at the time of examination) is 40 years, 56.1% are females. Maximal left ventricular wall thickness was less than 15 mm in 49.5% of genetically affected subjects, only in 9.7% of patients, the wall thickness exceeded 25 mm. The ECG was abnormal in the majority of affected subjects (78.8%). Congestive heart failure (CHF, NYHA class ≥ II) was present in 42.9% of subjects. Prognostic data were available for 30 affected families, 19 lamented sudden cardiac death within their families. In additional 31 index patients, sudden cardiac death, heart transplantation or an ICD implantation was reported on 11 patients. Watkins et al. (1995) overlooked a series of 67 subjects over the age of 16 years who had TnT mutations. He noted that 24% of these individuals did not fulfill the clinical diagnostic criteria of HCM. The risk for disease-related death, however, was high (sudden cardiac death, death related to CHF). Varnava et al. (2001) investigated histologically 75 hearts with HCM. Blood samples from relatives and/or affected patients (before death) were available in 50 cases, allowing genotyping. Mutations in the TNNT2 gene were found in 9/50 patients, 8 of the 9 patients died suddenly. The heart weight was less, but the degree of disarray was significantly more in those patients with a mutation of the TNNT2 gene as compared to mutations of other genes. Other authors confirmed this constellation "minor LVH and high risk for sudden cardiac death" particularly for the following mutations: Phe87Leu (Gimeno et al., 2009), Arg92Trp (Moolman et al., 1997), Ala104Val (Nakajima-Taniguchiet et al., 1997), and Lys273Glu (Fujino et al., 2002).

3.4 TNNI3
Reports on approx. 99 patients have been published so far (Kimura et al., 1997; Kokado et al., 2000; Mörner et al., 2000; Niimura et al., 2002; Richard et al., 2003; Van Driest et al., 2003; Mogensen et al., 2004; Arad et al., 2005b; Brito & Madeira, 2005; Doolan et al., 2005; Sheng et al., 2008). Table 5 summarizes the reports (41 families, 87 genetically affected subjects) which provided prognostic informations or some data on phenotype. The median age (at the time of examination) is 46 years, 55.1% are females. Maximal left ventricular wall thickness was less than 15 mm in 53.2% of genetically affected subjects, in none the wall thickness exceeded 25 mm. An abnormal ECG was observed in 90.5% of genetically affected patients. Congestive heart failure was present in 36.4% subjects. In 24 of 37 families, sudden cardiac death or cardiac arrest occurred.

3.5 TNNC1
Only six cases with mutations of the TNNC1 gene have been published so far (Hoffmann et al., 2001; Landstrom et al., 2008; Chung et al., 2011) (Table 6). The first missense mutation within the TNNC1 gene (Leu29Gln) was described by Hoffmann et al. (2001) in a 60 year-old man with a moderate LV hypertrophy, ECG abnormalities and heart failure. The number of cases is too low to characterize a typical phenotype. Three of the 6 cases underwent myectomie, in a 19 year-old man, sudden cardiac death occurred.

3.6 Prognosis in patients with mutations of the genes encoding cTnT and cTnI
Overall, patients with mutations within the gene encoding cardiac troponin T and I are characterized by minor/moderate left ventricular hypertrophy, the maximal wall thickness of the LV does exceed 25 mm in a small percentage only. Despite the presence of minor/moderate LV hypertrophy, the rate of abnormal ECGs is high (> 75%). Furthermore,

congestive heart failure is not an infrequent complication (35-40% of the genetically affected patients). The rate of sudden cardiac death/arrest appears to be very high (> 30% of index patients or in related family members). Whereas some mutations are associated with sudden cardiac death at any age (e.g. the Lys183 deletion mutation in he TNNI3 gene; Kokado et al., 2000), others are associated with disease-related death predominantly in older carriers (e.g. the Phe87Leu mutation within the TNNT2 gene; Gimeno et al., 2009), or at younger age (e.g. the Arg92Trp mutation within troponin T; Moolman et al., 1997). Of note, the degree of disarray of the myocytes may not parallel the magnitude of hypertrophy: Gambrin et al. (2008) described a 22 year old women who underwent cardiac transplantation for restrictive filling pattern and CHF. Histology revealed severe disarray in the absence of hypertrophy. Genetic analysis disclosed an Arg204His mutation in the TNNI3 gene.

The mechanism of sudden cardiac death in patients with HCM is still under debate (Ho, 2010 a,b). For many years, the ischemia hypothesis has been proposed, that is increased oxygen demand due to increased LV mass and wall stress, combined with reduced oxygen supply due to reduced capillary density and abnormal narrowed intramural coronary arteries. This balance may further deteriorate if myocardial bridging with systolic compression of epicardial coronary artery is present (Yetman et al., 1998). The ischemia hypothesis is supported by a study of Spirito et al. (2000). These authors investigated the relation between the magnitude of hypertrophy and mortality in 480 consecutive patients with HCM. Over a follow-up period of 6.5 years, 65 patients died (23 sudden death, 15 CHF-related, 27 noncardiac cause or stroke). The risk of sudden death increased progressively with the wall thickness (0 per 1000 person-years for a wall thickness ≤ 15 mm, up to 18.2 per 1000 person-years for those with a wall thickness ≥ 30 mm).

3.7 What we can learn from patients with troponin mutations

What can we learn from the patients with troponin mutations? One important message to the clinicians is that the risk of sudden cardiac death does not go along with the severity of left ventricular hypertrophy/wall thickness. Furthermore, sudden cardiac death may occur in all age groups with troponin mutations. These observations imply that other mechanisms than ischemia-triggered rhythm disturbances may account for the excessive risk of sudden cardiac death in this subgroup (and other subgroups?) of patients with HCM. In transgenic mice expressing the TnT-I79N (Ile79Asn) mutation, no ventricular hypertrophy or fibrosis was detected, but ventricular ectopy and the rate of stress-induced ventricular tachycardia were significantly increased (Knollmann et al, 2003). Baudenbacher et al. (2008) showed in this mouse model that the risk of developing ventricular tachycardia appears to be directly proportional to the degree of Ca^{2+} sensitization caused by different troponin T mutations (TnT-I79N, TnT-F110I, and TnT-R278C). They gave first evidence that reduction of Ca^{2+}-sensitivity (by blebbistatin) in myofilaments acts "antiarrhythmic". This work by Baudenbacher and coworkers clearly demonstrates that changes in the intracellular Ca^{2+}-sensor cardiac troponin are associated with arrhythmias, and histological/anatomical changes which do often later develop in the course of hypertrophic cardiomyopathy, are not a prerequisite for these life-threatening arrhythmias. In our laboratory, we studied the effects of the cTnI-R145G mutation on adrenergic signalling in isolated rat ventricular cardiomyocytes (Reis et al., 2008). This mutation hinders the transduction of the phosphorylation signal from troponin to the thin filament. Upon adrenergic stimulation of the cardiomyocytes, rates of shortening and relengthening were significantly suppressed.

his suppression was evident in response to ß$_2$- but not ß$_1$-adrenergic stimulation. These ata demonstrate that adrenoceptor-mediated signalling may be altered by troponin utations. Since sudden cardiac death in patients with HCM often occurs during exercise or hysical activity, thus conditions with increased sympathetic activity, altered adrenergic ignalling may be a potential player in the pathogenesis of life-threatening arrhythmias. Many other mechanism are currently under investigation, including the role of the myocyte nhancer factor 2, transforming growth factor, connective tissue factor, and periostin in the evelopment of hypertrophy, diastolic dysfunction, and myocardial scarring (Seidman & eidman, 2011); also altered intracellular calcium handling and abnormalities in myocardial nergetics are under discussion to participate in this complex phenotype (Ho, 2010a,b). despite obvious progress, the precise link between the molecular defect and the complex henotype HCM is still not understood.

Patients/ Family	Age/Sex	**Clinical**	**Presentation**				Prognosis	References
		Septum (mm)	Wall (mm)	LVH type+	ECG	CHF		
;er69Phe								
ำ=1 (9 ınrelated SCD) Area: U.K.	29 M	n.a.	n.a.	n.a.	n.a.	n.a.	SCD	Varnava et al., 2001
?ro77Leu								
ำ=1 (9 ınrelated SCD) Area: U.K.	37 M	n.a.	n.a.	n.a.	n.a.	n.a.	SCD	Varnava et al., 2001
Ile79Asn								
ำ=9 (1 family + ınrelated p.) Area: multi- •thnic/racial	n.a.	13.4±4 (n=4)	n.a.	n.a.	n.a.	n.a.	4 SCD in family	Watkins et al., 1995
ำ=1 (9 ınrelated SCD) Area: U.K.	16 M	n.a.	n.a.	n.a.	n.a.	n.a.	SCD	Varnava et al., 2001
ำ=9 (1 family) Area: U.S.A.	50 F[1]	n.a.	n.a.	n.a.	n.a.	+	DCM, death at age 64	Menon et al., 2008
	68 F	10	9	normal	+	+	DCM, death at age 73	
	66 F[1]	18	10	n.a.	+	+	-	
	46 M[1]	16	12	n.a.	+	+	mixed DCM/HCM	
	58 M[1]	12	10	normal	+	+	RCM type	
	53 F[1]	14	11	n.a.	+	+	RCM type	
	49 F[1]	16	9	n.a.	+	+	-	
	40 F[1]	24	8	n.a.	+	+	-	
	48 F	14	10	n.a.	-	-	-	

Patients/ Family	Age/Sex	Clinical Presentation						References
		Septum (mm)	Wall (mm)	LVH type+	ECG	CHF	Prognosis	
Asp86Ala								
n=1(389 unrelated p.) Area: U.S.A.	39 M	n.a.	30	n.a.	n.a.	+	-	Van Driest et al., 2003
Phe87Leu								
n=7 (1 family) Area: Spain	52 F	14	n.a.	n.a.	+	+	SCD in family	Gimeno et al., 2009
	39 M	13	n.a.	n.a.	+	+	"	
	40 F	14	n.a.	n.a.	+	+	", ICD	
	30 F	18	n.a.	n.a.	+	+	", ICD	
	30 M	27	n.a.	n.a.	+	-	"	
	29 F	25	n.a.	n.a.	+	+	"	
	9 M	12	n.a.	n.a.	+	-	"	
Arg92Gln								
n=1 (150 unrelated p.) Area: Toscana	23 M	29	n.a.	III	+	-	-	Thierfelder et al., 1994; Torricelli et al., 2003
n=32 (3 families + unrelated p.) Area : multi-ethnic/racial	n.a.	n.a.	15.0±6 (n=21)	n.a.	n.a.	n.a.	SCD in 11 p	Watkins et al., 1995
Arg92Trp								
n=18 (2 families) Area: South Africa	56 F	14	12	n.a.	+	n.a.	SCD in family	Moolman et al., 1997
	57 F	13	12	n.a.	+	n.a.	"	
	41 F	12	13	n.a.	+	n.a.	"	
	28 F	24	11	n.a.	+	n.a.	"	
	35 F	13.8	7.5	n.a.	-	n.a.	"	
	23 F	6	6	-	+	n.a.	"	
	21 M	normal	normal	-	+	n.a.	"	
	38 M	9	9	-	+	n.a.	"	
	35 F	8	8	-	+	n.a.	"	
	28 M	7	8	-	+	n.a.	"	
	47 F	7	7	-	-	n.a.	"	
	27 F	6	6	-	-	n.a.	"	
	9 F	4	4	-	-	n.a.	"	
	28 M	8.5	8.5	-	-	n.a.	"	
	15 F	5	5	-	-	n.a.	"	
	11 F	7	7	-	-	n.a.	"	
	34 F	18-20	11	n.a.	+	n.a.	"	
	56 F	8	7	-	+	n.a.	"	
n=1 (389 unrelated p.) Area : U.S.A.	27 F	n.a.	32	n.a.	n.a.	-	-	Van Driest et al., 2003
n=2(9 unrelated SCD) Area.U.K.	22 M	n.a.	n.a..	n.a.	n.a.	n.a.	SCD	Varnava et al., 2001
	6 F	n.a.	n.a.	n.a.	n.a.	+	transplant	

Patients/ Family	Age/Sex	Clinical Presentation					Prognosis	References
		Septum (mm)	Wall (mm)	LVH type+	ECG	CHF		
Arg92Leu								
n=1 (9 unrelated SCD) Area: U.K.	26 M	n.a.	n.a.	n.a.	n.a.	n.a.	SCD	Varnava et al., 2001
n=4 (1 family) Area: France	43 F	n.a.	19	n.a.	-	+	CHF at 44 y	Forissier et al., 1996
	23 M	n.a.	35	n.a.	+	+	n.a	
	20 F	n.a.	n.a.	apical	+	+	n.a.	
	45 F	n.a.	10	n.a.	+	-	n.a.	
Arg94Leu								
n=2 (9 unrelated SCD) Area: U.K.	17 M	n.a.	n.a.	n.a.	n.a.	n.a.	SCD	Varnava et al., 2001
	21 F	n.a.	n.a.	n.a.	n.a.	n.a.	SCD	
Ala104Val								
n=4 (1 family) Area: Japan	50 F	15	8	n.a.	+	+	SCD at age 50	Nakajima-Taniguchi et al., 1997
	36 F	17	6	n.a.	+	+	SCD at age 36	
	54 F	17	8	n.a.	+	+	ventricular tachycardia	
	33 F	20	12	n.a.	+	-	-	
Phe110Ile								
n=2 (1 family) Area : multi-ethnic/racial	n.a.	n.a.	17 (n=2)	n.a.	n.a.	n.a.	-	Watkins et al., 1995
n=16 (6 families) Area : Japan	38 F	27	17	III	+	-	-	Anan et al., 1998
	69 F	22	14	III	+	-	SCD in family	
	47 F	20	13	III	+	-	SCD in family	
	87 F	9	9	IV	+	-	-	
	48 M	10	10	IV	+	-	-	
	42 F	11	11	normal	-	-	-	
	64 M	23	10	II	+	-	-	
	70 M	20	11	II	+	-	-	
	47 F	13	13	III	+	-	-	
	45 M	12	10	normal	+	-	-	
	39 F	13	13	III	+	-	-	
	24 F	11	11	IV	+	-	-	
	56 F	19	11	II	+	-	SCD in family	
	53 M	15	13	III	+	-	"	
	31 F	21	12	II	+	-	"	
	28 F	10	10	normal	+	-	"	
Phe110Val								
n=3 (150 unrelated p.) Area: Italy	28 F	32	n.a.	III	+	-	-	Torricelli et al., 2003
	48 F	21	n.a.	III	+	n.a.	-	
	82 M	15	n.a.	II	+	n.a.	-	

Patients/ Family	Age/Sex	Clinical Presentation					Prognosis	References
		Septum (mm)	Wall (mm)	LVH type+	ECG	CHF		
Lys124Asn n=1 (71 unrelated p.) Area : China	41 F	n.a.	n.a.	LVH	n.a.	n.a.	-	An et al., 2004
Arg130Cys n=2 (150 unrelated p.) Area: Italy	55 M	23	n.a.	III	+	-	-	Torricelli et al., 2003
	58 F	13	n.a.	n.a.	+	-	-	
Glu160 n=32 (2 families +unrelated p.) Area : multi-ethnic/racial	n.a.	n.a.	17.5±5 (n=14)	n.a.	n.a.	n.a.	SCD in 14	Watkins et al., 1995
n=2 (150 unrelated p.) Area: Italy	50 F	20	n.a.	III	+	-	-	Torricelli et al., 2203
	55 M	22	n.a.	III	+	+	-	
Glu163Lys n=5(1 family + unrelated p.) Area. multi-ethnic/racial	n.a.	n.a.	19.8±8 (n=5)	n.a.	n.a.	n.a.	SCD in 0	Watkins et al., 1995
Ser179Phe n=1 (1 family) Area: Kuwait	17 M	25	11	n.a	+	-	SCD	Ho et al., 2000
Glu244Asp n=1 (1 family) Area: multi-ethnic/racial	n.a.	n.a.	n.a.	n.a.	n.a.	n.a.	SCD in 0	Watkins et al., 1995
Lys247Arg n=1 (30 unrelated p.) Area: Spain	60 F	23	n.a.	n.a.	n.a.	n.a.	-	Garcia-Castro et al., 2003
Intron 15 G1→A n=28 (1 family +unrelated p.) Area: multi-ethnic/racial	n.a.	n.a.	17.5±5 (n=17)	n.a.	n.a.	n.a.	SCD in 9	Watkins et al., 1995
n=1 (9 unrelated SCD) Area. U.K.	15 M	n.a.	n.a.	n.a.	n.a.	n.a.	SCD	Varnava et al., 2001
Asn271Ile 3 (1 family) Area: Spain	62 M	22	n.a.	n.a.	+	-	-	Gimeno et al., 2009
	36 M	14	n.a.	n.a.	+	-	-	
	31 F	9	n.a.	n.a.	-	-	-	

Patients/ Family	Age/Sex	Clinical Presentation					Prognosis	References
		Septum (mm)	Wall (mm)	LVH type+	ECG	CHF		
Lys273Glu								
n=8 (2 families) Area: Japan	58 F	7	8	n.a.	n.a.	n.a.	DCM features	Fujino et al., 2002
	32 F	23	7	asym.	n.a.	n.a	-	
	29 F	23	10	asym.	n.a.	n.a.	-	
	75 F	15	13	n.a.	n.a.	n.a.	SCD in family	
	78 F	15	11	asym.	n.a.	n.a.	"	
	75 F	16	9	asym.	n.a.	n.a.	"	
	49 F	20	9	asym	n.a.	n.a.	"	
	46 M	21	10	asym	n.a.	n.a.	"	
Arg278Cys								
n=3 (1 family + unrelated p.) Area: multi-ethnic/racial	n.a.	n.a.	16.3±6 (n=3)	n.a.	n.a.	n.a.	SCD in 1	Watkins et al., 1995
n=3(389 unrelated p.) Area: U.S.A.	57 M	n.a.	20	n.a.	n.a.	-	-	Van Driest et al.,, 2003
	66 M	n.a.	15	n.a.	n.a.	+	pacemaker	
	74 M	n.a.	23	n.a.	n.a.	+	TASH	
n=1 Area: U.K.	57 M	12	n.a.	n.a.	+	+	late onset HCM	Elliott et al., 1999
n=1 (30 unrelated p.) Area: Spain	60 F	22	n.a.	n.a.	n.a.	n.a.	-	Garcia-Castro et al., 2003
n=8 (2 families) Area: Spain	55 F	22	n.a.	n.a.	+	+	-	Gimeno et al., 2009
	59 M	22	n.a.	n.a.	+	+	-	
	27 M	12	n.a.	n.a.	-	-	-	
	30 M	10	n.a.	n.a.	-	-	-	
	29 M	10	n.a.	n.a.	-	-	-	
	21 M	40	n.a.	n.a.	+	+	ICD-Impl.	
	64 M	26	n.a.	n.a.	+	-	-	
	33 M	11	n.a.	n.a.	+	-	-	
n=6 (2 families) Area: Greek	40 M	20	11	asym	+	+	SCD in family	Theopistou et al., 2004
	71 F	13	12	conc.	+	+	"	
	41 M	10	8	normal	-	n.a.	"	
	38 M	10	10	normal	-	n.a.	"	
	14 F	7	8	normal	-	n.a.	"	
	13 M	22	11	asym.	+	-	SCD age 15	
n=1 (150 unrelated p.) Area: Italy	66 M	24	n.a.	III	+	+	-	Torricelli et al., 2003

Patients/ Family	Age/Sex	Clinical Presentation					Prognosis	References
		Septum (mm)	Wall (mm)	LVH type+	ECG	CHF		
Arg278Pro								
n=1 (389 unrelated p.) Area: U.S.A.	47 M	n.a.	19	n.a.	n.a.	+	ICD	Van Driest et al., 2003
n=1 (143 unrelated p.) Area : Greek	18 M	n.a.	n.a.	LVH	n.a.	n.a.	-	Miliou et al., 2005
Arg286Cys								
n=1 (143 unrelated p.) Area : Greek	26 F	n.a.	n.a.	LVH	n.a.	n.a.	-	Miliou et al., 2005
Arg286His								
n=2 (389 unrelated p.) Area: U.S.A.	49 M	n.a.	20	n.a.	n.a.	-	-	Van Driest et al., 2003
	39 M	n.a.	25	n.a.	n.a.	+	myectomy	

Table 4. Mutations in the TNNT2 Gene Associated with HCM

Number of affected patients is given (out of a group of unrelated HCM patients or families with HCM). Age=age at investigation if not otherwise noted; [1]age at diagnosis; n.a.=data not available; SCD=sudden cardiac death; DCM=dilated cardiomyopathy like-type; RCM=restrictive cardiomyopathy like-type; CHF=congestive heart failure; TASH=transcoronary septal ablation; ICD=internal automated defibrillator; area=living area of study patients. +Left ventricular hypertrophy (LVH) is classified according to according to Maron et al. (1981) type I=confined to the anterior segment of the ventricular septum, type II=involved anterior and posterior septum, type III=involvement of both the septum and the free wall of the left ventricle, and type IV=regions other than the basal and anterior septum (e.g. apical area).

Patients/Family	Age/Sex	Clinical Presentation					Prognosis	Reference
		Septum (mm)	Wall (mm)	LVH type+	ECG	CHF		
Arg21Cys								
n=1 (15 unrelated p.) Area: Europa	40 F	n.a.	n.a.	apical	n.a.	n.a.	SCD in family	Arad et al., 2005
Pro82Ser								
1 pt. with late-onset HCM Area: n.a.	> 40	n.a.	n.a.	LVH	+	+	n.a.	Niimura et al., 2002
Arg141Gln								
n=1 (389 unrelated p.) Area: U.S.A	41 M	n.a.	25	n.a.	n.a.	-	-	Van Driest et al., 2003
Arg145Gln								
n=1 (1 family) Area : U.K.	n.a.	21	n.a	apical	+	n.a.	n.a	Mogensen et al., 2004

Patients/Family	Age/Sex	Clinical Presentation					Prognosis	Reference
		Septum (mm)	Wall (mm)	LVH type+	ECG	CHF		
Ala157Val								
n=5 (3 families) Area : U.K.	n.a.	n.a.	n.a.	n.a.	+	n.a.	SCD in family	Mogensen et al., 2004
n=1 (1 family) Area: Portugal	24 M	n.a.	n.a.	LVH	*	*	SCD at age 44	Brito & Madeira, 2005
Arg162Gln								
n=7 (3 families) Area: U.K.	n.a.	n.a.	n.a.	n.a.	n.a.	n.a	SCD in family	Mogensen et al., 2004
n=2 (389 unrelated p.) Area: U.S.A.	76 F	n.a.	17	n.a.	n.a.	+	myectomy	Van Driest et al., 2003
	33 M	n.a.	19	n.a.	n.a.	+	SCD in family	
n=3 (1 family) Area: Australia	70 M	n.a.	n.a.	n.a.	n.a.	n.a.	n.a.	Doolan et al., 2005
	44 M	n.a.	10	normal	-	-	-	
	40 M	n.a.	10	normal	-	-	-	
Arg162Pro								
n=2 (1 family) Area: Australia	52 F	n.a.	9	normal.	-	-	-	Doolan et al., 2005
	25 F	n.a.	14	n.a.	+	-	cardiac arrest at age 21	
Ser166Phe								
n=3 (389 unrelated p.) Area: U.S.A.	48 F	n.a.	22	n.a.	n.a.	+	myectomy	Van Driest et al., 2003
	79 F	n.a.	14	n.a.	n.a.	+	myectomy	
	21 F	n.a.	17	n.a.	n.a.	+	myectomy	
n=1 (1 family) Area: U.K.	n.a.	19	n.a.	n.a.	+	n.a	-	Mogensen et al., 2004
Lys183Glu								
n=3 (1 family) Area: U.K.	n.a.	n.a.	n.a.	n.a.	+	n.a	-	Mogensen et al., 2004
Lys183del								
n=25 (7 families) Area: Japan	65 F	13	7	I/II	+	n.a.	SCD in family	Kokado et al., 2000
	61 F	17	12	I/II	+	n.a.	"	
	51 F	9	10	normal	+	n.a.	"	
	46 F	20	10	I/II	+	n.a.	"	
	36 F	16	8	I/II	+	n.a.	"	
	48 F	7	7	normal	+	n.a.	"	
	36 M	18	13	III	+	n.a.	"	
	33 F	21	9	I/II	+	n.a.	"	
	47 F	10	8	normal	+	n.a.	"	
	27 F	13	9	III	+	n.a.	"	
	8 M	5	5	normal	-	n.a.	"	
	85 M	14	10	I/II	+	n.a.	"	
	56 F	23	11	IV	+	n.a.	"	
	48 F	13	14	IV	+	n.a.	"	
	71 F	11	10	normal	+	n.a.	"	

Patients/Family	Age/Sex	Clinical Presentation					Prognosis	Reference
		Septum (mm)	Wall (mm)	LVH type+	ECG	CHF		
	49 M	5	9	normal	+	n.a.	"	
	24 F	20	11	I/II	+	n.a.	"	
	23 F	9	8	normal	+	n.a.	"	
	66 F	11	11	normal	+	n.a.	"	
	62 M	13	12	normal	+	n.a.	"	
	35 M	12	11	normal	-	n.a.	"	
	48 M	10	13	LVH	+	n.a.	"	
	24 M	13	10	LVH	+	n.a.	"	
	68 F	19	11	I/II	+	n.a.	"	
	78 F	22	13	I/II	+	n.a.	"	
Arg186Gln n=5 (2 families) Area: U.K.	n.a.	n.a.	n.a.	n.a.	n.a.	n.a	SCD in family	Mogensen et al., 2004
Asp196Asn n=4 (2 families) Area: U.K.	n.a.	n.a.	n.a.	n.a.	+	n.a	-	Mogensen et al., 2004
n=1 with late-onset HCM Area: n.a.	>40	n.a.	LVH	+	+	n.a.	n.a.	Niimura et al., 2002
Leu198Pro n=1 (1 family) Area: Australia	15 M	n.a.	22	n.a.	+	-	SCD at age 15	Doolan et al., 2005
Ser199Gly n=1 (1 family) Area: U.K.	n.a.	n.a.	n.a.	apical	+	n.a.	-	Mogensen et al., 2004
Ser199Asn n=8 (2 families) Area: U.K.	n.a.	n.a.	n.a.	n.a.	+	n.a.	SCD in family	Mogensen et al., 2004
n=1 (1 family) Area: Portugal	52 M	n.a.	n.a.	LVH	+	-	cardiac arrest at age 61	Brito & Madeira, 2005
Glu202Gly n=1 (1 family) Area: U.K.	n.a.	19	n.a.	n.a.	+	n.a.	-	Mogensen et al., 2004
Gly203Arg n=2 (1 family) Area: U.K.	n.a.	n.a.	n.a.	n.a.	+	n.a.	-	Mogensen et al., 2004
Gly203 frameshift n=4 (1 family) Area: Sweden	71 F	9	9	normal	+	+	-	Mörner et al., 2000
	61 M	15	8	LVH	+	-	-	
	64 M	16	14	LVH	+	-	-	
	27 F	8	7	normal	-	-	-	
Arg204His n=3 (1 family) Area: Australia	37 M	n.a.	17	n.a.	+	-	cardiac arrest at age 17	Doolan et al., 2005
	9 M	n.a.	7	normal	+	-	-	
	5 M	n.a.	5	normal	+	-	-	

Table 5. Mutations in the TNNI3 Gene Associated with HCM

Patients/ Family	Age/Sex	Clinical Presentation					Prognosis	Reference
		Septum (mm)	Wall (mm)	LVH type+	ECG	CHF		
Ala8Val n=1 (1025 unrelated p.) Area: U.S.A./ Caucasian	37M	18	n..a	n.a.	n.a.	+	myectomy	Landstrom et al., 2008
Leu29Gln n=1 Area: Germany	60 M	15	15	n.a.	+	+	n.a.	Hoffmann et al. ,2001
Cys84Tyr n=1 (1025 unrelated p.) Area: U.S.A./ Caucasian	17 M	19	n.a.	n.a.	n.a.	-	n.a.	Landstrom et al., 2008
Glu134Asp n=1 (1015 unrelated p.) Area: U.S.A./ Caucasian	22 F	26	n.a.	n.a.	n.a.	+	myectomy	Landstrom et al., 2008
Asp145Glu n=1 (1025 unrelated p.) Area: U.S.A./ Caucasian	58 M	22	n..a	n.a.	n.a.	+	myectomy	Landstrom et al., 2008
c.363dupG frameshift n=1(1 family) Area: U.S.A.	19 M	n.a.	n.a.	n.a.	n.a.	n.a.	SCD	Chung et al., 2011

Table 6. Mutations in the TNNC1 Gene Associated with HCM

4. References

Abbott, M. B., Gaponenko, V., Abusamhadneh, E., Finley, N., Li, G., Dvoretsky, A., Rance, M., Solaro, R. J. & Rosevear, P. R. (2000). Regulatory domain conformational exchange and linker region flexibility in cardiac troponin C bound to cardiac troponin I. *J. Biol. Chem.*, 275, pp. 20610-7

Abbott, M. B., Dong, W. J., Dvoretsky, A., DaGue, B., Caprioli, R. M., Cheung, H. C. & Rosevear, P. R. (2001). Modulation of cardiac troponin C-cardiac troponin I regulatory interactions by the amino-terminus of cardiac troponin I. *Biochemistry*, 40, pp. 5992-6001

An, F. S., Zhang, Y., Li, D. Q., Yang, X. S., Li L, Zhang, C, Yan, M.L., Wang, Y. & An, G. P. (2004). A novel missense mutation, K124N, in the troponin T gene of Chinese populations with hypertrophic cardiomyopathy. *Zhonghua Yi Xue Za Zhi*. 84(16), pp. 1340-3

Anan, R., Shono, H., Kisanuki, A., Arima, S., Nakao, S. &Tanaka, H. (1998). Patients with familial hypertrophic cardiomyopathy caused by a Phe110Ile missense mutation in the cardiac troponin T gene have variable cardiac morphologies and a favorable prognosis. *Circulation*, 98, pp. 391-7-3

Anderson, P. A., Malouf, N. N., Oakeley, A.E., Pagani, E. D. & Allen, P. D. (1991). Troponin T isoform expression in humans. A comparison among normal and failing adult heart, fetal heart, and adult and fetal skeletal muscle. *Circ. Res.*, 69(5), pp. 1226-33

Arad, M., Maron, B. J., Gorham, J. M., Johnson, W. H., Saul, J. P., Perez-Atayde, A. R., Spirito, P., Wright, G. B., Kanter, R.J., Seidman, C. E., Seidman, J. G. (2005a). Glycogen storage diseases presenting as hypertrophic cardiomyopathy. *N Engl J Med.*, 352(4), pp. 362-72

Arad, M., Penas-Lado, M., Monserrat, L., Maron, B. J., Sherrid, M., Ho, C. Y., Barr, S., Karim, A., Olson, T. M., Kamisago, M., Seidman, J. G. &, Seidman C. E. (2005b). Gene mutation in apical hypertrophic cardiomyopathy. *Circulation*, 112, pp. 2805-2811

Baudenbacher, F., Schober, T., Pinto, J.R., Sidorov, V.Y., Hilliard, F., Solaro, R. J., Potter, J. D. & Knollmann, B. C. (2008). Myofilament Ca2+ sensitization causes susceptibility to cardiac arrhythmia in mice. *J. Clin. Invest.*, 118(12), pp. 3893-903

Barta, J., Tóth, A., Jaquet, K., Redlich, A., Edes, I. & Papp, Z. (2003). Calpain-1-dependent degradation of troponin I mutants found in familial hypertrophic cardiomyopathy. *Mol Cell Biochem,.* 251(1-2), pp. 83-8

Baryshnikova, O. K., Li, M. X. & Sykes, B. D. (2008). Modulation of Cardiac Troponin C Function by the Cardiac-Specific N-Terminus of Troponin I: Influence of PKA Phosphorylation and Involvement in Cardiomyopathies. *J. Mol. Biol.*, 375(3), pp. 735-51

Biesiadecki, B. J., Chong, S. M., Nosek, T. M. & Jin, J. P. (2007). Troponin T core structure and the regulatory NH2-terminal variable region. *Biochemistry*, 46(5), pp. 1368-79

Braunwald, E. & Ebert, P. A. (1962). Hemodynamic alterations in idiopathic hypertrophic subaortic stenosis induced by sympathomimetic drugs. *Am. J. Cardiol.*, 10, pp. 489-95

Brito, D. & Madeira, H. (2005). Malignant mutations in hypertrophic cardiomyopathy: fact or fancy? *Rev. Port. Cardiol.*, 24(9), pp. 1137-46

Burhop, J., Rosol, M., Craig, R., Tobacman, L. S. & Lehman W. (2001). Effects of a cardiomyopathy-causing troponin t mutation on thin filament function and structure. *J. Biol. Chem.*, 276(23), pp. 20788-94

Cannan, C. R., Reeder, G. S., Bailey, K. R., Melton, L. J. & Gersh, B. J. (1995). Natural history of hypertrophic cardiomyo-pathy. A population-based study, 1976 through 1990. *Circulation*, 92, pp. 2488-95

Capek, P. & Skvor, J. (2006). Hypertrophic cardiomyoptahy. Molecular genetic analysis of exons 9 and 11 of the TNNT2 gene in Czech patients. *Methods Inf. Med.*, 45, pp. 169-72

Carballo, S., Robinson, P., Otway, R., Fatkin, D., Jongbloed, J. D., de Jonge, N., Blair, E., van Tintelen, J. P., Redwood, C. & Watkins, H. (2009). Identification and functional characterization of cardiac troponin I as a novel disease gene in autosomal dominant dilated cardiomyopathy. *Circ. Res.*, 105(4), pp. 375-82

Chandra, M., Tschirgi, M. L. & Tardiff, J. C. (2005). Increase in tension dependent ATP consumption induced by cardiac troponin T mutation. *AJP Heart*, 289(5), pp. H2112-9

Chong, P. C. & Hodges, R. S. (1982). Photochemical cross-linking between rabbit skeletal troponin and alpha-tropomyosin. Attachment of the photoaffinity probe N-(4-

azidobenzoyl-[2-3H]glycyl)-S-(2-thiopyridyl)-cysteine to cysteine 190 of alpha-tropomyosin. *J. Biol. Chem.*, 257(15), pp. 9152-60

Chung, W. K., Kitner, C. & Maron, B. J. (2011). Novel frameshift mutation in troponin C (TNNC1) associated with hypertrophic cardiomyopathy and sudden death. *Cardiol. Young*, Jan 25, epub ahead of print

Cooper, T. A. & Ordahl, C. P. (1985). A single cardiac troponin T gene generates embryonic and adult isoforms via developmentally regulated alternate splicing. *J. Biol. Chem.*, 260(20), pp. 11140-8

Davis, J. P. & Tikunova, S. B. (2008). Ca(2+) exchange with troponin C and cardiac muscle dynamics. *Cardiovasc. Res.*, 77(4), pp. 619-26. Review.

Davis, J. & Metzger, J. M. (2010). Combinatorial effects of double cardiomyopathy mutant alleles in rodent myocytes: a predictive cellular model of myofilament dysregulation in disease. *PLoS One*, 5(2), pp e9140

Deng, Y., Schmidtmann, A., Redlich, A., Westerdorf, B., Jaquet, K. & Thieleczek, R. (2001). Effects of phosphorylation and mutation R145G on human cardiac troponin I function. *Biochemistry*, 40(48), pp. 14593-602

Deng, Y., Schmidtmann, A., Kruse, S., Filatov, V., Heilmeyer, L. M. Jr., Jaquet, K. & Thieleczek, R. (2003). Phospho-rylation of human cardiac troponin I G203S and K206Q linked to familial hypertrophic cardiomyopathy affects actomyosin interaction in different ways. *J Mol Cell Cardiol.*, 35(11), pp. 1365-74

Doolan, A., Tebo, M., Ingles, J., Nguyen, L., Tsoutsman, T., Lam, L., Chiu, C., Chung, J., Weintraub, R. G., Semsarian, C. (2005). Cardiac troponin I mutations in Australian families with hypertrophic cardiomyopathy: clinical, genetic and functional consequences. *J Mol Cell Cardiol.*, 38(2), pp. 387-393

Dong, W. J., Xing, J., Villain, M., Hellinger, M., Robinson, J. M., Chandra, M., Solaro, R. J., Umeda, P. K. & Cheung, H. C. (1999). Conformation of the regulatory domain of cardiac muscle troponin C in its complex with cardiac troponin I. *J Biol Chem.*, 274(44), pp. 31382-90

Dong, W. J., Xing, J., Ouyang, Y., An, J. & Cheung, H. C. (2008). Structural kinetics of cardiac troponin C mutants linked to familial hypertrophic and dilated cardiomyopathy in troponin complexes. *J Biol Chem.*, 283(6), pp. 3424-32

Dweck, D., Hus, N. & Potter, J. D. (2008). Challeging current paradigm related to cardiomyopathies. *J Biol Chem.*, 283, pp. 33119-28

Ebashi, S. (1972). Calcium ions and muscle contraction. *Nature*, 240, pp. 217-8

Elliott, P. M, D'Cruz, L. & McKenna, W. J. (1999). Late-onset hypertrophic cardiomyopathy caused by a mutation in the cardiac troponin T gene. *N Engl J Med.*, 341, pp. 1855 (letter)

Elliott, P. M., Andersson, B., Arbustini, E., Bilinska, Z., Cecchi, F., Charron, P., Dubourg, O., Kühl, U., Maisch, B., McKenna, W. J., Monserrat, L., Pankuweit, S., Rapezzi, C., Seferovic, P., Tavazzi, L. & Keren, A. (2008). Classification of the cardiomyopathies: a position statement from the European Society Of Cardiology Working Group on myocardial and pericardial diseases. *Eur Heart J.*, 29, pp. 270-6

Elliott, P. M., McKenna, W. J. (2004). Hypertrophic cardiomyopathy. *Lancet*, 363, pp. 1881-91

Fatkin, D., Seidman, J. G. & Seidman, C. E. Hypertrophic cardiomyopathy. In: Willersen, J. T., Cohn, J. N., Wellens, H. J. J. & Holmes, D. R. (eds.) Cardiovascular Medicine, 3rd edition, 2007, pp. 1261-84

Feliciello, A., Gottesman, M. E. & Avvedimento, E. V. (2001). The biological functions of A-kinase anchor proteins. *J Mol Biol.,* 308(2), pp. 99-114

Feng, H. Z., Biesiadecki, B. J., Yu, Z. B., Hossain, M. M. & Jin, J. P. (2008). Restricted N-terminal truncation of cardiac troponin T: a novel mechanism for functional adaptation to energetic crisis. *J Physiol.,* 586(14), pp. 3537-50

Finley, N., Abbott, M. B., Abusamhadneh, E., Gaponenko, V., Dong, W., Gasmi-Seabrook, G., Howarth, J. W., Rance, M., Solaro, R. J., Cheung, H. C., Rosevear, P. R. (1999) NMR analysis of cardiac troponin C-troponin I complexes: effects of phosphorylation. *FEBS Lett.* 453,107-112.

Flicker, P. F., Phillips, G. N., Jr. & Cohen, C. (1982). Troponin and its interactions with tropomyosin. An electron microscope study. *J Mol Biol.,* 162(2), pp. 495-501

Forissier, J. F., Carrier, L., Farza, H., Bonne, G., Bercovici, J., Richard, P., Hainque, B., Townsend, P. J., Yacoub, M. H., Faure, S., Dubourg, O., Millaire, A., Hagege, A. A., Desnos, M., Komajda, M. & Schwartz, K. (1996). Codon 102 of the cardiac troponin T gene is a putative hot spot for mutations in familial hypertrophic cardiomyopathy. *Circulation,* 94, pp. 3069-3073

Foster, D. B., Noguchi, T., VanBuren, P., Murphy, A. M. & Van Eyk, J. E. (2003). C-terminal truncation of cardiac troponin I causes divergent effects on ATPase and force: implications for the pathophysiology of myocardial stunning. *Circ Res.,* 93, pp. 917-24

Frenneaux, M. P. (2004). Assessing the risk of sudden cardiac death in a patient with hypertrophic cardiomyopathy. *Heart,* 90, pp. 570-5

Fuchs, F. & Grabarek, Z. (2011). The Ca2+/Mg2+ sites of troponin C modulate crossbridge-mediated thin filament activation in cardiac myofibrils. *Biochem Biophys Res Commun.* 408(4), pp. 697-700

Fujino, N., Shimizu, M., Ino, H., Okeie, K., Yamaguchi, M., Yasuda, T., Kokado, H. & Mabuchi, H. (2001). Cardiac troponin T Arg92Trp mutation and progression from hypertrophic to dilated cardiomyopathy. *Clin Cardiol.,* 24(5), pp. 397-402

Fujino, N., Shiizu, M., Ino, H., Yamaguchi, M., Yasuda, T., Nagata, M., Konno, T. & Mabuchi, H. (2002). A novel mutation Lys273Glu in the cardiac troponin T gene shows high degree of penetrance and transition from hypertrophic to dilated cardiomyopathy. *Am J Cardiol.,* 89, 29-33

Galinska-Rakoczy, A., Engel, P., Xu, C., Jung, H., Craig, R., Tobacman, L. S. & Lehman, W. (2008). Structural basis for the regulation of muscle contraction by troponin and tropomyosin. *J Mol Biol.* , 379, pp. 929-35

Galińska, A., Hatch, V., Craig, R., Murphy, A. M., Van Eyk, J. E., Wang, C. L., Lehman, W. & Foster, D. B. (2010). The C terminus of cardiac troponin I stabilizes the Ca2+-activated state of tropomyosin on actin filaments. *Circ Res.,* 106(4), pp. 705-11

Gambarin, F. I., Tagliani, M. & Arbustini, E. (2008). Pure restrictive cardiomyopathy associated with cardiac troponin I gene mutation: mismatch between the lack of hypertrophy and the presence of disarray. *Heart,* 94(10), pp. 1257

Gaponenko, V., Abusamhadneh, E., Abbott, M. B., Finley, N., Gasmi-Seabrook, G., Solaro, R. J., Rance, M. & Rosevear, P. R. (1999) Effects of troponin I phosphorylation on conformational exchange in the regulatory domain of cardiac troponin C. *J. Biol. Chem.,* 274, pp. 16681-4 arcia-Castro, M., Ruguero, J. R., Batalla, A., Diaz-Molina, B., Gonzalez, P., Alvarez, V., Cortina, A., Cubero, G. I. & Coto, E. (2003). Hypertrophic cardiomyopathy: low frequency of mutations in the ß-myosin heavy chain (MYH7) and cardiac troponin T (TNNT2) genes among Spanish patients. *Clin Chem.*, 49(8), pp. 1279-85

asmi-Seabrook, G. M., Howarth, J. W., Finley, N., Abusamhadneh, E., Gaponenko, V., Brito, R. M., Solaro, R. J. & Rosevear, P. R. (1999). Solution structures of the C-terminal domain of cardiac troponin C free and bound to the N-terminal domain of cardiac troponin I. *Biochemistry*, 38(26), pp. 8313-22. Erratum in: *Biochemistry*. (1999) 38(43), pp. 14432

eisterfer-Lowrance, A. A, Kass, S., Tanigawa, G., Vosberg, H. P., McKenna, W., Seidman, C. E. & Seidman, J. G. (1990). A molecular basis for familial hypertrophic cardiomyopathy: a beta cardiac myoson heavy chain gene missense mutation. *Cell*, 62 (5), pp. 999-1006

imeno, J. R., Monserrat, L., Perez-Sanchez, I., Marin, F., Caballero, L., Hermida-Prieto, M., Castro, A. & Valdes, M. (2009). Hypertrophic cardiomyopathy: a study of the troponin-T gene in 127 Spanish families. *Rev Esp Cardiol.*, 62(12), pp. 1473-7

illis, T. E., Liang, B., Chung, F. & Tibbits, G. F. (2005). Increasing cardiomyocyte contractility with residues identified in trout troponin C. *Physiol Gen.*, 22, pp. 1-7

irolami, F., Ho, C. Y., Semsarian, C., Baldi, M., Will, M. L., Baldini, K., Torricelli, F., Yeates, L., Cecchi, F., Ackerman, M. J. & Olivotto, I. (2010). Clinical features and outcome of hypertrophic cardiomyopathy associated with triple sarcomere protein gene mutations. *J Am Coll Cardiol.*, 55(14), pp. 1444-53

omes, A. V., Guzman, G., Zhao, J. & Potter, J. D. (2002). Cardiac troponin T isoforms affect the Ca²⁺ sensitivity and inhibition of force development. Insights into the role of troponin T isoforms in the heart. *J Biol Chem.*, 277, pp. 35341–49

omes, A. V., Barnes, J. A., Harada, K. & Potter, J. D. (2004). Role of troponin T in disease. *Mol Cell Biochem.* ,263(1-2), pp. 115-29. Review.

omes, A. V. & Potter, J. D. (2004). Cellular and molecular aspects of familial hypertrophic cardiomyopathy caused by mutations in the cardiac troponin I gene. *Mol Cell Biochem.*, 263(1-2), pp. 99-114. Review.

omes, A. V. & Potter, J. D. (2004). Molecular and cellular aspects of troponin cardiomyopathies. *Ann N Y Acad Sci.* 1015, pp. 214-24. Review.

omes, A. V., Harada, K. & Potter, J. D. (2005). A mutation in the N-terminus of troponin I that is associated with hypertrophic cardiomyopathy affects the Ca2+-sensitivity, phosphorylation kinetics and proteolytic susceptibility of troponin. *J Mol Cell Cardiol.*, 39, pp. 754-5

omes, A. V., Venkatraman, G., Davis, J. P., Tikunova, S. B., Engel, P., Solaro, R. J. & Potter, J. D. (2004). Cardiac troponin T isoforms affect the Ca(2+) sensitivity of force development in the presence of slow skeletal troponin I: insights into the role of troponin T isoforms in the fetal heart. *J Biol Chem.*, 279(48), pp. 49579-87

usev, N. B, Dobrovolskii, A. B & Severin, S. E. (1980). Isolation and some properties of troponin T kinase from rabbit skeletal muscle. *Biochem J.*, 189(2), pp. 219-26

ernandez, O. M., Szczesna-Cordary, D., Knollmann, B. C., Miller, T., Bell, M., Zhao, J., Sirenko, S. G., Diaz, Z., Guzman, G., Xu, Y., Wang, Y., Kerrick, W. G. & Potter, J. D. (2005). F110I and R278C troponin T mutations that cause familial hypertrophic

cardiomyopathy affect muscle contraction in transgenic mice and reconstitute
human cardiac fibers. *J Biol Chem.*, 280(44):, pp. 37183-94

Hinkle, A. & Tobacman, L. S. (2003). Folding and function of the troponin tail domain
Effects of cardiomyopathic troponin T mutations. *J Biol Chem.*, 278(1), pp. 506-13

Ho, C. Y. (2010a). Hypertrophic cardiomyopathy: for Heart Failure Clinics. Genetics o
cardiomyopathy and heart failure. *Heart Fail Clin.*, 6(2), pp. 141-59

Ho, C. Y.(2010b). Is genotype clinically useful in predicting prognosis in hypertrophi
cardiomyopathy? Genetics and clinical destiny: improving care in hypertrophi
cardiomyopathy. *Circulation.*122, pp. 2430-40

Ho, C. Y., Lever, H. M., DeSanctis, R., Farver, C. F., Seidman, J. G. & Seidman, C. E. (2000)
Homozygous mutation in cardiac troponin T: implications for hypertrophi
cardiomyopthyy. *Circulation.* 102, pp. 1950-5

Ho, C. Y., Carlsen, C., Thune, J. J., Havndrup, O., Bundgaard, H., Farrohi, F., Rivero, J
Cirino, A. L, Andersen, P. S., Christiansen, M., Maron, B. J., Orav, E. J. & Kober, L
(2009). Echocardiographic strain imaging to assess early and late consequences o
sarcomere mutations in hypertrophic cardiomyopathy. *Circ Cardiovasc Genet.* 2, pp
314-21

Hoffmann, B., Schmidt-Traub, H., Perrot, A., Osterziel, K. J. & Gessner, R. (2001). Firs
mutation in cardiac troponin C, L29Q, in a patient with hypertrophi
cardiomyopathy. *Hum. Mutat.*, 17, pp. 524 only

Howarth, J. W., Meller, J., Solaro, R. J., Trewhella, J. & Rosevear, P. R. (2007)
Phosphorylation-dependent conformational transition of the cardiac specific N
extension of troponin I in cardiac troponin. *J. Mol. Biol.*, 373, pp. 706-22

James, J., Zhang, Y., Osinska, H., Sanbe, A., Klevitsky, R., Hewett, T. E. & Robbins, J. (2000)
Transgenic modeling of a cardiac troponin I mutation linked to familia
hypertrophic cardiomyopathy. *Circ Res.*, 87(9), pp. 805-11

Jaquet, K., Lohmann, K., Czisch, M., Holak, T., Gulati, J. & Jaquet, R. (1998). A model for th
function of the bisphos-phorylated heart-specific troponin-I N-terminus. *J Muscl
Res Cell Motil.*, 19(6), pp. 647-59

Jarcho, J. A., McKenna, W., Pare, J. A., Solomon, S. D, Holcombe, R. F, Dickie, S., Levi, T.
Donis-Keller, H., Seidman, J. G. & Seidman, C. E.(1989). Mapping a gene fo
familial hypertrophic cardiomyopathy to chromosome 14q1. *N Engl J Med.*, 321 (20)
pp. 1372-8

Javadpour, M. M, Tardiff, J. C, Pinz, I. & Ingwall, J. S. (2003). Decreased energetics in murin
hearts bearing the R92Q mutation in cardiac troponin T. *J Clin Invest.*, 112(5), pp
768-75

Jin, J. P. & Chong, S. M. (2010). Localization of the two tropomyosin-binding sites o
troponin T. *Arch Biochem Biophys.*, 500(2), pp. 144-50

Jin, J. P & Samanez, R. A. (2001). Evolution of a metal-binding cluster in the NH(2)-termina
variable region of avian fast skeletal muscle troponin T: functional divergence o
the basis of tolerance to structural drifting. *J Mol Evol.*, 52(2), pp. 103-16

Jin, J. P., Zhang, Z. & Bautista, J. A. (2008). Isoform diversity, regulation, and functiona
adaptation of troponin and calponin. *Crit Rev Eukaryot Gene Expr.*, 18(2), pp. 93-124
Review.

Kamisago, M., Sharma, S. D., DePalma, S. R., Solomon, S., Sharma, P., McDonough, B
Smoot, L., Mullen, M. P., Woolf, P. K., Wigle, E. D., Seidman, J. G. & Seidman, C. E

(2000). Mutations in sarcomeric protein genes as a cause of dilated cardiomyopathy. *N. Engl. J. Med.,* 343(23), pp. 1888-96

Kentish, J. C., McCloskey, D. T., Layland, J., Palmer, S., Leiden, J. M., Martin, A. F. & Solaro, R. J. (2001). Phosphorylation of troponin I by protein kinase A accelerates relaxation and crossbridge cycle kinetics in mouse ventricular muscle. *Circ. Res.* 88, pp. 1059-65

Keren, A., Syrris, P. & McKenna, W. J. (2008). Hypertrophic cardiomyopathy: the genetic determinants of clinical disease expression. *Nature Clin Pract.,* 5(3), pp. 158-68

Kimura, A., Harada, H., Park, J-E., Nishi, H., Satoh, M., Takahashi, M,, Hiroi, S., Sasaoka, T., Ohbuchi, N., Nakamura, T., Koyanagi, T., Hwang, T-H., Choo, J., Chung, K-S., Hasegawa, A., Nagai, R., Okazaki, O., Nakamura, H., Matsuzaki, M., Sakamoto, T., Toshima, H., Koga, Y., Imaizumi, T. & Sasazuki, T. (1997). Mutations in the cardiac troponin I gene associated with hypertrophic cardiomyopathy. Nature Genet., 16, pp. 379-82

Knollmann, B. C. & Potter, J. D. (2001). Altered regulation of cardiac muscle contraction by troponin T mutations that cause familial hypertrophic cardiomyopathy. *Trends Cardiovasc Med.,* 11(5), pp. 206-12

Knollmann, B. C., Blatt, S. A., Horton, K., de Freitas, F., Miller, T., Bell, M., Housmans, P. R., Weissman, N. J, Morad, M. &, Potter, J. D. (2001). Inotropic stimulation induces cardiac dysfunction in transgenic mice expressing a troponin T (I79N) mutation linked to familial hypertrophic cardiomyopathy. *J Biol Chem.,* 276(13), pp. 10039-48

Knollmann, B. C., Kirchhof, P., Sirenko, S. G., Degen, H., Greene, A. E., Schober, T., Mackow, J. C., Fabritz, L., Potter, J. D. & Morad, M. (2003). Familial hypertrophic cardiomyopathy-linked mutant troponin T causes stress-induced ventricular tachycardia and Ca2+-dependent action potential remodeling. *Circ Res.,* 92(4), pp. 428-36

Klues, H. G, Schiffers, A. & Maron, B. J. (1995). Phenotypic spectrum and patterns of left ventricular hypertrophy in hypertrophic cardiomyopathy: morphologic observations and significance as assessed by two-dimensional echocardiography in 600 patients. *J Am Coll Cardiol.,* 26(7), pp. 1699-1708

Kobayashi, T., Dong, W. J., Burkart, E. M., Cheung, H. C. & Solaro, R. J. (2004). Effects of protein kinase C dependent phosphorylation and a familial hypertrophic cardiomyopathy-related mutation of cardiac troponin I on structural transition of troponin C and myofilament activation. *Biochemistry,* 43 (20), pp. 5996-6004

Kobayashi, T. & Solaro, R. J. (2006). Increased Ca2+ affinity of cardiac thin filaments reconstituted with cardiomyopathy-related mutant cardiac troponin I. *J Biol Chem.,* 281(19), pp. 13471-7

Köhler, J., Chen, Y., Brenner, B., Gordon, A. M., Kraft, T., Martyn, D. A., Regnier, M., Rivera, A. J., Wang, C. K. & Chase, P. B. (2003). Familial hypertrophic cardiomyopathy mutations in troponin I (K183D, G203S, K206Q) enhance filament sliding. *Physiol Genomics,.* 14(2), pp. 117-28

Kofflard, M. J. M., ten Cate, F. J., van der Lee, C. & van Domburg, R. T. (2003). Hypertrophic cardiomyopathy in a large community-based population: clinical outcome and identification of risk factors for sudden death and clinical deterioration. *J Am Coll Cardiol.,* 41, pp. 987-93

Kokado, H., Shimizu, M., Yoshio, H., Ino, H., Okeie, K., Emoto, Y., Matsuyama, T., Yamaguchi, M., Ysuda, T., Fujino, N., Ito, H., Mabuchi, H. (2000). Clinical features of hypertrophic cardiomyopathy caused by a Lys183 deletion mutation in the cardiac troponin I gene. *Circulation*, 102, pp. 663-9

Konno, T., Shimizu, M., Ino, H., Fujino, N., Hayashi, K., Uchiyama, K., Kaneda, T., Inoue M., Masuda, E., Mabuchi, H. (2005). Phenotypic differences between electrocardiographic and echocardiographic determination of hypertrophic cardiomyopathy in genetically affected subjects. *J Intern Med.*, 258, pp. 216-24

Kruger, M., Zittrich, S., Redwood, C., Blaudeck, N., James, J., Robbins, J., Pfitzer, G. & Stehle R. (2005). Effects of the mutation R145G in human cardiac troponin I on the kinetics of the contraction-relaxation cycle in isolated cardiac myofibrils. *J Physiol.*, 564(Pt 2) pp. 347-57

Lam, L., Tsoutsman, T., Arthur, J. & Semsarian, C. (2010). Differential protein expression profiling of myocardial tissue in a mouse model of hypertrophic cardiomyopathy. *Mol Cell Cardiol.*, 48(5), pp. 1014-22

Landstrom, A. P. & Ackerman, M. J. (2010). Is genotype clinically useful in predicting prognosis in hypertrophic cardiomyopathy? Mutation type is not clinically useful in predicting prognosis in hypertrophic cardiomyopathy. *Circulation*, 122, pp. 2441 50

Landstrom, A. P., Parvatiyar, M. S., Pinto, J. R., Marquardt, M. L., Bos, J. M., Tester, D. J. Ommen, S. R., Potter, J. D. & Ackerman, M. J. (2008). Molecular and functional characterization of novel hypertrophic cardiomyopathy susceptibility mutations in TNNC1-encoded troponin C. *J Mol Cell Cardiol.*, 45, pp. 281-288

Lang, R., Gomes, A. V., Zhao, J., Housmans, P. R., Miller, T. & Potter, J. D. (2002). Functional analysis of a troponin I (R145G) mutation associated with familial hypertrophic cardiomyopathy. *J Biol Chem.*, 277(14), pp. 11670-8

Lassalle, M. W. (2010). Defective dynamic properties of human cardiac troponin mutations *Biosci Biotechnol Biochem.*, 74(1), pp. 82-91

Lechin, M., Quinones, M. A., Omran, A., Yu, Q. T., Rakowski, H., Wigle, D., Liew, C. C. Sole, M., Roberts, R. & Marian, A. J. (1995). Angiotensin-I conversing enzyme genotypes and left ventricular hypertrophy in patients with hypertrophic cardiomyopathy. *Circulation*, 92, pp. 1808-12

Li, M. X., Spyracopoulos, L. & Sykes, B. D. (1999). Binding of cardiac troponin-I147-163 induces a structural opening in human cardiac troponin-C. *Biochemistry*, 38(26), pp. 8289-98

Liang, B., Chung, F., Qu, Y., Pavlov, D., Gillis, T. E., Tikunova, S. B., Davis, J. P. & Tibbits, G. F. (2008). Familial hypertrophic cardiomyopathy- related cardiac troponin C mutation L29Q affects Ca2+ binding and myofilament contractility. *Physiol. Gen.*, 33, pp. 257-66

Liberthson, R. R.(1996). Sudden death from cardiac causes in children and young adults. N *Engl J Med.*, 334, pp. 1039-44

Lin, D., Bobkova, A., Homsher, E. & Tobacman, L. S. (1996). Altered cardiac troponin T in vitro function in the presence of a mutation implicated in familial hypertrophic cardiomyopathy. *J Clin Invest.* 97(12), pp. 2842-8

Lindhout, D. A., Li, M. X., Schieve, D. & Sykes, B. D. (2002). Effects of T142 phosphorylation and mutation R145G on the interaction of the inhibitory region of human cardiac troponin I with the C-domain of human cardiac troponin C. *Biochemistry*, 41(23), pp. 7267-74. Erratum in: *Biochemistry* (2003), 42(1), pp. 238

Lindhout DA, Boyko RF, Corson DC, Li MX & Sykes BD. (2005).The role of electrostatics in the interaction of the inhibitory region of troponin I with troponin C. *Biochemistry*, 44(45): 14750-9.

Lippi, G., Targher, G., Franchini, M. & Plebani, M. (2009). Genetic and biochemical heterogeneity of cardiac troponins: clinical and laboratory implications. *Clin Chem Lab Med.*, 47(10), pp. 1183-94

Marian, A. J. (2003). On predictors of sudden cardiac death in hypertrophic cardiomyopathy. *J Am Coll Cardiol.*, 41, pp. 994-6

Marian, A. J. (2010). Hypertrophic cardiomyopathy: from genetics to treatment. *Eur J Clin Invest.* 40(4), pp. 360-9

Marian, A. J., Yu, Q. T., Workman, R., Greve, G. & Roberts, R. (1993). Angiotensin-converting enzyme polymorphism in hypertrophic cardiomyopathy and sudden cardiac death. *Lancet*, 342, pp. 1085-6

Maron, B. J., Shirani, J., Poliac, L. C., Mathenge, R., Roberts, W. C. & Mueller, F. O. (1996). Sudden death in young competitive atheletes : clinical, demographic, and pathological profiles. *JAMA*, 276(3), pp. 199-204

Maron, B. J. (2003). Sudden death in young athletes. *N Engl J Med.*, 349,pp. 1064-75

Maron, B. J. & Roberts, W. C. (1979). Quantitative analysis of cardiac muscle cell disorganization in the ventricular septum of patients with hypertrophic cardiomyopathy. *Circulation*, 59, pp. 689-706

Maron, B. J., Gottdiener, J. S. & Epstein, S. E. (1981). Patterns and significance if distribution of left ventricular hypertrophy in hypertrophic cardiomyopathy. A wide angle, two dimensional echocardiographic study of 125 patients. *Am J Cardiol.*, 48(3), pp. 418-28

Maron, M. S., Olivotto, I., Zenovich, A. G., Link, M. S., Pandian, N. G., Kuvin, J. T., Nistri, S., Cecchi, F., Udelson, J. E. & Maron, B. J. (2006). Hypertrophic cardiomyoptahy is predominantly a disease of the left ventricular outflow tract obstruction. *Circulation*, 114, pp. 2232-9

Maron, B. J., Spirito, P., Wesley, Y. & Arce, J. (1986). Development and progression of left ventricular hypertrophy in children with hypertrophic cardiomyopathy. *N Engl J Med.*, 315(10), pp. 610-4

Menon, S. C., Michels, V. V., Pellikka, P. A., Ballew, J. D., Karst, M. L., Herron, K. J., Nelson, S. M., Rodeheffer, R. J. & Olson, T. M. (2008). Cardiac troponin T mutation in familial cardiomyopathy with variable remodeling and restrictive physiology. *Clin Genet.*, 74(5), pp. 445-54

Midde, K., Dumka, V., Pinto, J. R., Muthu, P., Marandos, P., Gryczynski, I., Gryczynski, Z., Potter J. D. & Borejdo, J. (2011). Myosin cross-bridges do not form precise rigor bonds in hypertrophic heart muscle carrying Troponin T mutations. *J Mol Cell Cardiol.*, Jun 12 [Epub ahead of print]

Miller, T., Szczesna, D., Housmans, P. R., Zhao, J., de Freitas, F., Gomes, A. V., Culbreath, L., McCue, J., Wang, Y., Xu, Y., Kerrick, W. G. & Potter, J. D. (2001). Abnormal contractile function in transgenic mice expressing a familial hypertrophic cardiomyopathy-linked troponin T (I79N) mutation. *J Biol Chem.*, 276(6), pp. 3743-55

Miliou, A., Anastasakis, A., D'Cruz, L. G., Theopistou, A., Rigopoulos, A., Rizos, I., Stamatelpoulos, S., Toutouzas, P., Stefanadis, C. (2005). Low prevalence of cardiac troponin T mutations in a Greek hypertrophic cardiomyopathy cohort. *Heart*, 91, pp. 966-7

Mittmann, K., Jaquet, K. & Heilmeyer, L. M., Jr. (1990). A common motif of two adjacent phosphoserines in bovine, rabbit and human cardiac troponin I. *FEBS Lett.*, 273(1-2), pp. 41-5

Mittmann, K., Jaquet, K. & Heilmeyer, L. M., Jr. (1992). Ordered phosphorylation of a duplicated minimal recognition motif for cAMP-dependent protein kinase present in cardiac troponin I. *FEBS Lett.*, 302(2), pp. 133-7

Mirza, M., Marston, S., Willott, R., Ashley, C., Mogensen, J., McKenna, W., Robinson, P., Redwood, C. & Watkins, H. (2005). Dilated cardiomyopathy mutations in three thin filament regulatory proteins result in a common functional phenotype. *J. Biol. Chem.*, 280, pp. 28498- 506

Mörner, S., Richard, P., Kazzam, E., Hainque, B., Schwartz, K., Waldenström, A. (2000). Deletion in he cardiac troponin I gene in a family from northern Sweden with hypertrophic cardiomyopathy. *J Mol Cell Cardiol.*, 32(3), pp. 521-5

Mogensen, J., Murphy, R. T., Kubo, T., Bahl, A., Moon, J. C., Klausen, I. C., Elliot, P. M., McKenna, W. J. (2004). Frequency and clinical expression of cardiac troponin I mutations in 748 consecutive falilies with hypertrophic cardiomyopathy. *J Am Coll Cardiol.*, 44, pp. 2315-25

Mogensen, J., Murphy, R. T., Shaw, T., Bahl, A., Redwood, C., Watkins, H., Burke, M., Elliott, P. M. & McKenna, W. J. (2004). Severe disease expression of cardiac troponin C and T mutations in patients with idiopathic dilated cardiomyopathy. J. Am. Coll. Cardiol., 44, pp. 2033-40

Monserrat, L., Gimeno-Blanes, J. R., Marin, F., Hermida-Prieto, M., Garcia-Honrubia, A., Perez, I., Fernandez, I., de Nicolas, R., de la Morena, G., Paya, E., Yague, J. & Egido, J.(2007).Prevalence of Fabry disease in a cohort of 508 unrelated patients with hypertrophic cardiomyopathy. *J Am Coll Cardiol.*, 50(25), 2399-403

Montgomery, D. E., Wolska, B. M., Pyle, W. G., Roman, B. B., Dowell, J. C., Buttrick, P. M., Koretsky, A. P., Del Nido, P. & Solaro, R. J. (2002). alpha-Adrenergic response and myofilament activity in mouse hearts lacking PKC phosphorylation sites on cardiac TnI. *Am J Physiol Heart Circ Physiol.*, 282(6), pp. H2397-405

Moolman, J. C., Corfield, V. A., Posen, B., Ngumbela, K., Seidman, C., Brink, P. A., & Watkins, H. (1997). Sudden death due to troponin T mutations. *J Am Coll Cardiol.*, 29, pp. 549-55.

Morris, E. P. & Lehrer, S. S. Troponin-tropomyosin interactions. Fluorescence studies of the binding of troponin, troponin T, and chymotryptic troponin T fragments to specifically labeled tropomyosin. *Biochemistry* 23, 2214-20.

Mukherjea, P., Tong, L., Seidman, J. G., Seidman, C. E. & Hitchcock-DeGregory, S. E. (1999). Altered regulatory function of two familial hypertrophic cardiomyopathy troponin T mutants. *Biochemistry*, 38(49), pp. 13296-301

Murakami, K., Stewart, M., Nozawa, K,, Tomii, K., Kudou, N., Igarashi, N., Shirakihara, Y., Wakatsuki, S., Yasunaga, T. & Wakabayashi, T. (2008). Structural basis for tropomyosin overlap in thin (actin) filaments and the generation of a molecular swivel by troponin-T. *Proc Natl Acad Sci U.S.A.* 105(20), pp. 7200-5

Murphy, R. T., Mogensen, J., Shaw, A., Kubo, T., Hughes, S. & McKenna, W, J. (2009). Novel mutation in cardiac troponin I in recessive idiopathic dilated cardiomyopathy. *Circ Res.*, 105(4), pp. 375-82

Nagueh, S. F., Bachinski, L. L., Meyer, D., Hill, R., Zoghbi, W. A., Tam, J. W., Quinones, M. A., Roberts, R., Marian, A. J. (2001). Tissue Doppler imaging consistently detects myocardial abnormalities in patients with hypertrophic cardiomyopathy and provides a novel means for an early diagnosis before and independently of hypertrophy. *Circulation*, 104(2), pp. 128-30

Nakajima-Taniguchi, C., Matsui, H., Fujio, Y, Nagata, S, Kishimoto T, Yamauchi-Takihara, K. (1997). Novel missense mutation in cardiac troponin T gene found in Japanese patient with hypertrophic cardiomyopathy. *J Mol Cell Cardiol.*, 29, 839-43

Nakaura, H., Yanaga, F., Ohtsuki, I. & Morimoto, S. (1999). Effects of missense mutations Phe110Ile and Glu244Asp in human cardiac troponin T on force generation in skinned cardiac muscle fibers. *J Biochem.*, 126(3), pp. 457-60

Narolska, N. A., Piroddi, N., Belus, A., Boontje, N. M., Scellini, B., Deppermann, S., Zaremba, R., Musters, R. J., dos Remedios, C., Jaquet, K., Foster, D. B., Murphy, A. M., van Eyk, J. E., Tesi, C., Poggesi, C., van der Velden, J. & Stienen, G. J. (2006). Impaired diastolic function after exchange of endogenous troponin I with C-terminal truncated troponin I in human cardiac muscle. *Circ Res.*, 99(9), pp. 1012-20

Niimura, C., Patton, K. K., McKenna, W. J., Soults, J., Maron, B. J., Seidman, J. G. & Seidman, C. E. (2002). Sarcomere protein gene mutations in hypertrophic cardiomyopathy of the elderly. *Circulation*, 105, 446-51

Nguyen, L., Chung, J., Lam, L., Tsoutsman, T. & Semsarian, C. (2006). Abnormal cardiac response to exercise in a murine model of familial hypertrophic cardiomyopathy. *J Mol Cell Cardiol.*, 41(4), pp. 623-32

Ohtsuki, I. (1979). Molecular Arrangement of Troponin-T in the Thin Filament. *J. Biochem.*, 86(2), pp. 491-7

Olivotto, I., Maron, B. S., Adabag, A. S., Casey, S. A., Vargiu, D., Link, M. S., Udelson, S. E, Cecchi, F. & Maron, B. J. (2005). Gender- related differences in the clinical presentation and outcome of hypertrophic cardiomyopathy. *J. Am Coll Cardiol.*, 46(3), pp. 480-7

Ommen, S. R., Nishimura, R. A., Appelton, C. P., Miller, F. A., Oh, J. K., Redfield, M. M. & Tajik, A. J. (2000). Clinical utility of Doppler echocardiography and tissue Doppler imaging in the estimation of left ventricular filling pressures: a comparative simultaneous Doppler-catheterization study.*Circulation*, 102, pp. 1788-94

Palm, T., Graboski, S., Hitchcock-DeGregori, S. E., Greenfield, N. J. (2001). Disease-causing mutations in cardiac troponin T: identification of a critical tropomyosin-binding region. *Biophys J.*, 81(5), 2827-37. Erratum in *Biophys. J.* (2002) 82(5), pp. 2826

Paul, D. M., Morris, E. P., Kensler, R. W. & Squire, J. M. (2009). Structure and orientation of troponin in the thin filament. *J Biol Chem.*, 284(22), pp. 15007-15.

Paulus, W. J., Tschöpe, C., Anderson, J. E., Rusconi, C., Flachskampf, F. A., Rademakers, F. E., Marino, P., Smiseth, O. A., De Keulenaer, G., Leite-Moreira, A. F., Borbely, A., Edes, I., Handoko, M. L., Heymans, S., Pezzali, N., Pieske, B., Dickstein, K., Fraser, A. G. & Brutsaert, D. L. (2007). How to diagnose diastolic heart failure: a consensus statement on the diagnosis of heart failure with normal left ventricular ejection fraction by the Heart Failure and Echocardiography Associations of the Europea Society of Cardiology. *Eur Heart J.,* 28, pp. 2539-50

Parvatiyar, M. S., Pinto, J. R., Dweck, D. & Potter, J. D. (2010). Cardiac troponin mutation and restrictive cardiomyopathy. *J Biomed Biotechnol.,* 2010, 350706. Review.

Pearlstone, J. R. & Smillie, L. B. (1983) Effects of troponin-I plus-C on the binding c troponin-T and its fragments to alpha-tropomyosin. Ca^{2+} sensitivity an cooperativity. *J. Biol. Chem.,* 258, pp. 2534-42

Perry, S. V. (1998). Troponin T: genetics, properties and function. *J Muscle Res Cell Motil.,* 1$ pp. 575-602

Pinto, J. R., Parvatiyar, M. S., Jones, M. A., Liang, J. & Potter, J. D. (2008). A troponin mutation that causes infantile restrictive cardiomyopathy increases Ca2+ sensitivit of force development and impairs the inhibitory properties of troponin. *J. Bio Chem.,* 283(4), pp. 2156-66

Pinto, J. R., Parvatiyar, M. S., Jones, M. A., Liang, J., Ackerman, M. J. & Potter, J. D. (2009). functional and structural study of troponin C mutations related to hypertrophi cardiomyopathy. *J Biol Chem.,* 284(28), pp. 19090-100

Pinto, J. R., Reynaldo, D.P., Parvatiyar, M. S., Dweck, D., Liang, J., Jones, M. A., Sorenson, M M. & Potter, J. D. (2011a). Strong cross-bridges potentiate the Ca(2+) affinit changes produced by hypertrophic cardiomyopathy cardiac troponin C mutants i myofilaments: a fast kinetic approach. *J Biol Chem.,* 286(2), pp. 1005-13

Pinto, J. R., Yang, S.W., Hitz, M.P., Parvatiyar, M.S., Jones, M.A., Liang,J., Kokta, V., Talajic M., Tremblay, N., Jaeggi, M., Andelfinger, G. & Potter, J. D. (2011). Fetal cardia troponin isoforms rescue the increased Ca2+ sensitivity produced by a nove double deletion in cardiac troponin T linked to restrictive cardiomyopathy: clinical, genetic, and functional approach. *J Biol Chem.,* 286(23), pp. 20901-12

Pinto, Y. M., Wilde, A. M., van Rijsingen, I. A. W., Christaans, I., Lekanne, Deprez, R. H. & Elliot, P. M. (2011). Clinical utility gene card for: hypertrophic cardiomyopath (type 1-4). *Eur J Hum Genet.,* epub ahead of print.

Pirani, A., Xu, C., Hatch, V., Craig, R., Tobacman, L. S. & Lehman, W. (2005). Single particl analysis of relaxed and activated muscle thin filaments. *J Mol Biol.,* 346, pp. 761-72

Redwood, C., Lohmann, K., Bing, W., Esposito, G. M., Elliott, K., Abdulrazzak, H., Knott A., Purcell, I., Marston, S. & Watkins, H. (2000). Investigation of a truncated cardia troponin T that causes familial hypertrophic cardiomyopathy. Ca(2+) regulator properties of reconstituted thin filaments depend on the ratio of mutant to wild type protein. *Circ Res.,* 86(11), pp. 1148-52

Reiffert, S. U., Jaquet, K., Heilmeyer, L. M., Jr., Ritchie, M. D., Geeves, M. A. (1996) Bisphosphorylation of cardiac troponin I modulates the Ca(2+)-dependent bindin of myosin subfragment S1 to reconstituted thin filaments. *FEBS Lett.,* 384(1), 43-7

Reis, S., Littwitz, C., Preilowski, S., Mügge, A., Stienen, G. J., Pott, L. & Jaquet, K. (2008) Expression of cTnI-R145G affects shortening properties of adult ra cardiomyocytes. *Pflugers Arch.,* 457(1), pp. 17-24

Revera, M., Van der Merwe, L., Heradien, M., Goosen, A., Corfield, V. A., Brink, P. A. & Moolman-Smook, J. C. (2007). Long-term follow-up of R403WMYH7 anc R92WTNNT2 HCM families: mutations determine left ventricular dimensions bu not wall thickness during disease progression. *Cardiovasc J Afr.,* 18(3), pp. 146-53

Richard, P., Charron, P., Carrier, L., Ledeuil, C., Cheav, T., Picherau, C., Benaiche, A., Isnard, R., Dubourg, O., Burban, M., Gueffet, J. P., Millaire, A., Desnos, M., Schwartz, K., Hainque, B. & Komajda, M. for the EUROGENE Heart Failure Project: Hypertrophic cardiomyopathy. (2003). Distribution of disease genes, spectrum of mutations, and implications for a molecular diagnosis strategy. Circulation., 107, pp. 2227-32

Risnik, V. V. & Gusev, N. B. (1984). Some properties of the nucleotide-binding site of troponin T kinase-casein kinase type II from skeletal muscle. Biochim Biophys Acta., 790(2), pp. 108-16

Robinson, P., Griffiths, P. J., Watkins, H. & Redwood, C. S. (2007). Dilated and hypertrophic cardiomyopathy mutations in troponin and alpha-tropomyosin have opposing effects on the calcium affinity of cardiac thin filaments. Circ Res., 101(12), 1266-73

Rust, E. M., Albayya, F. P. & Metzger, J. M. (1999). Identification of a contractile deficit in adult cardiac myocytes expressing hypertrophic cardiomyopathy-associated mutant troponin T proteins. J Clin Invest., 103(10), 1459-67

Sadayappan, S., Finley, N., Howarth, J. W., Osinska, H., Klevitsky, R., Lorenz, J. N., Rosevear, P. R. & Robbins, J. (2008). Role of the acidic N' region of cardiac troponin I in regulating myocardial function. FASEB J., 22(4), pp. 1246-57

Sakthivel, S., Finley, N. L., Rosevear, P. R., Lorenz, J. N., Gulick, J., Kim, S., VanBuren, P., Martin, L. A. & Robbins, J. (2005). In vivo and in vitro analysis of cardiac troponin I phosphorylation. J. Biol. Chem. 280, pp. 703-14

Sakamoto, T., Tei, C., Murayama, M., Ischiyasu, H. & Hada, Y. (1976). Giant negative T-wave inversion as a manifestation of asymmetric apical hypertrophy of the left ventricle: echocardiographic and ultrasonocardiotomography. Jpn Heart J., 17(5), pp. 611-29

Schmidtmann, A., Lohmann, K. & Jaquet, K. (2002). The interaction of the bisphosphorylated N-terminal arm of cardiac troponin I-A 31P-NMR study. FEBS Lett., 513(2-3), pp. 289-93

Schmidtmann, A., Lindow, C., Villard, S., Heuser, A., Mügge, A., Gessner, R., Granier, C. & Jaquet, K. (2005). Cardiac troponin C-L29Q, related to hypertrophic cardiomyopathy, hinders the transduction of the protein kinase A dependent phosphorylation signal from cardiac troponin I to C. FEBS J., 272(23), 6087-97

Sia, S. K., Li, M. X., Spyracopoulos, L., Gagné, S. M., Liu, W., Putkey, J. A. & Sykes, B. D. (1997). Structure of cardiac muscle troponin C unexpectedly reveals a closed regulatory domain. J Biol Chem., 272(29), pp. 18216-21

Sirenko, S. G., Potter, J. D. & Knollmann, B. C. (2006). Differential effect of troponin T mutations on the inotropic responsiveness of mouse hearts--role of myofilament Ca2+ sensitivity increase. J Physiol. 575(Pt 1), pp. 201-13

Seidman, C. E. & Seidman, J. G. (2011). Identifying sarcomere gene mutations in hypertrophic cardiomyopathy. A personal history. Circ Res. 108, pp. 743-50

Semsarian, C., French, J., Trent, R. J., Richmond, D. R. & Jeremy, R. W. (1997). The natural history of left ventricular wall thickening in hypertrophic cardiomyopathy. Aust NZ J Med., 27(1), 51-58

Sheng, H. Z., Shan, Q. J., Wu, X. & Cao, K. J. (2008). Cardiac troponin I gene mutation (Asp127Tyr) in a Chinese patient with hypertrophic cardiomyopathy). Zhonghua Xin Xue Guan Bing Za Zhi. 36(12): 1063-5

Spirito, P., Bellone, P., Harris, K. M., Bernabo, P., Bruzzi, P. & Maron, B. J. (2000). Magnitude of left ventricular hypertrophy and risk of sudden death in hypertrophic cardiomyopathy. *N Engl J Med.*, 342(24), pp. 1778-85

Smith, L., Greenfield, N. J. & Hitchcock-DeGregori, S. E. (1999). Mutations in the N- and D-helices of the N-domain of troponin C affect the C-domain and regulatory function. *Biophys J.*, 76(1 Pt 1), pp. 400-8

Solaro, R. J. & Kobayashi, T. (2011). Protein Phosphorylation and signal transduction in cardiac filaments. *J. Biol. Chem.*, 286(12), pp. 9935-40

Stelzer, J. E., Patel, J. R., Olsson, M. C., Fitzsimons, D. P., Leinwand, L. A. & Moss, R. L. (2004). Expression of cardiac troponin T with COOH-terminal truncation accelerates cross-bridge interaction kinetics in mouse myocardium. *AJP Heart*, 287(4), pp. H1756-61

Sumandea, M. P., Pyle, W. G., Kobayashi, T., de Tombe, P. P. & Solaro, R. J. (2003). Identification of a functionally critical protein kinase C phosphorylation residue of cardiac troponin T. *J Biol Chem.*, 278(37), pp. 35135-44. Review.

Sumandea, C. A., Garcia-Cazarin, M. L., Bozio, C. H., Sievert, G. A., Balke, C. W. & Sumandea, M. P. (2011). Cardiac troponin T, a sarcomeric AKAP, tethers protein kinase A at the myofilaments. *J Biol Chem.* 286(1), pp. 530-41

Sweeney, H. L., Feng, H. S., Yang, Z. & Watkins, H. (1998). Functional analyses of troponin T mutations that cause hypertrophic cardiomyopathy: insights into disease pathogenesis and troponin function. *Proc Natl Acad Sci U S A.*, 95(24), 14406-10

Swiderek, K., Jaquet, K., Meyer, H. E., Schächtele, C., Hofmann, F. & Heilmeyer, L. M., Jr. (1990). Sites phosphorylated in bovine cardiac troponin T and I. Characterization by 31P-NMR spectroscopy and phosphorylation by protein kinases. *Eur J Biochem.*, 190(3), 575-82

Szczesna, D., Zhang, R., Zhao, J., Jones, M., Guzman, G., Potter, J. D. (2000). Altered regulation of cardiac muscle contraction by troponin T mutations that cause familial hypertrophic cardiomyopathy. *J Biol Chem.*, 275(1), pp. 624-30

Tachampa, K., Wang, H., Farman, G. P. & de Tombe, P. P. (2007). Cardiac troponin I threonine 144: role in myofilament length dependent activation. *Circ Res.*, 101(11), pp. 1081-3

Takeda, S., Yamashita, A., Maeda, K. & Maéda, Y. (2003). Structure of the core domain of human cardiac troponin in the Ca(2+)-saturated form. *Nature*, 424(6944), pp. 35-41

Tester, D. J., Ackeman, M. J. (2011). Genetic testing for potentially lethal, highly treatable inherited cardiomyopathies/channelopathies in clinical practice. *Circulation*, 123, 1021-37

Theopistou, A., Anastasakis, A., Miliou, A., Rigopoulos, A., Toutouzas, P. & Stefanadis, C. (2004). Clinical features of hypertrophic cardiomyopathy caused by an Arg278Cys missense mutation in the cardiac troponin T gene. *Am J Cardiol.*, 94, 246-9

Thierfelder, L., Watkins, H., MacRae, C., Lamas, R., Mc Kenna, W., Vosberg, H. P., Seidman, J. G. & Seidman, C. E. (1994). Alpha-tropomyosin and cardiac troponin T mutations cause familial hypertrophic cardiomyopathy: a disease of the sarcomere. *Cell*, 77(5), 701-12

Tobacman, L. S. (1988). Structure-function studies of the amino-terminal region of bovine cardiac troponin T. *J Biol Chem.*, 263(6), 2668-72

Torricellli, F., Girolami, F., Olivotto, I., Passerini, I., Frusconi, S., Vardiu, D., Richard, P. & Cecchi, F. (2003). Prevalence and clinical profile of troponin T mutations among patients with hypertrophic cardiomyopathy in Tuscany. *Am J Cardiol.*, 92, pp. 1358-62

Townsend, P. J., Barton, P. J., Yacoub, M. H. & Farza, H. (1995). Molecular cloning of human cardiac troponin T isoforms: expression in developing and failing heart. *J Mol Cell Cardiol.*, 27(10), pp. 2223-36

Turnbull, L., Hoh, J. F., Ludowyke, R. I. & Rossmanith, G. H. (2002). Troponin I phosphorylation enhances crossbridge kinetics during beta-adrenergic stimulation in rat cardiac tissue. *J. Physiol.*, 542, pp. 911-20

Tsoutsman, T., Chung, J., Doolan, A., Nguyen, L., Williams, I.A., Tu, E., Lam, L., Bailey, C. G., Rasko, J. E., Allen, D. G. & Semsarian, C. (2006). Molecular insights from a novel cardiac troponin I mouse model of familial hypertrophic cardiomyopathy. *J Mol Cell Cardiol.*, 41(4), pp. 623-32

Tsoutsman, T., Bagnall, R. D. & Semsarian, C. (2008). Impact of multiple gene mutations in determining the severity of cardiomyopathy and heart failure. *Clin Exp Pharmacol Physiol.*, 35(11), pp. 1349-57. Review.

Tsoutsman, T., Kelly, M., Ng, D. C., Tan, J. E., Tu, E., Lam, L., Bogoyevitch, M. A., Seidman, C. E., Seidman, J. G. & Semsarian, C. (2008). Severe heart failure and early mortality in a double-mutation mouse model of familial hypertrophic cardiomyopathy. *Circulation*, 117(14), pp. 1820-31

Vahebi, S., Kobayashi, T., Warren, C. M., de Tombe, P. P. & Solaro, R. J. (2005). Functional effects of rho-kinase-dependent phosphorylation of specific sites on cardiac troponin. *Circ Res.*, 96(7), pp. 740-7

van der Velden, J., Papp, Z., Zaremba, R., Boontje, N. M., de Jong, J. W., Owen, V. J., Burton, P. B., Goldmann, P., Jaquet, K. & Stienen, G. J. (2003) Increased Ca2+-sensitivity of the contractile apparatus in end-stage human heart failure results from altered phosphorylation of contractile proteins. *Cardiovasc Res.*, 57(1), pp. 37-47

Van Driest, S. L., Ellsworth, E. G., Ommen, S. R., Tajik, J., Gersh, B. J. & Ackerman, M. J. (2003). Prevalence and spectrum of thin filament mutations in an outpatient referral population with hypertrophic cardiomyopathy. *Circulation*, 108, pp. 445-51

Varnava, A. M., Elliot, P. M., Baboonian, C., Davison, F., Davies, M. J. & McKenna, W. J. (2001). Hypertrophic cardiomyopathy. Histological features of sudden death in cardiac troponin T disease. *Circulation*, 104, pp. 1380-4

Venkatraman, G., Gomes, A. V., Kerrick, W. G. & Potter J. D. (2005). Characterization of troponin T dilated cardiomyopathy mutations in the fetal troponin isoform. *J Biol. Chem.*, 280(18), pp. 17584-92

Wang, P., Zou, Y., Fu, C. Y., Zhou, X. & Hui, R. (2005). MYBPC3 polymorphism is a modifier for expression of cardiac hypertrophy in patients with hypertrophic cardiomyopathy. *Biochem Biophys Res Comm.*, 329(2), pp. 796-9

Ward, D. G., Brewer, S. M., Cornes, M. P. & Trayer, I. P. (2003) .A cross-linking study of the N-terminal extension of human cardiac troponin I. *Biochemistry*, 42, pp. 10324-32

Ward, D. G., Brewer, S. M., Gallon, C. E., Gao, Y., Levine, B. A., Trayer & I. P. (2004). NMR and mutagenesis studies on the phosphorylation region of human cardiac troponin I. *Biochemistry*, 43, pp. 5772-81

Ward, D. G., Brewer, S. M., Calvert, M. J., Gallon, C. E., Gao, Y. & Trayer, I. P. (2004). Characterization of the interaction between the N-terminal extension of human cardiac troponin I and troponin C. *Biochemistry*, 43, pp. 4020-7

Watkins, H., McKenna, W. J, Thierfelder, L., Suk, H. J., Anan, R., O'Donoghue, A., Spirito, P., Matsumori, A., Moravec, C. S., Seidman, J. G. & Seidman, C. E. (1995). Mutations in the genes for cardiac troponin T and α-tropomyosin in hypertrophic cardiomyopathy. *N Engl J Med.*, 332, pp. 1058-64

Watkins, H., Ashrafian, H. & Redwood, C. (2011). Inherited cardiomyopathies. *N Engl J Med.*, 364, pp. 1643-56

Wen, Y., Pinto, J. R., Gomes, A. V., Xu, Y., Wang, Y., Wang, Y., Potter, J. D. & Kerrick, W. G. (2008). Functional consequences of the human cardiac troponin I hypertrophic cardiomyopathy mutation R145G in transgenic mice. *J Biol Chem.*, 283(29), pp. 20484-94

Westermann, D., Knollmann, B. C., Steendijk, P., Rutschow, S., Riad, A., Pauschinger, M., Potter, J. D., Schultheiss, H. P. & Tschöpe, C. (2006). Diltiazem treatment prevents diastolic heart failure in mice with familial hypertrophic cardiomyopathy. *Eur J Heart Fail.*, 8(2), pp. 115-21

White, S. P., Cohen, C. & Phillips, G. N., Jr. (1987). Structure of co-crystals of tropomyosin and troponin. *Nature*, 325(6107), pp. 826-8

Xu, C., Wie, M., Su, B., Hua, X. W., Zhang, G. W., Xue, X. P., Pan, C. M., Liu, R., Sheng, Y., Lu, Z. G., Jin, L. R. & Song, H. D. (2008). Ile90Met, a novel mutation in the cardiac troponin T gene for familial hypertrophic cardiomyopathy in a Chinese pedigree. *Genet Res.*, 90(5), pp. 445-50

Yanaga, F., Morimoto, S. & Ohtsuki, I. (1999). Ca2+ sensitization and potentiation of the maximum level of myofibrillar ATPase activity caused by mutations of troponin T found in familial hypertrophic cardiomyopathy. *J Biol Chem.*, 274(13), pp. 8806-12

Yetman, A. T., McCrindle, B. W., MacDonald, C., Freedom, R. M. & Gow, R.(1998). Myocardial bridging in children with hypertrophic cardiomyopathy – a risk factor for sudden death. *N Engl J Med.*, 339, pp. 1201-9

Zhang R, Zhao J & Potter JD. (1995). Phosphorylation of both serine residues in cardiac troponin I is required to decrease the Ca2+ affinity of cardiac troponin C. *J Biol Chem,*. 270(51), pp. 30773-80

Zhang, Z., Biesiadecki, B. J. & Jin, J. P. (2006). Selective deletion of the NH$_2$-terminal variable region of cardiac troponin T in ischemia reperfusion by myofibril-associated mu-calpain cleavage. *Biochemistry*, 45, pp. 11681–94

8

Cardiomyopathies Associated with Myofibrillar Myopathies

Lilienbaum Alain[1] and Vernengo Luis[2]

[1]Univ. Paris Diderot-Paris 7, Unit of Functional and Adaptive Biology (BFA)
affiliated with CNRS (EAC4413), Laboratory of Stress
and Pathologies of the Cytoskeleton, Paris
[2]Clinical Unit, Department of Genetics, Faculty of Medicine,
University of the Republic, Montevideo
[1]France
[2]Uruguay

1. Introduction

The aim of this chapter is to describe cardiomyopathies associated with myofibrillar myopathies (MFM, OMIM 601419). Myofibrillar myopathies are a group of heterogeneous neuromuscular disorders usually characterized by a severe myopathy, and generally associated with cardiomyopathy in 15% to 30% of the affected individuals. These familial or sporadic muscle disorders are characterized morphologically by focal disintegration of the myofibrils and abnormal ectopic accumulation of multiple proteins due to their degradation. The six genes that are held responsible so far for this clinically heterogenous, genetically heterogenous and morphologically homogeneous disorders are desmin, αB-crystallin, myotilin, LDB3 (ZASP), FLNC and BAG3. In the first part of the chapter the normal function in skeletal and cardiac muscles of the six genes will be discussed as well as physiopathological consequences of their mutations. The second part will describe how proteins encoded by these genes, together with main contractile proteins such as actin, tropomyosin, myosin, troponin, integrate into functional sarcomeric structures, which in turn determine the main cardiac functions : force generation, force transmission, nervous influx conduction, energy metabolism. Special emphasis will be put on a dynamic point of view, including protein turnover, protein quality control, with the involvement of ubiquitin-proteasome and autophagic systems. The third part gives a view of the latest insight of the clinical and therapeutic perspectives.

2. Clinical manifestations of myofibrillar myopathies

Myofibrillar myopathies represent a group of muscular dystrophies, generally associated with cardiomyopathy. They present specific but not always identical morphologic features. Because aggregates present desmin with other proteins, it has been called desmin-related myopathy.

2.1 Clinical and histopathological features of DRMs

Diagnosis is based on clinical observations of patients and histologic studies usin, histochemistry and electron microscopy. Common symptoms of the disease are weaknes and atrophy of the distal muscles of the lower limbs which progress to the hands and arms then the trunk, neck and face. Wasting, muscle stiffness, cramps can also be found. Th myopathy may progress to facial, cervical, velopharyngeal, truncal and respiratory muscles The vast majority of MFM patients have an adult onset of their progressive muscl symptoms (Goldfarb et al., 2004). Cardiomyopathy is associated in 15 to 30 % of the affecte individuals. However, in some patients, the cardiomyopathy may precede the muscl weakness. Therefore, distal muscle involvement, cardiomyopathy and periphera neuropathy are important clinical clues, although they are not present in all patients (Bar e al., 2004; Finsterer & Stollberger, 2008; Schroder et al., 2007).

2.1.1 Skeletal

The abnormal size of muscular fibers, with few atrophic fibers, are the characteristics of th disorder. These fibers present amorphous, granular or hyaline deposits that vary in shap and size. As abnormal fibers can be focally distributed, the symptomatic changes may b missed in small samples. Many abnormal fibers show alteration in oxidative enzyme activity, which are diminished or absent. Reduced oxidative activity is often associated wit the presence of hyaline structures, and conversely, enhanced activity around the large inclusions. Some muscular fibers harbor small to large vacuoles containing membranou materials. Many hyaline structures are stained blue or blue-red with Trichome or intensivel stained with Congo red, which is an important diagnostic feature of MFM biopsie (Schroder & Schoser, 2009).

Immunohistochemical studies reveal accumulations of desmin, myotilin, dystrophin sarcoglycans, actin, plectin, gelsolin, filamin C, syncoilin, Bag3, synemin, αB-crystallin Hsp27 and DNAJB2. Additional pathologic markers may be observed, including phosphorylated tau proteins, β amyloids, ubiquitin, glycoxidation and lipoxidation can b found, more specifically in desmin- and myotilin-opathies (Selcen, 2011).

Electron microscopy shows a marked disorganization of the myofibrils ultrastructure beginning at the Z-disc. Accumulation of dense materials is found in the close proximity o the Z-disc. In patients with desmin, αB-crystallin or Bag3 mutations, small pleiomorphi dense structures or granulofilamentous materials are found between the myofibrils. At late stages, Z-disc are disintegrated and sarcomeres disorganized, a prelude to myofibril dislocation (Goldfarb & Dalakas, 2009). Electromyogram (EMO) studies of affected muscle reveal myopathic motor units potentials and abnormal electrical irritability, often wit myotonic discharges (Schroder & Schoser, 2009).

2.1.2 Cardiac

All the genes cited in paragraph 2.3 cause cardiomyopathy. In 15 to 30 % of patients, th disorder presents with cardiomyopathy. There are also cases with only cardiomyopathi signs without skeletal muscle involvement. In advanced stages of the disease cardiomyopathies develop in up to 60 % of the patients. MFM-associated atrioventricula conduction blocks can be associated with dilated (17 %), restricted (12 %), or hypertrophic (%) cardiomyopathy (van Spaendonck-Zwarts et al., 2010). When the cardiac muscle i involved, impaired conduction, arrhythmia, cardiac hypertrophy or dilation, secondar alvular insufficiency, intracardial formation of thrombi and heart failure can be observed. The least severe cases are caused by myotilin mutations. Atrioventricular conduction bnormalities may occur, and require urgent implantation of permanent pacemaker. This eature of MFMs can be attributed to the fact that the conduction system is rich in desmin Finsterer & Stollberger, 2008; Goldfarb & Dalakas, 2009).

.1.3 Respiratory

As the diaphragm is the main muscle involved in the respiratory cycle, progressive espiratory muscle impairment can occur, sometimes at early stages. Respiratory nsufficiency can therefore be a major cause of disability and death with hypoventilation and ultimately respiratory failure, caused for example by mutations A357P, L370P in the lesmin gene, or P209L in the BAG3 gene. Respiratory muscle weakness leads to a restrictive entilatory failure when there is a mutation on the genes causing any of the myopathies xcept on ZASPopathy in which respiratory muscle involvement has not yet been described Goldfarb & Dalakas, 2009).

.2 Inheritance

The majority of cases follow an autosomal dominant mode of inheritance, and very few an autosomal recessive pattern. However, a significant number of MFMs shows sporadic lisease manifestation.

.2.1 Autosomal dominant mode

80 % of families with MFMs present an autosomal dominant pattern of inheritance, mostly vith full penetrance (Goldfarb & Dalakas, 2009). Depending on the mutation, however, hese facts can be modulated: for example, in families with the I451M mutation in the lesmin gene, incomplete penetrance was demonstrated for the first time (Li et al., 1999). It is not possible, however, to link a specific mutation of the affected genes to clinical signs, although certain mutations are more frequently associated with specific signs. For example, he desmin A350P mutation predisposes male patients to higher risks of sudden cardiac leath (Walter et al., 2007), as it is also the case for men and women in mutations p.E114del and N116S of the segment 1A of the desmin gene (Klauke et al., 2010; Vernengo et al., 2010).

.2.2 Autosomal recessive mode

n a restricted number of families (6%), mutations are autosomal recessive (Goldfarb & Dalakas, 2009). The disease generally develops in childhood with severe clinical symptoms Goldfarb et al., 2004). This is the case, for example, of the deletion A173_G179del of 21 nucleotides in the 1B helical segment of desmin (Muñoz-Marmol et al., 1998). Another ntriguing report indicate two mutations A360P and N393I in the desmin protein, which are not pathogenic in heterozygous state, but give rise to a highly aggressive cardioskeletal myopathy when combined in the same child (Goldfarb et al., 1998). There is also a case reported for αB-crystallin (mutation S21AfsX24) (Selcen, 2011).

2.2.3 Modifying genes

Lamin A/C mutations have been involved in muscular dystrophies but can also lead to completely different pathologies, depending on the mutations involved. A patient with a combination of Lamin A/C A644C and desmin V469M mutations developed severe muscl weakness and complete heart block, requiring heart transplantation (Muntoni et al., 2006) Lamin A/C and desmin networks are supposed to be indirectly connected (Costa et al. 2004), and therefore may interact in the development of the disease. As individuals from th same family are diversely affected by the disease, one can suspect their individual histor (practice of sport) or differential genetic background. The question of the identity o modifying genes remains, however, largely unresolved.

2.3 Molecular genetics
So far, six genes have been formally identified and are held responsible for MFMs associate with cardiomyopathy, but for around 80 % of the patients, the disease still awaits molecular diagnosis (Selcen, 2011). Schröder et al. include FHL1 and plectin in MFM causing genes (Schröder, 2009). The knowledge of the structure and function of the alread identified genes is, therefore, a prerequisite for the understanding of human MFMs.

2.3.1 Desmin
The human *DES* gene (NM_001927.3), on chromosome 2q35, comprises nine exons within a 8.4 kb region that encodes a 470 amino acids (53 kDa) muscle-specific protein (Li et al. 1989). Desmin belongs to the family of type III intermediate filaments (IF) proteins, whicl polymerize into 10 nm filaments, a size intermediate between thick (15 nm) and thin (5-nm) filaments. Desmin is synthetized only in cardiac, skeletal and smooth muscle (Lazarides & Hubbard, 1976 ; Paulin & Li, 2004). It is organized into three domains, a highl conserved α helical core of 303 amino acids residues flanked by globular N- and C- termina structures. The helical structure, called the rod domain, is interrupted by three shor polypeptide linkers (L1, L12, L2), which determine four consecutive helical segments (1A 1B, 2A, 2B). Desmin is more abundant in heart muscle (2% of total proteins) of mammal than in their skeletal muscle (0.35%) (Paulin et al., 2004). It forms a three-dimensiona scaffold around the myofibrillar Z-disc, and interconnects the entire contractile apparatu with the subsarcolemmal cytoskeleton and the nuclei (Lazarides & Hubbard, 1976). Desmi also forms longitudinal connections between the peripheries of successive Z-discs and alon the plasma membrane. In addition, desmin IFs bind and participate to the location o mitochondria. In the heart, desmin is particularly abundant in Purkinje conduction fibers and at intercalated discs, where it forms a double-banded structure (Thornell & Eriksson 1981). Since the first description of desminopathy by Goldfarb et al. (Goldfarb et al., 1998 and Muñoz-Marmol et al. (Muñoz-Marmol et al., 1998), more than 50 mutations (45 missenses, 4 in frame deletions, 1 exon skipping, 2 single nucleotide insertion with premature termination) have been described (Klauke et al., 2011; Selcen, 2011; var Spaendonck-Zwarts et al., 2010).
Studies of DES-knockout mice have shown that defects develop in skeletal, smooth and cardiac muscle after birth, principally characterized by a loss of lateral alignment and anchorage of myofibrils, swollen mitochondria and loss of nuclear shape. The heart develop a myopathy with impaired force generation, increased diastolic pressure with thicker ventricle walls (Li et al., 1996; Milner et al., 1996). Few transgenic mice have beer described. With the Arg173_Glu179del desmin mutant transgene, aggregates containing desmin and other cytoskeletal proteins have been found in the heart (Wang et al., 2001a). A clear explanation of the molecular pathogenesis remains to be found.

Misfolded desmin molecules escape regular degradation mechanisms and accumulate with other proteins as aggregates. Cellular transfection studies have demonstrated that aggregates inhibit the proteasome system (Liu et al., 2006). In general, aggregates may accumulate through an active transport mechanism into perinuclear bodies called aggresomes (Johnston et al., 1998). Aggregates and proteasome impairement trigger autophagy (macroautophagy) as a mechanism of cellular cleaning (Tannous et al., 2008a), but recent studies have shown that this process is stalled at least with the desmin S13F mutant used in these studies (Wong et al., 2008).

.3.2 αB-crystallin

AlphaB-crystallin is a small heat shock protein (shSP) of 20 kDa that assembles into 500 – 800 kDa homo and heterodimers with other shSPs. It is encoded by the CRYAB gene (NM_001885.1), a three-exon gene on chromosome 11 (11q21-23) in human beings. αB-crystallin proteins contain a conserved α crystallin domain (residues 67 to 149), surrounded by a N-terminal domain and a C-terminal extension (residues 149 – 175) (Ganea, 2001; MacRae, 2000). αB-crystallin is abundantly expressed, together with αA-crystallin and other similar shSPs in the lens where it prevents cataract formation (Horwitz, 2003). It is also found in other tissues, with the highest level in cardiac and skeletal muscles (Iwaki et al., 1990; Sax & Piatigorsky, 1994). In these tissues, αB-crystallin is localized to the Z-disc, and its expression is induced after stress (Golenhofen et al., 2004; Lutsch et al., 1997). αB-crystallin is known to act as a molecular chaperone of desmin, actin, tubulin and several other soluble molecules (Goldfarb & Dalakas, 2009). αB-crystallin expression reduces aggregate formation, both *in vitro* and *in vivo*, and is supposed to help neosynthetized desmin proteins by avoiding their aggregation (Bennardini et al., 1992).

The first identification of a MFM case due to a heterozygous missense mutation in the αB-crystallin gene (R120G) was reported in 1998 (Vicart et al., 1998). Since then 9 other mutations have been discovered. Some patients develop also a familial cataract. The only knock-out model is deleted for both αB-crystallin and HspB2 (MKBP) genes because of their close proximity on the chromosome (Brady et al., 2001). CRYAB/HspB2 null mouse heart display poorer functional recovery, high cell death rate, increased stiffness and poor relaxation of myocardium following ischemia / reperfusion. In these mice, mitochondrial permeability transition and calcium uptake were increased in cardiomyocytes (Morrison et al., 2004). In contrast, overexpression of WT αB-crystallin delays or suppresses cardiac hypertrophic response to pressure overload (Kumarapeli et al., 2008). In addition, transgenic mice with cardiac-specific expression of R120G mutant αB-crystallin develop cardiomyopathy in three months and die of heart failure in six – seven months. Just as it is the case of the desmin mutations causing MFMs, αB-crystallinopathies present cytoplasmic aggregates that include desmin, αB-crystallin and several other proteins (Wang et al., 2001b).

.3.3 Myotilin

Myotilin is a 57 kDa protein that is predominantly expressed in skeletal muscle and more weakly in the heart (Salmikangas et al., 1999). The human gene (NM_001135940) is located at the locus 5q31. The N-terminal region contains serine-rich and hydrophobic stretches, and the C-terminal half two immunoglobulin-(Ig)-like domains. The Ig-like domains are required for the formation of antiparallel myotilin dimers. Myotilin is located at the Z-disc where it binds to α-actinin, the main component of the Z-disc, and to filamin C at the periphery. Myotilin also cross-links actin filaments and plays a role in the alignment of myofibrils (Salmikangas et al., 2003). The involvement of myotilin was detected in the yea. 2000 as a missense mutation (T57I) and was identified as limb-girdle muscular dystrophy 1A (LGMD1A) (Hauser et al., 2000). Since then, six new myotilin mutations were identified in eight unrelated patients of the Mayo Clinic MFM cohort. The LGDM1A pathology is therefore a MFM (Selcen & Engel, 2004). Cardiac involvement was found in a subset of patients. While myotilin deletion in mice does not lead to obvious abnormalities, transgenic mice expressing the T57I mutant reproduce morphological and functional features of human myotilinopathies (Garvey et al., 2006). As for desmin, abnormal accumulation of many proteins occur in myotilinopathies.

2.3.4 ZASP

ZASP (Z band Alternatively Spliced PDZ motif-containing protein), also called Oracle or Cypher, is expressed predominantly in cardiac and skeletal muscles (Faulkner et al., 1999). The ZASP gene, called LDB3 (NM_001080114), situated on chromosome 10 (10q22.3-q23.2), encompasses 16 exons, and splice variants exist in cardiac and skeletal muscles, each expressing 3 distincts variants. All ZASP isoforms have a N- terminal PDZ (PSD-95/SAP90, ZO-1 proteins) domain important for interaction with other proteins and a ZASP-like motif (ZM) needed for the interaction with α-actinin. The largest isoforms have three C-terminal LIM (LIN-11, Isl1m, MEC-3 proteins) domains that interact with Protein kinases C (PKCs) (Zhou et al., 1999). ZASP proteins were shown to localize at the Z disc (Klaavuniemi & Ylanne, 2006). The first case of ZASPopathy causing MFM was described in 2005 in 11 MFM patients carrying heterozygous missense mutations (Selcen & Engel, 2005). There was a cardiac involvement in 3 of these 11 patients. Mutations in ZASP was also shown to be responsible for dilated cardiac myopathy, and left-ventricle non compaction (Vatta et al., 2003). Knockout mice for ZASP develop skeletal and cardiac myopathy with fragmented Z-discs (Zheng et al. 2009).

2.3.5 Filamin C

Filamin C (γ-filamin or Filamin 2) belongs to a family of high molecular weight cytoskeletal proteins, expressed in skeletal and cardiac muscle, in contrast to an ubiquitous expression of filamin A and B. Filamin C (NM_001127487) is a 48-exon gene (280 aminoacids) on chromosome 7 (7q32) which belongs to the filamin family of actin-binding proteins that are involved in the reshaping of the actin cytoskeleton and it is associated to myotilin. The amino terminal domain contains an actin-binding domain, followed by a semiflexible rod comprising 24 Ig-like folds, serving as interface for interaction with numerous filamin-binding proteins (van der Flier & Sonnenberg, 2001). Homodimers of Filamin C are involved in the organization of actin filaments and serve as a scaffold for signaling proteins. They link the Z-disc to the sarcolemma by interacting with Z-disc proteins and sarcoglycans in costameres (Thompson et al., 2000). The Ig-like domain 20 also binds to myotilin, and may represent a Z disc targeting motif (van der Ven et al., 2000). The nonsense mutation W2710X was identified in 2005 in patients presenting MFM signs, associated with cardiomyopathy, respiratory insufficiency and peripheral europathy (Vorgerd et al., 2005). Life expectancy is shortened in patients who have utations in the filamin C gene because of cardiomyopathy and the involvement of the espiratory muscles. Cataract and peripheral neuropathy can also occur thus emonstrating that there is a multisystem involvement. Filamin C is expressed before ormation of myotubules and is required for a proper muscle development (van der Ven t al., 2000).

3.6 BAG3

AG3 (Bcl-2 associated athanogen 3), which gene (NM_004281) is situated on hromosome 10 (10q25.2-q26.2), encodes a 535 aminoacid protein. It is a complex ochaperone which principally mediates interaction with Hsp70, Hsc70 and Bcl-2, an ntiapoptotic protein, through its C-terminal BAG domain. The proline-rich domain iteracts with the WW-domain (~35–40 amino acid residues including two highly onserved tryptophan (W) residues separated by 20–23 amino acids) that interacts with roteins implicated in signal transduction (Takayama & Reed, 2001). BAG3 forms a stable omplex with HspB8 (Hsp22) and therefore participates to the degradation, via utophagy, of misfolded and aggregated proteins (Carra et al., 2008a). The first case of AG3 mutation causing MFM was described in 2009 (P209L) in exon 3 (Selcen et al., 2009). ll patients presented a childhood onset with severe progressive muscle weakness and trophy, associated with large left atrium, pulmonary and mitral regurgitation with a estrictive cardiomyopathy pattern. There is also bilateral diaphragm paralysis, reduced orced vital capacity and respiratory insufficiency. Patients have a rigid spine and capular winging. The progression of illness was found rapid when compared to other IFM mutations, and was linked to a significant level of apoptosis (8 % of nuclei). The unction of BAG3 is to stabilize myofibril structure through F-actin. When it is mutated here is myofibril disruption and destabilization of the Z-disk structure under mechanical tress. Knockout mice for BAG3 results in a rapidly-developing myopathy with early ethality and apoptotic features, suggesting a role for BAG3 in supporting cytoskeletal onnections between the Z-disc and myofibrils under mechanical stress (Homma et al., 006).

4 Conclusion

IFMS are muscular dystrophies with specific, but not always identical morphologic eatures. All six genes causing MFMs with cardiac involvement identified so far encode roteins (Figure 1) that are related to the Z-disc. It is therefore important to study the Z-disc, vhich appears increasingly more complex. In fact, it is subjected to an exquisitely fine-tuned rocess of proteins quality control and protein turnover, and is involved in a mechanism of nechanosensing and signaling. These two important functions will be detailed in the ollowing part.

. Integrative biology of myofibrillar myopathies-involved genes

o understand how MFMs develop, it is necessary to describe how muscles are depending n the optimal functioning of the products of the genes described above. For that purpose, his part will develop how the different partners of the muscular structure interact with each thers, in a static as well as in a dynamic point of view.

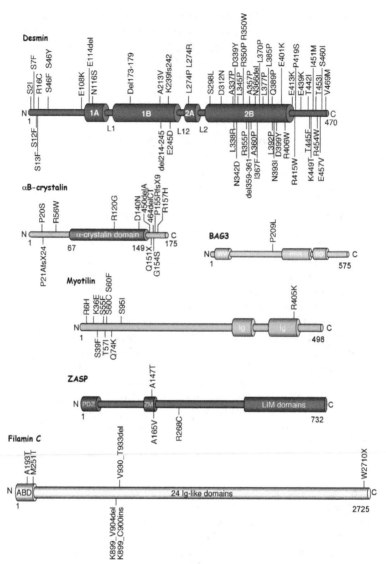

Fig. 1. Schematic representation and localization of mutations in the six proteins involved in myofibrilar myopathies.

N, C: respectively aminoterminal and carboxyterminal extremities. Numbers indicate the aminoacid position in the molecule. 1A, 1B, 2A, 2B are the helical domains of desmin. L1 L12, L2 are the non-helical linkers. WW: tryptophan-conserved domain interacting with proline-rich regions. PRR: Proline-rich region, interacting with WW domains. BD: BAG domain. Ig: immunoglobulin-like domain. PDZ: PSD-95 / SAP90 / ZO-1 proteins common domain. ZM: ZASP-like motif. LIM domains: LIN-11 / Isl1m / MEC-3 proteins common domain. ABD: Actin-binding domain. Ig-like domains: immunoglobulin-like domain.

.1 The smallest contractile unit: The sarcomere

'he myocardium is composed of an assembly of a number of interconnecting, branching .bers, or short cells, separated at their end by the intercalated disk. The fibers contain .umerous fibrils, composed of a regular repeating structure termed the "sarcomere" (Figure A) (Sonnenblick, 1968). The sarcomere is the basic and fundamental unit of striated muscles. Jnderstanding the structure-function relationship linking the structure of the sarcomere to the •hysiology of normal or pathologic heart is therefore essential to understand myofibrillar 1yopathies development. Sarcomeres are distinguished by the striated distribution of their •roteins, visible in light microscopy as three major bands, called A, I and Z (Figure 2B). A •ands contain thick filaments of myosin and proteins that bind to myosin. The I band omprise thin actin filaments and proteins that bind actin. In the middle of the A is the "M •and" also called "M line". The middle part of the I band is the "Z band", also called the "Z line" •r "Z disk". The basic contractile system is the well known actin-myosin tandem. Two heavy 1yosin chains are associated to two light chains and form a globular part. Actin filaments, the hin structure, are composed of a double helix of G-actin (a globular molecule of 46 kDa) •olymerized into a chain (Lehninger et al., 2005). αB-crystallin as chaperone molecule, ₁yotilin and filamin C as scaffolding molecules, are known to interact with actin.

.2 Force transmission

'he first important role of Z-discs is passive transmission of tension through the Z-disc tructural assembly. When a mutation occurs, like in MFM, the mechanism that maintains ixed Z-disc may go awry. In addition, Z-disc proteins allow to transmit force and ensure nechanical coupling between sarcomeres and the sarcolemma via the costameres. Three of our filaments systems of the sarcomere, filamentous F-actin, titin and nebulin/nebulette, nteract with the Z-disc structure. Two proteins participate to the cardiac sacomeric ytoskeleton: titin and nebulette (Figure 2B).

'itin is a giant 3 MDa elastic protein that spans half sarcomeres from Z-disc to M-band, thus orming a continuous structure from one end of the sarcomere to the other, with consecutive itins. Titin can be considered as a giant bidirectional spring responsible for the generation •f passive retraction force in mechanically stretched cardiac myocytes (Granzier & Labeit, .004). Stiffness of titin can be adjusted during development and diseases through a shift in he expression ratio of the two main titin isoforms in cardiac sarcomeres (Lahmers et al., :004; Opitz et al., 2004; Warren et al., 2004). Titin binds to more than 20 structural, •ontractile or signaling molecules, and therefore plays a role as major integrating omponent in the mechanosensory complexes associated to the sarcomeres.

Nebulette is a 107 kDa nebulin homologue present in the cardiac muscle Z-disc. It is omposed of only 22 nebulin motifs (compared to up to 185 in nebulin), and contains a 1ebulin-like C terminus, mediating Z-disc localization (Moncman & Wang, 1995). At •resent, however, its molecular function in cardiac myocytes is still unclear.

The backbone of the Z-disc consists of layers of α-actinin aligned in an antiparallel fashion. n muscle, it cross-links actin filaments of opposite polarity originating from adjacent arcomeres (Stromer & Goll, 1972) and provides anchors for the binding of actin thin ilaments, as well as titin and nebulin/nebulette (Otey & Carpen, 2004). Myotilin and ZASP nteract with α-actinin, and myotilin is linked to filamin C, thus creating a network of •roteins at the Z-disc.

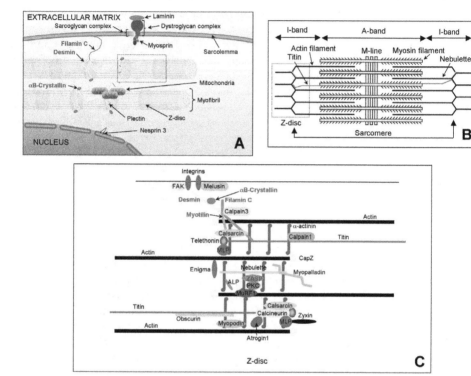

Fig. 2. Schematic representation of the general organization of muscular fibers (A), sarcomere (B) and schematic localization of the major proteins involved in the cardiac Z-disc structure (C).

Figure 2B represents the enlarged dotted rectangle in figure 2A, and Figure 2C the enlarged representation of the dotted rectangle in Figure 2B. Names in red and bold correspond to proteins involved in myofibrillar myopathies, excepted for Bag3 which is not represented. Not all proteins participating to the Z-disc structure or signaling are represented, due to the complexity of this structure. For more details, see text. Figure C is adapted from Frank et al., 2006.

Another essential component is CapZ, a heterodimer composed of α and β subunits which caps the barbed ends of actin filaments. CapZ is proposed to regulate actin dynamics at the barbed end, thereby anchoring the thin filament system to the Z-disc (Schafer et al., 1996).

he costameres are multiproteic complexes which link the marginal Z-discs at their rcumferences to the sarcolemma, the specialized membrane of the individual myofibers. ostameres have been described as transmitters of contractile force to the sarcolemma and xtracellular matrix. This lateral force transmission ensures identical sarcomere length, ereby minimizing shear stress. However, desmin, filamin C, dystrophin, sarcoglycans, tegrins, melusin and focal adhesion kinases have been involved in its structure (reviewed Bloch et al., 2002).

any other proteins (myopalladin, obscurin, Enigma, telethonin, zyxin, ...) participate to the -disc structure (Table 1), but their study is beyond the scope of this review (reviewed in rank et al., 2006). The six genes held responsible for MFM are involved at various degrees Z-disc structure and force transmission (Figure 2C). Desmin forms a continuous network at maintains a spatial relationship between the contractile apparatus and other structural ements of the cells, and is believed to provide maintenance of structural integrity, force ansmission, mechanosignaling, and resistance to external mechanical stress. Myotilin nstitutes the core of a network of proteins, including actin, α-actinin and filamin C, that re part of the force transmission mechanism. In turn, filamin C provides a scaffold for gnaling proteins at the Z-disc, and may be part of a mechanosensing device.

3 Energy metabolism

this part, we will focus on specific effects of the alteration of genes causing MFMs on nergy in muscle. The main effects have been studied on the localization and function of itochondria. Structural studies of intracellular arrangements of mitochondria into nctional complexes with myofibrils and sarcoplasmic reticulum demonstrate their nportance in mitochondrial oxydative activity and membrane permeability (Andrienko et ., 2003; Appaix et al., 2003). There are findings with pathological respiratory chain enzyme ctivities in patients with MFM (Reimann et al., 2003). Desmin intermediate filaments (IFs) ight participate in mitochondrial positioning to areas of high energy demand, respiratory nction, and calcium cycling in cardiac and skeletal muscle (Capetanaki, 2002).

4 Dynamic view of the sarcomere

hile often described as a static structure, the sarcomere is actually dynamic and undergoes nstant turnover, allowing to adapt to physiological changes while still maintaining its nction. New factors have been identified that play a role in the regulation of protein quality ntrol in the sarcomere, including chaperones that mediate the assembly of sarcomere mponents and ubiquitin ligases that control their specific degradation. The Z-disc has dditional important roles as it houses or anchors many additional proteins, which have arious roles, including stretch sensing and signaling or protein quality control. The Z-disc can erefore be considered as a nodal point in signaling and disease (reviewed in Frank et al., 06). In MFMs, the Z-discs are abnormal, the arrangements of myofibrils are in disarray, or ggregates of proteins are present, often near the Z-disc. The highly ordered arrangements of roteins in the sarcomere, which persists even as contractile force is generated, suggest that inding interactions between Z-disc proteins are strong and very stable (Sanger & Sanger, 08). Thus, the continual remodelling of the cardiac sarcomere allows efficient adaptation to hysiological stresses, including exercice or metabolic variations, but also initial efficient daptation to starting pathologies such as ischemic heart disease and myofibrillar myopathies. ince this dynamic turnover is the basis of homeostatic mechanism of sarcomere maintenance, is essential to better understand it.

Cardiomyopathies: Pathophysiology and Genetic

NAME	Size (kDa)	BINDING	FUNCTION	REMARKS
Obscuring	868	M-line, calmodulin, titin	Rho-GEF domain signaling	Giant protein
Myopalladin	145	Nebulette, α-actinin cadiac ankyrin repeat proteins (CARP)	Intra-Z-disc meshwork binds nebulette (directly) and titin (via α-actinin) to actin, CARP signaling ?	Palladin familly
ALP	39	Spectrin repeats of α-actinin	enhances cross-linking actin to α-actinin	PDZ and LIM domain protein 3 (PDLIM3)
Enigma	50	Ret kinase, actin, insulin receptor β tropomyosin	anchor for LIM proteins	PDLIM7
ENH	64	α-actinin 2, PKCε (brain)	hypertrophic program	PDLIM5
CLP36	36	α-actinin 2, Clik1 kinase	stress fibers control, FA	PDLIM1
Zyxin	61	binds actin to MLP α-actinin	close to Z-disc and FAK signalling / antiapoptotic	LIM protein family Nucleoplasmic shuttling
MLP	21	α-actinin, telethonin calcineurin, β spectrin	cardiac stretch receptor and mechanosignalling, negative regulator of cardiac hypertrophy	Nucleoplasmic shuttling
Telethonin	19	Titin N-terminus K+ channels, calsarcin	cardiomyocytes passive tension	negative regulator of myostatin = T-Cap
Calsarcin	27 – 32 *	Calcineurin, α-actinin telethonin, Filamin C, α-actinin	crosslinks Z-disc and Ca²⁺/ calcineurin signalling, inhibits hypertrophic genes sensor for biomechanical stress	= synaptopodin-2
Myopodin	118 – 136 *	α-actinin colocalization	multiadaptor protein ?	nucleoplasmic shuttling

Table 1. Proteins involved in the Z-disc structure as well as in Z-disc signaling, and not detailed in the text.

Other structural and signaling molecules are described paragraphs 3.1, 3.2 and paragraph 3.4.6, respectively. ALP: Actinin-associated LIM Protein. PDZ: PSD-95 / SAP90 / ZO-1 proteins common domain. LIM domains: LIN-11 / Isl1m / MEC-3 proteins common domain. ENH: Enigma Homologue protein. MLP: Muscle LIM Protein. FA: Focal Adhesion. FAK: Focal Adhesion Kinase. PKC: Protein Kinase C.

4.1 Main contractile protein turnover

he following half-lives have been estimated in myocytes:
ctin: 7 to 10 days (Zak, 1977).
[yosin: 5 to 8 days (Martin et al., 1977).
ropomyosin: 7 to 10 days (Zak, 1977).
roponin: 3 to 5 days (Michele et al., 1999).
tin is subjected to a "rapid" turnover, with a half-life estimated to be 3 days in myocytes
ong et al., 1996).

4.2 Protein quality control: Role of chaperone molecules

ultiple endogenous pathways are engaged in restoring cellular homeostasis, among
hich one of the best characterized mechanism involves protein folding by the heat-shock
mily of stress proteins (HSP), also termed chaperones. There are several families of
olecular chaperones present in the cytoplasm of mammalian cells, including Hsp90,
[sp70, TCP1 (CCT, TriC) and small HSP (shSPs). Members of the Hsp90 family are the
ost abundant chaperones located in the cytosol in non-stressed cells which are inducible
ith stress.
[sp70 and Hsc70 (Hsp70 cognate protein) are major players in cardiomyocyte
rotection: the induction of HSP70 by ischemia, and conversely, overexpression of Hsp70
r Hsc70 promotes substantial cardioprotective benefits (Donnelly et al., 1992; Hutter et
l., 1994).
haperonin TRiC requires additional components, such as Hsp40, to stimulate the Hsc70
TPase for protein folding, and is required for folding of actin and tubulin *in vivo*.
nlike Hsp70, small HSPs, including αB-crystallin, Hsp27, Hsp22 and Hsp20 cannot bind
or hydrolyze ATP, and are not able to refold proteins, but can buffer them against
ggregation (Merck et al., 1993). αB-crystallin represents a substantial fraction of adult heart
tal soluble proteins (1 to 3 %) (Kato et al., 1991). The highest level of αB-crystallin
xpression in muscles has been found in the cardiac conduction fibers (Leach et al., 1994).
revious studies indicate that αB-crystallin is highly soluble and localized in the cytosolic
action in unstimulated cardiac myocytes. Heat or ischemia triggers rapid translocation of
B-crystallin into the cytoskeletal and nuclear fraction and specific interactions at the Z-disc
Neufer et al., 1998). HspB8 (Hsp22) and HspB6 (Hsp20) are also expressed in striated
yogenic lineages with high oxidative capacity, such as the heart and type I skeletal muscle
bers (Depre et al., 2002).
ISP molecules are assisted by co-chaperones which perform a variety of tasks, including
odulation of ATPase activity (DNAJ), substrate protein binding and release (BAG : Bcl-2
Associated athanoGene), protein folding (Hsp40 family), assembly, and translocation or
egradation (CHIP : Carboxyterminus of Hsp70 Interacting Protein). Co-chaperones also
ind substrate proteins to modulate folding in a substrate-specific manner (reviewed in
Villis & Patterson, 2010). Among many proteins (more than 40 Co-chaperones), only
naJ, BAG-1, Hop and CHIP have been described in the heart. pDJA1 (DnaJ-like
olecule) expression is restricted to cardiomyocytes. Its levels increase four-fold after
eperfusion (Depre et al., 2003). BAG-1 is able to inhibit apoptosis and to induce
utophagy by interacting with Hsc70, stimulated after ischemia / reperfusion injury
Townsend et al., 2004). The BAG-3 isoform participates in the induction of
acroautophagy in association with HspB8 (Gurusamy et al., 2009). Another protein,

CHIP, plays a role as cochaperone of Hsp70 and in the ubiquitin-proteasome system as a ubiquitin ligase. CHIP may exert a critical function in shuttling damaged and oxydize proteins into autophagic pathways after ischemia / reperfusion injury (Zhang et al., 2005 Increased cochaperone expression in the heart has been found to be cardioprotective i ischemia (Benjamin & McMillan, 1998).

During assembling of the sarcomere, molecular chaperones are needed for the correc folding, assembly and prevention of aggregation. Two molecular chaperone Gim (prefoldin) and TriC (TCP-1 Ring Complex) have been found to play a synergistic rol during synthesis and incorporation of actin filaments into the sarcomere. In contrast t actin, myosin cannot self-assemble without additional factors, including chaperones suc as Unc45, Hsp90 and Hsp70. The assembly of desmin requires the chaperone αB crystallin, to prevent its misfolding and aggregation (Bennardini et al., 1992). αB crystallin also interacts with titin and actin. These data suggest a highly cooperativ relationship between various chaperones during the assembly of the actin filaments i the sarcomere.

In animal models with targeted deletion of muscle-specific chaperone proteins, there is clear evidence of sarcomere disorganization. Cardiac chaperones such as Hsp70, αB crystallin and HspB8 levels are increased during the development of cardia hypertrophy. Hsp27 and αB-crystallin can protect cardiomyocytes against ischemi damages (Martin et al., 1997). Increase in HspB8 expression also results in the re expression of the foetal gene program characteristic of cardiac hypertrophy (Depre et al 2002). The protective role of Hsp22 in ischemia / reperfusion injury appears to be due t its function in activating autophagy, which is critical during the course of this type c injury (Carra et al., 2008b).

3.4.3 The specific ubiquitin – Proteasome system in the sarcomere

The ubiquitin-proteasome system (UPS) recognizes specific proteins and target them fo degradation. Ubiquitin ligases recognize proteins to be degraded and interact with E (activating) and E2 (conjugating) enzymes to create poly-ubiquitin chains on th substrate. Poly-ubiquitin chains are then recognized by the 20S proteasome prior t degradation. Several ubiquitin ligases integrated to the sarcomere have been identified the MuRF family proteins (MuRF1, MuRF2 and MuRF3), MAFbx / atrogin-1 an MDM2.

MuRF1 is found mainly in the M-line of the sarcomere where it interacts with the gian protein titin. MuRF1 specifically recognizes and degrades troponin I. MuRF1 and MuRF are reported to interact with troponin T, myosin light chain 2, myotilin and telethonin While single deletion of either MuRF1 or MuRF2 allows a normal development, cardia hypertrophy develop in mice lacking both genes (Witt et al., 2008). MuRF1 and MuRF3 als interact together with the E2 enzyme to degrade β / slow myosin heavy chains in the heart Mice lacking both proteins develop a hypertrophic cardiomyopathy and skeletal muscl myopathy (Fielitz et al., 2007). MuRF1 may preferentially poly-ubiquitinate oxydize proteins as previous results suggest it (Zhao et al., 2007). Therefore, MuRF1, in cooperatio with MuRF2 and MuRF3 may ensure protein quality control by detecting damaged protein to allow continuous optimal functions of the cardiac sarcomere (reviewed in Willis et al 2009).

additional ubiquitin ligases are also playing important roles in sarcomere maintenance: CHIP, which plays a role as co-chaperone of Hsp70 and as ubiquitin ligase has been recognized as an important factor involved in ischemia / reperfusion injury in the heart Zhang et al., 2005).

MAFbx / atrogin-1 was first identified as an ubiquitin ligase involved in skeletal muscle atrophy (Bodine et al., 2001), possibly by regulating cardiac hypertrophy genes (Li et al., 2007).

MDM-2 is a critical regulator of apoptosis through its ubiquitin-dependent degradation of ARC (Apoptosis Repressor with Caspase recruitment domain). It interacts and mediates telethonin degradation in a proteasome-dependent manner (Tian et al., 2006). Its specific role in the maintenance of sarcomere has to be further explored.

.4.4 Calpain degradation

The highly integrative organization of the sarcomere does not allow direct degradation of the integrated proteins. Predigestion by proteases such as calpains which are embedded in the sarcomeric structure is therefore required. Calpains are a group of calcium-dependent, non-lysosomal cystein proteases expressed ubiquitously in all cells. Calpains are involved in a variety of cellular processes such as cell-cycle control and cell fusion (Goll et al., 2003). Calpain 1 has been found tightly associated to titin in a calcium-dependent manner. It is required to allow the dissociation of sarcomere proteins from the assembled myofibrils before the ubiquitin proteasome system is able to degrade them (Dargelos et al., 2008; Jackman & Kandarian, 2004). When calpains are inhibited in the heart, protein aggregation occur, ubiquitin ligases such as MuRF1 and MAFbx / atrogin-1 are no longer efficient in mediating proteasome-dependent degradation, and autophagy is increased. However, increased levels of calpain 1 in cardiomyocytes of transgenic models lead to cell lysis, cardiac hypertrophy, inflammation and ultimately heart failure (Galvez et al., 2007). These findings are consistent with a critical role of the calpain system in protein quality control in the heart.

.4.5 Sarcomere maintenance and autophagy

Autophagy is a process for protein degradation that uses lysosomal hydrolases working at acidic pH. Autophagy begins with the formation of isolation membrane (phagophore). The phagophore then elongates and engulfs a portion of the cytoplasm to form a mature autophagosome, which then fuses with lysosomes to form autolysosomes. Autophagy removes damaged organelles such as mitochondria and aggregates of misfolded or damaged proteins (Beau et al., 2011). Autophagy-mediated degradation also contributes to the maintenance of the sarcomere (Portbury et al., 2011). In cardiomyocytes, autophagy occurs at the basal level and can be further induced by physiological or pathological conditions such as starvation, haemodynamic stress, ischemia / reperfusion, proteotoxicity, and toxins (Gustafsson & Gottlieb, 2008). Inhibition of autophagy leads to global disorganization of the sarcomere, mitochondrial aggregation, with ventricular dilation, cardiac hypertrophy and contractile dysfunction in adult animal models (Nakai et al., 2007). When autophagy is inactivated, there is an increase in poly-ubiquitinated proteins, as well as in proteasome activity, which suggest that despite its compensatory increase in activity, the UPS may be rapidly overwhelmed by the accumulation of toxic proteins (Bennett et al., 2005). Conversely, inhibition of proteasome activity leads to the accumulation of poly-ubiquitinated proteins and activation of autophagy (Tannous et al., 2008b). These result suggest, therefore, an essential role of cooperativeness between UPS and autophagy in maintaining protein quality control in the heart. Cell signaling pathways, such as PI3K , Akt, and transcription factors like FOXO3 have just begun to be involved as essential mediators in coordinating the proteasomal and lysosomal systems. In addition, shHSP and co-chaperones, like the Hsp22 – BAG3 complex activate autophagy, while BAG1 / BAG3 ratio is important to the balance between proteasomal to autophagic degradation (reviewed in Willis et al., 2009).

3.4.6 Physiological signaling and stress signals

An essential component of cardiac signaling is a process termed mechanotransduction which translates a mechanical stress into a transcriptional response, and may constitute on of the most important stimuli leading to cardiac hypertrophy. Z-disc-associated protein appear to play a critical role in this process (Frank et al., 2008). Mechanosignaling results in increased rate of protein synthesis, alteration of cell shape and increased expression of gene that are normally expressed predominantly during fetal life. Nodal points o mechanotransduction are found along the cardiac sarcomere, notably in the Z-disc, I-band and M-band regions (reviewed in Frank et al., 2006). It has been found that separate directional pathways are implicated by static transverse and longitudinal forces applied to cardiomyocytes to activate distinct cell signaling pathways. The mains involved are foca adhesion kinases (FAK), proteins kinase C (PKC) and integrins:

FAK is the primary effector of integrin signaling, and is localized to costameres in myocyte. (Tornatore et al., 2011). Mechanical stress leads to disruption of FAK interaction with myosin heavy chain at the A-band to Z-disc, costameres and nuclei. Cyclic stretch induces a FAK-mediated activation of JNK and c-jun as well as of MEF2 (Nadruz et al., 2005). FAK appears therefore to play a critical function in hypertrophy, triggered in biomechanical a well as pharmacological models.

PKCε is a modulator of cardiac hypertrophy that belongs to the groups of "unconventional PKCs which do not require Ca^{2+} for their activation (Dorn & Force, 2005). PKCε translocate to the Z-disc in cardiomyocytes upon stimulation, in particular by mechanical stress, or in pressure overload (Gu & Bishop, 1994). PKCε is necessary for cardiac hypertrophy induced by G protein receptors coupled agonists (Iwata et al., 2005). CapZ also plays a role in PKC signaling, which subsequent effects on cardiac contractility. Anchors to the Z-disc for PKCε are also provided by ZASP which links them to α-actinin through binding either to PDZ or LIM domains.

Other molecules, including PDE5A (PhosphoDiEsterase 5A), PCAF (P300/CBP Associated Factor), Zyxin, myopodin and HDAC4, ArgBP2, localize to the Z-disc, A-bands and I-band of myocardial tissue, were found to shuttle between the sarcomere and the nucleus, and modulate the signaling pathways involved in cardiomyopathies (rewieved in Frank & Frey 2011).

Strains on cultured cardiomyocytes also increases FAK activity and PKCε, which lead to the activation of the Rho/ROCK GTPases/kinase pathway, for which substantial evidences support a role in myofibrillogenesis (Franchini et al., 2000; Torsoni et al., 2003). One of the target of PKCε is the muscle actin capping protein for the barbed end of the actin filamen (Schafer et al., 1994). Myocyte contractility, through titin and T-cap may also regulate muscle LIM proteins (MLP) shuttling to and from the nucleus, that may play a further role in myocyte remodeling and hypertrophy, and is required for adaptation to hypertrophic stimuli (Iwata et al., 2005).

Integrins are transmembrane proteins which transduce signals from the extracellular matrix to the inner cell space and conversely. In the myocardium, integrin signalling plays an important role in mediating hypertrophic signals converging on the kinases Erk 1/2, PKC (Heidkamp et al., 2003), p38 MAPK (Aikawa et al., 2002) or JNK (Zhang et al., 2003). Among the proteins binding to integrins upon signaling, were identified the Integrin-Linked Kinase (ILK), FAK and Melusin.

ILK is a serine/threonine kinase. Its specific cardiac deletion in mice leads to dilated cardiomyopathy (DCM) and sudden death, while cardiac-restricted overexpression of ILK induces cardiac hypertrophy via activation of Erk 1/2 and p38 MAPK, indicating a function in hypertrophic signaling (Bendig et al., 2006; Lu et al., 2006).

Melusin is transiently upregulated in the heart upon pressure overload. Deletion of the Melusin gene show DCM and contractile dysfunction upon stress only, while overexpression leads to pathological hypertrophy (Brancaccio et al., 2003; De Acetis et al., 2005).

The Calcineurin / NFAT pathway is modulated by proteins like CIB1/ MLP/Calsarcin/LMDC1 that play a pivotal role in the mediation of pathologic cardiac hypertrophy (Frey et al., 2004). Calcineurin is linked to the Z-disc via calsarcin and MLP, and directly binds to the L-Type Calcium Channel, the major mediator of calcium influx in cardiomyocytes. Calcineurin activates by dephosphorylation the NFAT (Nuclear Factor of Activated T cells) transcription factors family, one of the major mediators of cardiac hypertrophy and remodelling.

PKA and PKG (cGMP-dependent protein kinase-G) are bound to titin. PKA is stimulated by β-adrenergic stimulation by catecholamines, while PKG is stimulated by nitric oxide and the natriuretic peptide (Wong & Fiscus, 2010). PKA can phosphorylate troponin-I, myosin-binding protein C and titin (Yamasaki et al., 2002; Yang et al., 2001; Zakhary et al., 1999).

4. From healthy to failing heart : Etiology and studies of myofibrilar cardiomyopathies

4.1 Diagnosis

As MFM refers to a group of genetically distinct disorders, common morphologic features observed on muscles are determinant. The following clinical findings should direct the diagnosis to a myofibrillar myopathy.

4.1.1 Clinical signs

Most patients with MFM show progressive muscle weakness. A small proportion of patients show paresthesias, muscle atrophy, stiffness or aching, cramps, dyspnea or dysphagia, or mild facial weakness. In about one third of the cases, the weakness is predominantly distal, in another third it is more proximal than distal, and in the other third it is mixed. In some patients, however, the cardiomyopathy may precede the muscle weakness.

Cardiomyopathy is a "classical" feature in MFM and may precede, coincide or follow the skeletal muscle weakness. Cardiomyopathy includes arrhythmogenic type (with atrio-ventricular blocks, supraventricular and ventricular ectopic beats and tachycardia), hypertrophic, dilated or restrictive features (reviewed in Ferrer & Olive, 2008; Goldfarb & Dalakas, 2009; Schroder & Schoser, 2009; Selcen, 2011).

Serum creatine kinase (CK) is variable, sometimes elevated. Differences depending on th causal gene have been reported (Schroder & Schoser, 2009):

DES, CRYAB and MYOT: normal up to 5 fold (reported maximal 15 fold for MYOT)
FLNC: normal up to 10 fold
ZASP: normal up to 6 fold
BAG3: 3 up to 15 fold

4.1.2 Histopathology

Muscle histology is essential and reveals characteristic features:
- Amorphous, hyaline or granular materials stained by trichrome.
- hyaline structures intensely positive for Congo red staining.
- significant decrease of oxidative enzyme activity in many abnormal fibers regions.
- small vacuoles in a variable number of fibers.

Immunohistochemistry performed on frozen sections (paraformaledehyde-fixed (4%)) from biopsies show abnormal ectopic expression of desmin, αB-crystallin, myotilin and dystrophin (Claeys et al., 2009; Schroder & Schoser, 2009; Selcen, 2011).

4.1.3 Electromyography

Electromyography (EMG) should be performed to confirm the histopathological data. EMG reveals abnormal electrical irritability often with myotonic discharges. The motor uni potentials are mostly myopathic, sometimes in combination with neurogenic feature (Schroder & Schoser, 2009).

4.1.4 Electron microscopy

Electron microscopy of muscles showing progressive myofibrillar degeneration revea abnormalities starting from the Z-disc area: streaming, defects in stacking, accumulation o granulo-filamentous dense materials, sarcomere disintegration, dislocated membranous materials, autophagic vacuoles, abnormal accumulation or location of mitochondria Ultrastructural observation may allow to differentiate between granulofilamentous accumulation, "sandwich" formation, filamentous bundles, floccular thin filaments, tubular filamentous accumulations, and early apoptotic changes, to allow to direct diagnostic efforts toward the type of gene causing the MFM (Claeys et al., 2008).

4.2 Clinical perspectives and therapeutic considerations

There is currently no specific treatment for myofibrillar myopathies, nor clinical trial investigations (to the best of our knowledge).

MFM share protein aggregation with other aggregate-prone diseases, such as Alzheimer's Parkinson's and Huntington's diseases. Accumulation of toxic β-amyloid oligomers impairment of the ubiquitin proteasome system, alteration of the efficiency of the autophagic process have also been reported in studies about these diseases (Aguzzi & O'Connor, 2010). Several treatments have been set up and are currently tested for clinical trials, and may possibly be studied in the case of myofibrillar myopathies. However, caution should be taken because reducing the formation of aggregates may not directly allow to the cure of the disease (Sanbe et al., 2005).

Curcumin, a polyphenol naturally occurring in plant products, has been shown to inhibit α-synuclein aggregates formation involved in Parkinson's disease (Pandey et al., 2008).

nother way to reduce aggregates formation is to activate HSP, which may favour refolding
r degradation of mutant proteins, or folding of the WT proteins expressed in the normal
lele. Non-steroidal anti-inflammatory drugs, prostaglandins (Amici et al., 1992), Celastrol
Westerheide et al., 2004) or Geranylgeranylacetone (Sanbe et al., 2009) have been shown to
ctivate the heat shock response. However, it is probably not judicious to induce αB-
rystallin if this gene is mutated.

ctivators of the autophagic pathway of degradation have been reported and could
onstitute a way to clear aggregates from the cardiomyocytes. Among many compounds
ctually tested, one can cite starvation, rapamycin, wortmanin, trehalose, etc (Sarkar &
ubinsztein, 2008).

ntioxydant agents, such as vitamin C, N-acetyl cysteine, ROS trapping agents like phenyl-
J-tert-butylnitrone may also help to reduce aggregates formation, or help to their
egradation (Squier, 2001).

. Conclusion

here has been considerable improvement in the understanding of myofibrillar myopathies
ince they were first reported in 1978 (Fardeau et al., 1978). New avenues of discoveries
ave just opened with concepts of protein quality control, involving chaperone molecules,
ie ubiquitine proteasome system, and macroautophagy. Moreover, the sarcomere is not
nly seen now as a passive force generator, but also as a mechanosensor which signals to the
ucleus and to the whole muscular fiber, and activates specific programs of renewal of
arcomeric proteins, in case of damages. These new findings will help to integrate more
omponents of the muscle physiology, and to understand how they are modified when
1FM-causing genes are mutated. However, only 20 % of MFM have found a "culprit" gene,
o it may be necessary to analyze other Z-disc-specific structural, quality control or signaling
enes to find new candidates responsible for MFMs.

. Acknowledgment

Ve thank Sabrina Pichon and Patrick Vicart for careful reading of the manuscript. This work
vas supported by grants from Association Française contre les Myopathies (AFM) and
CNRS (A.L).

. References

A. Aguzzi & T. O'Connor. (2010) Protein aggregation diseases: pathogenicity and
    therapeutic perspectives. Nat Rev Drug Discov, Vol.9, No.3, pp. 237-48
t. Aikawa, T. Nagai, S. Kudoh, Y. Zou, M. Tanaka, M. Tamura, H. Akazawa, H. Takano, R.
    Nagai & I. Komuro. (2002) Integrins play a critical role in mechanical stress-
    induced p38 MAPK activation. Hypertension, Vol.39, No.2, pp. 233-8
C. Amici, L. Sistonen, M. G. Santoro & R. I. Morimoto. (1992) Antiproliferative
    prostaglandins activate heat shock transcription factor. Proc Natl Acad Sci U S A,
    Vol.89, No.14, pp. 6227-31
'. Andrienko, A. V. Kuznetsov, T. Kaambre, Y. Usson, A. Orosco, F. Appaix, T. Tiivel, P.
    Sikk, M. Vendelin, R. Margreiter & V. A. Saks. (2003) Metabolic consequences of

functional complexes of mitochondria, myofibrils and sarcoplasmic reticulum in muscle cells. *J Exp Biol*, Vol.206, No.Pt 12, pp. 2059-72

F. Appaix, A. V. Kuznetsov, Y. Usson, L. Kay, T. Andrienko, J. Olivares, T. Kaambre, P. Sik, R. Margreiter & V. Saks. (2003) Possible role of cytoskeleton in intracellular arrangement and regulation of mitochondria. *Exp Physiol*, Vol.88, No.1, pp. 175-90

H. Bar, S. V. Strelkov, G. Sjoberg, U. Aebi & H. Herrmann. (2004) The biology of desmin filaments: how do mutations affect their structure, assembly, and organisation? *Struct Biol*, Vol.148, No.2, pp. 137-52

I. Beau, M. Mehrpour & P. Codogno. (2011) Autophagosomes and human diseases. *Int Biochem Cell Biol*, Vol.43, No.4, pp. 460-4

G. Bendig, M. Grimmler, I. G. Huttner, G. Wessels, T. Dahme, S. Just, N. Trano, H. A. Katus, M. C. Fishman & W. Rottbauer. (2006) Integrin-linked kinase, a novel component of the cardiac mechanical stretch sensor, controls contractility in the zebrafish heart. *Genes Dev*, Vol.20, No.17, pp. 2361-72

I. J. Benjamin & D. R. McMillan. (1998) Stress (heat shock) proteins: molecular chaperones in cardiovascular biology and disease. *Circ Res*, Vol.83, No.2, pp. 117-32

F. Bennardini, A. Wrzosek & M. Chiesi. (1992) Alpha B-crystallin in cardiac tissue. Association with actin and desmin filaments. *Circ Res*, Vol.71, No.2, pp. 288-94

E. J. Bennett, N. F. Bence, R. Jayakumar & R. R. Kopito. (2005) Global impairment of the ubiquitin-proteasome system by nuclear or cytoplasmic protein aggregates precedes inclusion body formation. *Mol Cell*, Vol.17, No.3, pp. 351-65

R. J. Bloch, Y. Capetanaki, A. O'Neill, P. Reed, M. W. Williams, W. G. Resneck, N. C. Porter & J. A. Ursitti. (2002) Costameres: repeating structures at the sarcolemma of skeletal muscle. *Clin Orthop Relat Res*, No.403 Suppl, pp. S203-10

S. C. Bodine, E. Latres, S. Baumhueter, V. K. Lai, L. Nunez, B. A. Clarke, W. T. Poueymirou, F. J. Panaro, E. Na, K. Dharmarajan, Z. Q. Pan, D. M. Valenzuela, T. M. DeChiara, T. N. Stitt, G. D. Yancopoulos & D. J. Glass. (2001) Identification of ubiquitin ligases required for skeletal muscle atrophy. *Science*, Vol.294, No.5547, pp. 1704-8

J. P. Brady, D. L. Garland, D. E. Green, E. R. Tamm, F. J. Giblin & E. F. Wawrousek. (2001) AlphaB-crystallin in lens development and muscle integrity: a gene knockout approach. *Invest Ophthalmol Vis Sci*, Vol.42, No.12, pp. 2924-34

M. Brancaccio, L. Fratta, A. Notte, E. Hirsch, R. Poulet, S. Guazzone, M. De Acetis, C. Vecchione, G. Marino, F. Altruda, L. Silengo, G. Tarone & G. Lembo. (2003) Melusin, a muscle-specific integrin beta1-interacting protein, is required to prevent cardiac failure in response to chronic pressure overload. *Nat Med*, Vol.9, No.1, pp. 68-75

Y. Capetanaki. (2002) Desmin cytoskeleton: a potential regulator of muscle mitochondria behavior and function. *Trends Cardiovasc Med*, Vol.12, No.8, pp. 339-48

S. Carra, S. J. Seguin & J. Landry. (2008a) HspB8 and Bag3: a new chaperone complex targeting misfolded proteins to macroautophagy. *Autophagy*, Vol.4, No.2, pp. 237-9

S. Carra, S. J. Seguin, H. Lambert & J. Landry. (2008b) HspB8 chaperone activity toward poly(Q)-containing proteins depends on its association with Bag3, a stimulator of macroautophagy. *J Biol Chem*, Vol.283, No.3, pp. 1437-44

. G. Claeys, M. Fardeau, R. Schroder, T. Suominen, K. Tolksdorf, A. Behin, O. Dubourg, B. Eymard, T. Maisonobe, T. Stojkovic, G. Faulkner, P. Richard, P. Vicart, B. Udd, T. Voit & G. Stoltenburg. (2008) Electron microscopy in myofibrillar myopathies reveals clues to the mutated gene. *Neuromuscul Disord,* Vol.18, No.8, pp. 656-66

. G. Claeys, P. F. van der Ven, A. Behin, T. Stojkovic, B. Eymard, O. Dubourg, P. Laforet, G. Faulkner, P. Richard, P. Vicart, N. B. Romero, G. Stoltenburg, B. Udd, M. Fardeau, T. Voit & D. O. Furst. (2009) Differential involvement of sarcomeric proteins in myofibrillar myopathies: a morphological and immunohistochemical study. *Acta Neuropathol,* Vol.117, No.3, pp. 293-307

1. L. Costa, R. Escaleira, A. Cataldo, F. Oliveira & C. S. Mermelstein. (2004) Desmin: molecular interactions and putative functions of the muscle intermediate filament protein. *Braz J Med Biol Res,* Vol.37, No.12, pp. 1819-30

. Dargelos, S. Poussard, C. Brule, L. Daury & P. Cottin. (2008) Calcium-dependent proteolytic system and muscle dysfunctions: a possible role of calpains in sarcopenia. *Biochimie,* Vol.90, No.2, pp. 359-68

1. De Acetis, A. Notte, F. Accornero, G. Selvetella, M. Brancaccio, C. Vecchione, M. Sbroggio, F. Collino, B. Pacchioni, G. Lanfranchi, A. Aretini, R. Ferretti, A. Maffei, F. Altruda, L. Silengo, G. Tarone & G. Lembo. (2005) Cardiac overexpression of melusin protects from dilated cardiomyopathy due to long-standing pressure overload. *Circ Res,* Vol.96, No.10, pp. 1087-94

. Depre, M. Hase, V. Gaussin, A. Zajac, L. Wang, L. Hittinger, B. Ghaleh, X. Yu, R. K. Kudej, T. Wagner, J. Sadoshima & S. F. Vatner. (2002) H11 kinase is a novel mediator of myocardial hypertrophy *in vivo. Circ Res,* Vol.91, No.11, pp. 1007-14

. Depre, L. Wang, J. E. Tomlinson, V. Gaussin, M. Abdellatif, J. N. Topper & S. F. Vatner. (2003) Characterization of pDJA1, a cardiac-specific chaperone found by genomic profiling of the post-ischemic swine heart. *Cardiovasc Res,* Vol.58, No.1, pp. 126-35

. J. Donnelly, R. E. Sievers, F. L. Vissern, W. J. Welch & C. L. Wolfe. (1992) Heat shock protein induction in rat hearts. A role for improved myocardial salvage after ischemia and reperfusion? *Circulation,* Vol.85, No.2, pp. 769-78

3. W. Dorn, 2nd & T. Force. (2005) Protein kinase cascades in the regulation of cardiac hypertrophy. *J Clin Invest,* Vol.115, No.3, pp. 527-37

1. Fardeau, J. Godet-Guillain, F. M. Tome, H. Collin, S. Gaudeau, C. Boffety & P. Vernant. (1978) [A new familial muscular disorder demonstrated by the intra-sarcoplasmic accumulation of a granulo-filamentous material which is dense on electron microscopy (author's transl)]. *Rev Neurol (Paris),* Vol.134, No.6-7, pp. 411-25

3. Faulkner, A. Pallavicini, E. Formentin, A. Comelli, C. Ievolella, S. Trevisan, G. Bortoletto, P. Scannapieco, M. Salamon, V. Mouly, G. Valle & G. Lanfranchi. (1999) ZASP: a new Z-band alternatively spliced PDZ-motif protein. *J Cell Biol,* Vol.146, No.2, pp. 465-75

. Ferrer & M. Olive. (2008) Molecular pathology of myofibrillar myopathies. *Expert Rev Mol Med,* Vol.10, e25

. Fielitz, M. S. Kim, J. M. Shelton, S. Latif, J. A. Spencer, D. J. Glass, J. A. Richardson, R. Bassel-Duby & E. N. Olson. (2007) Myosin accumulation and striated muscle myopathy result from the loss of muscle RING finger 1 and 3. *J Clin Invest*, Vol.117 No.9, pp. 2486-95

J. Finsterer & C. Stollberger. (2008) Primary myopathies and the heart. *Scand Cardiovasc* Vol.42, No.1, pp. 9-24

S. Fong, S. J. Hamill, M. Proctor, S. M. Freund, G. M. Benian, C. Chothia, M. Bycroft &] Clarke. (1996) Structure and stability of an immunoglobulin superfamily domain from twitchin, a muscle protein of the nematode Caenorhabditis elegans. *J Mol Bio* Vol.264, No.3, pp. 624-39

K. G. Franchini, A. S. Torsoni, P. H. Soares & M. J. Saad. (2000) Early activation of the multicomponent signaling complex associated with focal adhesion kinase induced by pressure overload in the rat heart. *Circ Res*, Vol.87, No.7, pp. 558-65

D. Frank, C. Kuhn, H. A. Katus & N. Frey. (2006) The sarcomeric Z-disc: a nodal point in signalling and disease. *J Mol Med*, Vol.84, No.6, pp. 446-68

D. Frank, C. Kuhn, B. Brors, C. Hanselmann, M. Ludde, H. A. Katus & N. Frey. (2008) Gen expression pattern in biomechanically stretched cardiomyocytes: evidence for a stretch-specific gene program. *Hypertension*, Vol.51, No.2, pp. 309-18

D. Frank & N. Frey. (2011) Cardiac Z-disc signaling network. *J Biol Chem*, Vol.286, No.12, pp 9897-904

N. Frey, T. Barrientos, J. M. Shelton, D. Frank, H. Rutten, D. Gehring, C. Kuhn, M. Lutz, B Rothermel, R. Bassel-Duby, J. A. Richardson, H. A. Katus, J. A. Hill & E. N. Olson (2004) Mice lacking calsarcin-1 are sensitized to calcineurin signaling and show accelerated cardiomyopathy in response to pathological biomechanical stress. *Na Med*, Vol.10, No.12, pp. 1336-43

A. S. Galvez, A. Diwan, A. M. Odley, H. S. Hahn, H. Osinska, J. G. Melendez, J. Robbins, R A. Lynch, Y. Marreez & G. W. Dorn, 2nd. (2007) Cardiomyocyte degeneration with calpain deficiency reveals a critical role in protein homeostasis. *Circ Res*, Vol.100 No.7, pp. 1071-8

E. Ganea. (2001) Chaperone-like activity of alpha-crystallin and other small heat shock proteins. *Curr Protein Pept Sci*, Vol.2, No.3, pp. 205-25

S. M. Garvey, S. E. Miller, D. R. Claflin, J. A. Faulkner & M. A. Hauser. (2006) Transgeni mice expressing the myotilin T57I mutation unite the pathology associated with LGMD1A and MFM. *Hum Mol Genet*, Vol.15, No.15, pp. 2348-62

L. G. Goldfarb, K. Y. Park, L. Cervenakova, S. Gorokhova, H. S. Lee, O. Vasconcelos, J. W Nagle, C. Semino-Mora, K. Sivakumar & M. C. Dalakas. (1998) Missense mutation in desmin associated with familial cardiac and skeletal myopathy. *Nat Gene* Vol.19, No.4, pp. 402-3

L. G. Goldfarb, P. Vicart, H. H. Goebel & M. C. Dalakas. (2004) Desmin myopathy. *Brain* Vol.127, No.Pt 4, pp. 723-34

L. G. Goldfarb & M. C. Dalakas. (2009) Tragedy in a heartbeat: malfunctioning desmin causes skeletal and cardiac muscle disease. *J Clin Invest*, Vol.119, No.7, pp. 1806-13

N. Golenhofen, M. D. Perng, R. A. Quinlan & D. Drenckhahn. (2004) Comparison of the small heat shock proteins alphaB-crystallin, MKBP, HSP25, HSP20, and cvHSP in heart and skeletal muscle. *Histochem Cell Biol*, Vol.122, No.5, pp. 415-25

. E. Goll, V. F. Thompson, H. Li, W. Wei & J. Cong. (2003) The calpain system. *Physiol Rev,* Vol.83, No.3, pp. 731-801

. L. Granzier & S. Labeit. (2004) The giant protein titin: a major player in myocardial mechanics, signaling, and disease. *Circ Res,* Vol.94, No.3, pp. 284-95

. Gu & S. P. Bishop. (1994) Increased protein kinase C and isozyme redistribution in pressure-overload cardiac hypertrophy in the rat. *Circ Res,* Vol.75, No.5, pp. 926-31

. Gurusamy, I. Lekli, M. Gherghiceanu, L. M. Popescu & D. K. Das. (2009) BAG-1 induces autophagy for cardiac cell survival. *Autophagy,* Vol.5, No.1, pp. 120-1

.. B. Gustafsson & R. A. Gottlieb. (2008) Recycle or die: the role of autophagy in cardioprotection. *J Mol Cell Cardiol,* Vol.44, No.4, pp. 654-61

. A. Hauser, S. K. Horrigan, P. Salmikangas, U. M. Torian, K. D. Viles, R. Dancel, R. W. Tim, A. Taivainen, L. Bartoloni, J. M. Gilchrist, J. M. Stajich, P. C. Gaskell, J. R. Gilbert, J. M. Vance, M. A. Pericak-Vance, O. Carpen, C. A. Westbrook & M. C. Speer. (2000) Myotilin is mutated in limb girdle muscular dystrophy 1A. *Hum Mol Genet,* Vol.9, No.14, pp. 2141-7

. C. Heidkamp, A. L. Bayer, B. T. Scully, D. M. Eble & A. M. Samarel. (2003) Activation of focal adhesion kinase by protein kinase C epsilon in neonatal rat ventricular myocytes. *Am J Physiol Heart Circ Physiol,* Vol.285, No.4, pp. H1684-96

. Homma, M. Iwasaki, G. D. Shelton, E. Engvall, J. C. Reed & S. Takayama. (2006) BAG3 deficiency results in fulminant myopathy and early lethality. *Am J Pathol,* Vol.169, No.3, pp. 761-73

Horwitz. (2003) Alpha-crystallin. *Exp Eye Res,* Vol.76, No.2, pp. 145-53

. M. Hutter, R. E. Sievers, V. Barbosa & C. L. Wolfe. (1994) Heat-shock protein induction in rat hearts. A direct correlation between the amount of heat-shock protein induced and the degree of myocardial protection. *Circulation,* Vol.89, No.1, pp. 355-60

. Iwaki, A. Kume-Iwaki & J. E. Goldman. (1990) Cellular distribution of alpha B-crystallin in non-lenticular tissues. *J Histochem Cytochem,* Vol.38, No.1, pp. 31-9

. Iwata, A. Maturana, M. Hoshijima, K. Tatematsu, T. Okajima, J. R. Vandenheede, J. Van Lint, K. Tanizawa & S. Kuroda. (2005) PKCepsilon-PKD1 signaling complex at Z-discs plays a pivotal role in the cardiac hypertrophy induced by G-protein coupling receptor agonists. *Biochem Biophys Res Commun,* Vol.327, No.4, pp. 1105-13

. W. Jackman & S. C. Kandarian. (2004) The molecular basis of skeletal muscle atrophy. *Am J Physiol Cell Physiol,* Vol.287, No.4, pp. C834-43

. A. Johnston, W. C. L. & R. R. Kopito. (1998) Aggresomes: a cellular response to misfolded proteins. *J. Cell. Biol.,* Vol.143, No.7, pp. 1883-1898

. Kato, H. Shinohara, N. Kurobe, Y. Inaguma, K. Shimizu & K. Ohshima. (1991) Tissue distribution and developmental profiles of immunoreactive alpha B crystallin in the rat determined with a sensitive immunoassay system. *Biochim Biophys Acta,* Vol.1074, No.1, pp. 201-8

. Klaavuniemi & J. Ylanne. (2006) Zasp/Cypher internal ZM-motif containing fragments are sufficient to co-localize with alpha-actinin--analysis of patient mutations. *Exp Cell Res,* Vol.312, No.8, pp. 1299-311

. Klauke, S. Kossmann, A. Gaertner, K. Brand, I. Stork, A. Brodehl, M. Dieding, V. Walhorn, D. Anselmetti, D. Gerdes, B. Bohms, U. Schulz, E. Zu Knyphausen, M.

Vorgerd, J. Gummert & H. Milting. (2010) De novo desmin-mutation N116S i. associated with arrhythmogenic right ventricular cardiomyopathy. *Hum Mol Genet* Vol.19, No.23, pp. 4595-607

A. R. Kumarapeli, H. Su, W. Huang, M. Tang, H. Zheng, K. M. Horak, M. Li & X. Wang (2008) Alpha B-crystallin suppresses pressure overload cardiac hypertrophy. *Circ Res*, Vol.103, No.12, pp. 1473-82

S. Lahmers, Y. Wu, D. R. Call, S. Labeit & H. Granzier. (2004) Developmental control of titin isoform expression and passive stiffness in fetal and neonatal myocardium. *Circ Res*, Vol.94, No.4, pp. 505-13

E. Lazarides & B. D. Hubbard. (1976) Immunological characterization of the subunit of the 100 A filaments from muscle cells. *Proc Natl Acad Sci U S A*, Vol.73, No.12, pp. 4344 8

I. H. Leach, M. L. Tsang, R. J. Church & J. Lowe. (1994) Alpha-B crystallin in the norma human myocardium and cardiac conducting system. *J Pathol*, Vol.173, No.3, pp 255-60

A. L. Lehninger, D. L. Nelson & M. M. Cox (2005) *Principles of biochemistry* (4th), W.H Freeman, 9780716743392,

D. Li, T. Tapscoft, O. Gonzalez, P. E. Burch, M. A. Quinones, W. A. Zoghbi, R. Hill, L. L Bachinski, D. L. Mann & R. Roberts. (1999) Desmin mutation responsible fo: idiopathic dilated cardiomyopathy. *Circulation*, Vol.100, No.5, pp. 461-4

H. H. Li, M. S. Willis, P. Lockyer, N. Miller, H. McDonough, D. J. Glass & C. Patterson (2007) Atrogin-1 inhibits Akt-dependent cardiac hypertrophy in mice via ubiquitin dependent coactivation of Forkhead proteins. *J Clin Invest*, Vol.117, No.11, pp. 3211 23

Z. Li, E. Colucci-Guyon, M. Pincon-Raymond, M. Mericskay, S. Pournin, D. Paulin & C Babinet. (1996) Cardiovascular lesions and skeletal myopathy in mice lacking desmin. *Dev Biol*, Vol.175, No.2, pp. 362-6

Z. L. Li, A. Lilienbaum, G. Butler-Browne & D. Paulin. (1989) Human desmin-coding gene complete nucleotide sequence, characterization and regulation of expression during myogenesis and development. *Gene*, Vol.78, No.2, pp. 243-54

J. Liu, Q. Chen, W. Huang, K. M. Horak, H. Zheng, R. Mestril & X. Wang. (2006) Impairmen of the ubiquitin-proteasome system in desminopathy mouse hearts. *Faseb J*, Vol.20 No.2, pp. 362-4

H. Lu, P. W. Fedak, X. Dai, C. Du, Y. Q. Zhou, M. Henkelman, P. S. Mongroo, A. Lau, H Yamabi, A. Hinek, M. Husain, G. Hannigan & J. G. Coles. (2006) Integrin-linkec kinase expression is elevated in human cardiac hypertrophy and induces hypertrophy in transgenic mice. *Circulation*, Vol.114, No.21, pp. 2271-9

G. Lutsch, R. Vetter, U. Offhauss, M. Wieske, H. J. Grone, R. Klemenz, I. Schimke, J. Stahl & R. Benndorf. (1997) Abundance and location of the small heat shock proteins HSP2E and alphaB-crystallin in rat and human heart. *Circulation*, Vol.96, No.10, pp. 3466-76

T. H. MacRae. (2000) Structure and function of small heat shock/alpha-crystallin proteins established concepts and emerging ideas. *Cell Mol Life Sci*, Vol.57, No.6, pp. 899-913

. F. Martin, M. Rabinowitz, R. Blough, G. Prior & R. Zak. (1977) Measurements of half-life of rat cardiac myosin heavy chain with leucyl-tRNA used as precursor pool. *J Biol Chem*, Vol.252, No.10, pp. 3422-9

L. Martin, R. Mestril, R. Hilal-Dandan, L. L. Brunton & W. H. Dillmann. (1997) Small heat shock proteins and protection against ischemic injury in cardiac myocytes. *Circulation*, Vol.96, No.12, pp. 4343-8

. B. Merck, P. J. Groenen, C. E. Voorter, W. A. de Haard-Hoekman, J. Horwitz, H. Bloemendal & W. W. de Jong. (1993) Structural and functional similarities of bovine alpha-crystallin and mouse small heat-shock protein. A family of chaperones. *J Biol Chem*, Vol.268, No.2, pp. 1046-52

. E. Michele, F. P. Albayya & J. M. Metzger. (1999) Thin filament protein dynamics in fully differentiated adult cardiac myocytes: toward a model of sarcomere maintenance. *J Cell Biol*, Vol.145, No.7, pp. 1483-95

. J. Milner, G. Weitzer, D. Tran, A. Bradley & Y. Capetanaki. (1996) Disruption of muscle architecture and myocardial degeneration in mice lacking desmin. *J Cell Biol*, Vol.134, No.5, pp. 1255-70

. L. Moncman & K. Wang. (1995) Nebulette: a 107 kD nebulin-like protein in cardiac muscle. *Cell Motil Cytoskeleton*, Vol.32, No.3, pp. 205-25

. E. Morrison, R. J. Whittaker, R. E. Klepper, E. F. Wawrousek & C. C. Glembotski. (2004) Roles for alphaB-crystallin and HSPB2 in protecting the myocardium from ischemia-reperfusion-induced damage in a KO mouse model. *Am J Physiol Heart Circ Physiol*, Vol.286, No.3, pp. H847-55

. M. Muñoz-Marmol, G. Strasser, M. Isamat, P. A. Coulombe, Y. Yang, X. Roca, E. Vela, J. L. Mate, J. Coll, M. T. Fernandez-Figueras, J. J. Navas-Palacios, A. Ariza & E. Fuchs. (1998) A dysfunctional desmin mutation in a patient with severe generalized myopathy. *Proc Natl Acad Sci U S A*, Vol.95, No.19, pp. 11312-7

. Muntoni, G. Bonne, L. G. Goldfarb, E. Mercuri, R. J. Piercy, M. Burke, R. B. Yaou, P. Richard, D. Recan, A. Shatunov, C. A. Sewry & S. C. Brown. (2006) Disease severity in dominant Emery Dreifuss is increased by mutations in both emerin and desmin proteins. *Brain*, Vol.129, No.Pt 5, pp. 1260-8

V. Nadruz, Jr., M. A. Corat, T. M. Marin, G. A. Guimaraes Pereira & K. G. Franchini. (2005) Focal adhesion kinase mediates MEF2 and c-Jun activation by stretch: role in the activation of the cardiac hypertrophic genetic program. *Cardiovasc Res*, Vol.68, No.1, pp. 87-97

. Nakai, O. Yamaguchi, T. Takeda, Y. Higuchi, S. Hikoso, M. Taniike, S. Omiya, I. Mizote, Y. Matsumura, M. Asahi, K. Nishida, M. Hori, N. Mizushima & K. Otsu. (2007) The role of autophagy in cardiomyocytes in the basal state and in response to hemodynamic stress. *Nat Med*, Vol.13, No.5, pp. 619-24

. D. Neufer, G. A. Ordway & R. S. Williams. (1998) Transient regulation of c-fos, alpha B-crystallin, and hsp70 in muscle during recovery from contractile activity. *Am J Physiol*, Vol.274, No.2 Pt 1, pp. C341-6

. A. Opitz, M. C. Leake, I. Makarenko, V. Benes & W. A. Linke. (2004) Developmentally regulated switching of titin size alters myofibrillar stiffness in the perinatal heart. *Circ Res*, Vol.94, No.7, pp. 967-75

C. A. Otey & O. Carpen. (2004) Alpha-actinin revisited: a fresh look at an old player. Ce Motil Cytoskeleton, Vol.58, No.2, pp. 104-11

N. Pandey, J. Strider, W. C. Nolan, S. X. Yan & J. E. Galvin. (2008) Curcumin inhibit aggregation of alpha-synuclein. Acta Neuropathol, Vol.115, No.4, pp. 479-89

D. Paulin, A. Huet, L. Khanamyrian & Z. Xue. (2004) Desminopathies in muscle disease. Pathol, Vol.204, No.4, pp. 418-27

D. Paulin & Z. Li. (2004) Desmin: a major intermediate filament protein essential for th structural integrity and function of muscle. Exp Cell Res, Vol.301, No.1, pp. 1-7

A. L. Portbury, M. S. Willis & C. Patterson. (2011) Tearin' up my heart: proteolysis in th cardiac sarcomere. J Biol Chem, Vol.286, No.12, pp. 9929-34

J. Reimann, W. S. Kunz, S. Vielhaber, K. Kappes-Horn & R. Schroder. (2003) Mitochondria dysfunction in myofibrillar myopathy. Neuropathol Appl Neurobiol, Vol.29, No.1, pp 45-51

P. Salmikangas, O. M. Mykkanen, M. Gronholm, L. Heiska, J. Kere & O. Carpen. (1999 Myotilin, a novel sarcomeric protein with two Ig-like domains, is encoded by candidate gene for limb-girdle muscular dystrophy. Hum Mol Genet, Vol.8, No.7 pp. 1329-36

P. Salmikangas, P. F. van der Ven, M. Lalowski, A. Taivainen, F. Zhao, H. Suila, R. Schroder P. Lappalainen, D. O. Furst & O. Carpen. (2003) Myotilin, the limb-girdle muscula dystrophy 1A (LGMD1A) protein, cross-links actin filaments and control sarcomere assembly. Hum Mol Genet, Vol.12, No.2, pp. 189-203

A. Sanbe, H. Osinska, C. Villa, J. Gulick, R. Klevitsky, C. G. Glabe, R. Kayed & J. Robbins (2005) Reversal of amyloid-induced heart disease in desmin-related cardiomyopathy. Proc Natl Acad Sci U S A, Vol.102, No.38, pp. 13592-7

A. Sanbe, T. Daicho, R. Mizutani, T. Endo, N. Miyauchi, J. Yamauchi, K. Tanonaka, C. Glab & A. Tanoue. (2009) Protective effect of geranylgeranylacetone via enhancement c HSPB8 induction in desmin-related cardiomyopathy. PLoS One, Vol.4, No.4, pp e5351

J. M. Sanger & J. W. Sanger. (2008) The dynamic Z bands of striated muscle cells. Scienc signaling, Vol.1, pe37

S. Sarkar & D. C. Rubinsztein. (2008) Small molecule enhancers of autophagy fo neurodegenerative diseases. Mol Biosyst, Vol.4, No.9, pp. 895-901

C. M. Sax & J. Piatigorsky. (1994) Expression of the alpha-crystallin/small heat-shoc protein/molecular chaperone genes in the lens and other tissues. Adv Enzymol Rela Areas Mol Biol, Vol.69, 155-201

D. A. Schafer, Y. O. Korshunova, T. A. Schroer & J. A. Cooper. (1994) Differentia localization and sequence analysis of capping protein beta-subunit isoforms o vertebrates. J Cell Biol, Vol.127, No.2, pp. 453-65

D. A. Schafer, P. B. Jennings & J. A. Cooper. (1996) Dynamics of capping protein and acti assembly in vitro: uncapping barbed ends by polyphosphoinositides. J Cell Bio Vol.135, No.1, pp. 169-79

R. Schroder, A. Vrabie & H. H. Goebel. (2007) Primary desminopathies. J Cell Mol Mea Vol.11, No.3, pp. 416-26

. Schroder & B. Schoser. (2009) Myofibrillar myopathies: a clinical and myopathological guide. *Brain Pathol*, Vol.19, No.3, pp. 483-92

). Selcen & A. G. Engel. (2004) Mutations in myotilin cause myofibrillar myopathy. *Neurology*, Vol.62, No.8, pp. 1363-71

). Selcen & A. G. Engel. (2005) Mutations in ZASP define a novel form of muscular dystrophy in humans. *Ann Neurol*, Vol.57, No.2, pp. 269-76

). Selcen, F. Muntoni, B.K. Burton, E. Pegoraro, C. Sewry, A.C. Bite & E. Engel. (2009) Mutation in BAG3 causes severe dominant chilhood muscular dystrophy. *Ann. Neurol.* Vol.65, No.3, pp. 83-89

). Selcen. (2011) Myofibrillar myopathies. *Neuromuscul Disord*, Vol.21, No.3, pp. 161-71

. H. Sonnenblick. (1968) Correlation of myocardial ultrastructure and function. *Circulation*, Vol.38, No.1, pp. 29-44

'. C. Squier. (2001) Oxidative stress and protein aggregation during biological aging. *Exp Gerontol*, Vol.36, No.9, pp. 1539-50

Λ. H. Stromer & D. E. Goll. (1972) Studies on purified -actinin. II. Electron microscopic studies on the competitive binding of -actinin and tropomyosin to Z-line extracted myofibrils. *J Mol Biol*, Vol.67, No.3, pp. 489-94

. Takayama & J. C. Reed. (2001) Molecular chaperone targeting and regulation by BAG family proteins. *Nat Cell Biol*, Vol.3, No.10, pp. E237-41

'. Tannous, H. Zhu, J. L. Johnstone, J. M. Shelton, N. S. Rajasekaran, I. J. Benjamin, L. Nguyen, R. D. Gerard, B. Levine, B. A. Rothermel & J. A. Hill. (2008a) Autophagy is an adaptive response in desmin-related cardiomyopathy. *Proc Natl Acad Sci U S A*, Vol.105, No.28, pp. 9745-50

'. Tannous, H. Zhu, A. Nemchenko, J. M. Berry, J. L. Johnstone, J. M. Shelton, F. J. Miller, Jr., B. A. Rothermel & J. A. Hill. (2008b) Intracellular protein aggregation is a proximal trigger of cardiomyocyte autophagy. *Circulation*, Vol.117, No.24, pp. 3070-8

'. G. Thompson, Y. M. Chan, A. A. Hack, M. Brosius, M. Rajala, H. G. Lidov, E. M. McNally, S. Watkins & L. M. Kunkel. (2000) Filamin 2 (FLN2): A muscle-specific sarcoglycan interacting protein. *J Cell Biol*, Vol.148, No.1, pp. 115-26

.. E. Thornell & A. Eriksson. (1981) Filament systems in the Purkinje fibers of the heart. *Am J Physiol*, Vol.241, No.3, pp. H291-305

.. F. Tian, H. Y. Li, B. F. Jin, X. Pan, J. H. Man, P. J. Zhang, W. H. Li, B. Liang, H. Liu, J. Zhao, W. L. Gong, T. Zhou & X. M. Zhang. (2006) MDM2 interacts with and downregulates a sarcomeric protein, TCAP. *Biochem Biophys Res Commun*, Vol.345, No.1, pp. 355-61

Γ. F. Tornatore, A. P. Dalla Costa, C. F. Clemente, C. Judice, S. A. Rocco, V. C. Calegari, L. Cardoso, A. C. Cardoso, A. Goncalves, Jr. & K. G. Franchini. (2011) A role for focal adhesion kinase in cardiac mitochondrial biogenesis induced by mechanical stress. *Am J Physiol Heart Circ Physiol*, Vol.300, No.3, pp. H902-12

Λ. S. Torsoni, S. S. Constancio, W. Nadruz, Jr., S. K. Hanks & K. G. Franchini. (2003) Focal adhesion kinase is activated and mediates the early hypertrophic response to stretch in cardiac myocytes. *Circ Res*, Vol.93, No.2, pp. 140-7

'. A. Townsend, R. I. Cutress, C. J. Carroll, K. M. Lawrence, T. M. Scarabelli, G. Packham, A. Stephanou & D. S. Latchman. (2004) BAG-1 proteins protect cardiac myocytes from simulated ischemia/reperfusion-induced apoptosis via an alternate mechanism c cell survival independent of the proteasome. *J Biol Chem*, Vol.279, No.20, pp. 20723 8

A. van der Flier & A. Sonnenberg. (2001) Structural and functional aspects of filamins *Biochim Biophys Acta*, Vol.1538, No.2-3, pp. 99-117

P. F. van der Ven, W. M. Obermann, B. Lemke, M. Gautel, K. Weber & D. O. Furst. (2000) Characterization of muscle filamin isoforms suggests a possible role of gamma filamin/ABP-L in sarcomeric Z-disc formation. *Cell Motil Cytoskeleton*, Vol.45, No.2 pp. 149-62

K. van Spaendonck-Zwarts, L. van Hessem, J. D. Jongbloed, H. E. de Walle, Y. Capetanak A. J. van der Kooi, I. M. van Langen, M. P. van den Berg & J. P. van Tintelen. (2010 Desmin-related myopathy: a review and meta-analysis. *Clin Genet*, PMID: 2071879.

M. Vatta, B. Mohapatra, S. Jimenez, X. Sanchez, G. Faulkner, Z. Perles, G. Sinagra, J. H. Lir T. M. Vu, Q. Zhou, K. R. Bowles, A. Di Lenarda, L. Schimmenti, M. Fox, M. A Chrisco, R. T. Murphy, W. McKenna, P. Elliott, N. E. Bowles, J. Chen, G. Valle & A. Towbin. (2003) Mutations in Cypher/ZASP in patients with dilate cardiomyopathy and left ventricular non-compaction. *J Am Coll Cardiol*, Vol.42 No.11, pp. 2014-27

L. Vernengo, O. Chourbagi, A. Panuncio, A. Lilienbaum, S. Batonnet-Pichon, F. Bruston, F Rodrigues-Lima, R. Mesa, C. Pizzarossa, L. Demay, P. Richard, P. Vicart & M. M Rodriguez. (2010) Desmin myopathy with severe cardiomyopathy in a Uruguayan family due to a codon deletion in a new location within the desmin 1A rod domain *Neuromuscul Disord*, Vol.20, No.3, pp. 178-87

P. Vicart, A. Caron, P. Guicheney, Z. Li, M. C. Prevost, A. Faure, D. Chateau, F. Chapon, F Tome, J. M. Dupret, D. Paulin & M. Fardeau. (1998) A missense mutation in the alphaB-crystallin chaperone gene causes a desmin-related myopathy. *Nat Genet* Vol.20, No.1, pp. 92-5

M. Vorgerd, P. F. van der Ven, V. Bruchertseifer, T. Lowe, R. A. Kley, R. Schroder, H Lochmuller, M. Himmel, K. Koehler, D. O. Furst & A. Huebner. (2005) A mutation in the dimerization domain of filamin c causes a novel type of autosomal dominant myofibrillar myopathy. *Am J Hum Genet*, Vol.77, No.2, pp. 297-304

M. C. Walter, P. Reilich, A. Huebner, D. Fischer, R. Schroder, M. Vorgerd, W. Kress, C. Born B. G. Schoser, K. H. Krause, U. Klutzny, S. Bulst, J. R. Frey & H. Lochmuller. (2007 Scapuloperoneal syndrome type Kaeser and a wide phenotypic spectrum of adult onset, dominant myopathies are associated with the desmin mutation R350P. *Brain* Vol.130, No.Pt 6, pp. 1485-96

X. Wang, H. Osinska, G. W. Dorn, 2nd, M. Nieman, J. N. Lorenz, A. M. Gerdes, S. Witt, T Kimball, J. Gulick & J. Robbins. (2001a) Mouse model of desmin-related cardiomyopathy. *Circulation*, Vol.103, No.19, pp. 2402-7

X. Wang, H. Osinska, R. Klevitsky, A. M. Gerdes, M. Nieman, J. Lorenz, T. Hewett & J Robbins. (2001b) Expression of R120G-alphaB-crystallin causes aberrant desmin and alphaB-crystallin aggregation and cardiomyopathy in mice. *Circ Res*, Vol.89 No.1, pp. 84-91

. M. Warren, P. R. Krzesinski, K. S. Campbell, R. L. Moss & M. L. Greaser. (2004) Titin isoform changes in rat myocardium during development. *Mech Dev*, Vol.121, No.11, pp. 1301-12

D. Westerheide, J. D. Bosman, B. N. Mbadugha, T. L. Kawahara, G. Matsumoto, S. Kim, W. Gu, J. P. Devlin, R. B. Silverman & R. I. Morimoto. (2004) Celastrols as inducers of the heat shock response and cytoprotection. *J Biol Chem*, Vol.279, No.53, pp. 56053-60

1. S. Willis, J. C. Schisler, A. L. Portbury & C. Patterson. (2009) Build it up-Tear it down: protein quality control in the cardiac sarcomere. *Cardiovasc Res*, Vol.81, No.3, pp. 439-48

1. S. Willis & C. Patterson. (2010) Hold me tight: Role of the heat shock protein family of chaperones in cardiac disease. *Circulation*, Vol.122, No.17, pp. 1740-51

. C. Witt, S. H. Witt, S. Lerche, D. Labeit, W. Back & S. Labeit. (2008) Cooperative control of striated muscle mass and metabolism by MuRF1 and MuRF2. *Embo J*, Vol.27, No.2, pp. 350-60

. S. Wong, J. M. Tan, W. E. Soong, K. Hussein, N. Nukina, V. L. Dawson, T. M. Dawson, A. M. Cuervo & K. L. Lim. (2008) Autophagy-mediated clearance of aggresomes is not a universal phenomenon. *Hum Mol Genet*, Vol.17, No.16, pp. 2570-82

C. Wong & R. R. Fiscus. (2010) Essential roles of the nitric oxide (NO)/cGMP/protein kinase G type-Ialpha (PKG-Ialpha) signaling pathway and the atrial natriuretic peptide (ANP)/cGMP/PKG-Ialpha autocrine loop in promoting proliferation and cell survival of OP9 bone marrow stromal cells. *J Cell Biochem*, PMID: 21190199

. Yamasaki, Y. Wu, M. McNabb, M. Greaser, S. Labeit & H. Granzier. (2002) Protein kinase A phosphorylates titin's cardiac-specific N2B domain and reduces passive tension in rat cardiac myocytes. *Circ Res*, Vol.90, No.11, pp. 1181-8

. Yang, T. E. Hewett, R. Klevitsky, A. Sanbe, X. Wang & J. Robbins. (2001) PKA-dependent phosphorylation of cardiac myosin binding protein C in transgenic mice. *Cardiovasc Res*, Vol.51, No.1, pp. 80-8

. Zak. (1977) Metabolism of myofibrillar proteins in the normal and hypertrophic heart. *Basic Res Cardiol*, Vol.72, No.2-3, pp. 235-40

. R. Zakhary, C. S. Moravec, R. W. Stewart & M. Bond. (1999) Protein kinase A (PKA)-dependent troponin-I phosphorylation and PKA regulatory subunits are decreased in human dilated cardiomyopathy. *Circulation*, Vol.99, No.4, pp. 505-10

. Zhang, Z. Xu, X. R. He, L. H. Michael & C. Patterson. (2005) CHIP, a cochaperone/ubiquitin ligase that regulates protein quality control, is required for maximal cardioprotection after myocardial infarction in mice. *Am J Physiol Heart Circ Physiol*, Vol.288, No.6, pp. H2836-42

. Zhang, C. Weinheimer, M. Courtois, A. Kovacs, C. E. Zhang, A. M. Cheng, Y. Wang & A. J. Muslin. (2003) The role of the Grb2-p38 MAPK signaling pathway in cardiac hypertrophy and fibrosis. *J Clin Invest*, Vol.111, No.6, pp. 833-41

. J. Zhao, Y. B. Yan, Y. Liu & H. M. Zhou. (2007) The generation of the oxidized form of creatine kinase is a negative regulation on muscle creatine kinase. *J Biol Chem*, Vol.282, No.16, pp. 12022-9

M. Zheng, H. Cheng, X. Li, J. Zhang, L. Cui, K. Ouyang, L. Han, T. Zhao, Y. Gu, N. D Dalton, M. L. Bang, K. L. Peterson & J. Chen. (2009) Cardiac-specific ablation o Cypher leads to a severe form of dilated cardiomyopathy with premature death *Hum Mol Genet,* Vol.18, No.4, pp. 701-13

Q. Zhou, P. Ruiz-Lozano, M. E. Martone & J. Chen. (1999) Cypher, a striated muscle restricted PDZ and LIM domain-containing protein, binds to alpha-actinin-2 and protein kinase C. *J Biol Chem,* Vol.274, No.28, pp. 19807-13

9

Functional Consequences of Mutations in the Myosin Regulatory Light Chain Associated with Hypertrophic Cardiomyopathy

Priya Muthu, Wenrui Huang,
Katarzyna Kazmierczak and Danuta Szczesna-Cordary
University of Miami Miller School of Medicine, Miami, FL,
USA

. Introduction

amilial hypertrophic cardiomyopathy (FHC) is an autosomal dominant disease haracterized by left ventricular wall thickening, myofilament disarray and abnormal chocardiography findings. Molecular genetic studies have defined FHC as a disease of the arcomere caused by mutations in all major sarcomeric proteins, such as β-myosin heavy hain (44%), myosin binding protein C (35%), regulatory light chain (2%), essential light hain (1.6%), α-tropomyosin (2.5%), troponin T (7%), troponin I (5%), troponin C (~1%), α-ctin (1%), and titin (<1%) (Alcalai et al., 2008). .lthough mutations in the regulatory light chain (RLC) of myosin are rare, they are of reat significance given the importance of RLC for muscle contraction and heart function. he RLC plays an essential structural and functional role by supporting the architecture of ιe myosin neck region and fine-tuning the kinetics of the actin-myosin interaction Morano, 1999; Szczesna, 2003). As shown in **Fig. 1**, the RLC wraps around the α-helical eck region of the myosin head by binding to a 35 amino acid IQ motif in the myosin eavy chain (MHC) (Rayment et al., 1993). This domain of MHC is anticipated to act as a ²ver arm, amplifying small conformational changes that originate at the catalytic site into ιrge movements thus allowing myosin to generate motion and force (Geeves & Holmes, 005; Lowey et al., 1993). Furthermore, this neck region has been proposed to serve as the ompliant element of the myosin cross-bridge with the RLC contributing to the stiffness of ιe lever arm (Howard & Spudich, 1996; Pant et al., 2009). Two functionally important omains of the RLC molecule include its Ca^{2+}-Mg^{2+} binding site, comprised of the N-²rminal helix-loop-helix EF-hand Ca^{2+} binding motif, and a highly conserved N-terminal hosphorylatable serine constituting a myosin light chain kinase (MLCK)-dependent hosphorylation site. he N-terminal divalent cation-binding site of the RLC is thought to be occupied by Mg^{2+} √hen muscles are in the relaxed state and may become partially saturated with Ca^{2+}, .epending on the length of the $[Ca^{2+}]$ transient (Robertson et al., 1981). The MLCK hosphorylation site of RLC is also of great structural and functional importance. 'hosphorylation of this site in smooth muscle activates contraction (Hartshorne & Mrwa, 982; Small & Sobieszek, 1977; Sobieszek, 1977). In skeletal and cardiac muscle, Ca^{2+}-

calmodulin (CaM) activated MLCK phosphorylation of RLC modulates contraction b
increasing the Ca²⁺ sensitivity and the level of force and also by modulating the kinetics c
force generating myosin cross-bridges (for review see (Kamm & Stull, 2011)). Of particula
importance, the phosphorylation of RLC has been shown to regulate the function c
myosin in the heart (Morano, 1999; Szczesna, 2003). Attenuation of RLC phosphorylatio
was demonstrated to lead to ventricular myocyte hypertrophy with histological evidenc
of necrosis and fibrosis (Ding et al., 2010). Recent results from Szczesna-Cordary's la
shown that RLC phosphorylation plays an essential role not only in the physiologica
performance of the heart, but also helps to maintain normal cardiac function in th
diseased myocardium (Muthu et al., 2011). At the level of protein, the phosphorylation c
RLC at Ser-15 was shown to alter the secondary structure (α-helical content) and Ca²
binding affinity of the human ventricular RLC protein (Szczesna et al., 2001). At the leve
of myofilaments, RLC phosphorylation was demonstrated to result in a significantl
decreased distance between the myosin heads and actin filaments bringing them closer t
each other (Colson et al., 2010)

Myosin cross-bridge

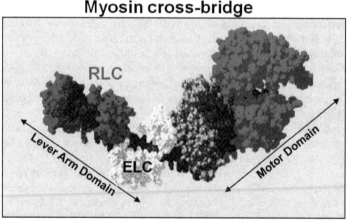

Fig. 1. Schematic representation of the myosin head (cross-bridge) containing regulatory
(RLC, labeled in magenta) and essential (ELC, labeled in yellow) light chains. Indicated
are 1) motor domain, and 2) lever arm (Rayment et al., 1993).

1.1 FHC-linked mutations in the regulatory light chain (RLC)

To date, eight single point mutations and two intron alternative splicing mutations in th
MYL2 gene encoding for the human ventricular RLC (Swiss-Prot: P10916) have bee
identified to cause FHC (**Fig. 2**). They are A13T (alanine to threonine), F18L (phenylalanin
to leucine), E22K (glutamic acid to lysine), N47K (asparagine to lysine), R58Q (arginine t
glutamine), P95A (proline to alanine), K104E (lysine to glutamic acid), D166V (aspartic aci
to valine), IVS5-2 (a A>G transversion in intron 5 that leads to a premature terminatio
codon), and IVS6-1 (a G>C transversion in the acceptor splice site of intron 6).
The A13T mutation arises from a replacement of alanine, an uncharged and nonpolar amin
acid by threonine, an uncharged but polar amino acid. The mutation was first discovered in a
American patient (Poetter et al., 1996) and was later found in a Danish proband diagnose

ith hypertrophic cardiomyopathy (HCM). Two of his family members were found to be
eterozygous for the mutation (Andersen et al., 2001). The proband, 42 years old, suffered
om exercise-induced dyspnoea and had pronounced septal hypertrophy, diastolic filling
onormities but no significantly increased left ventricular outflow tract. One of the family
embers, the mother of the proband, was diagnosed with HCM late in life and died at the age
f 72; while the other, 10 years old, showed no sign of HCM. In 2005, another proband
arrying the A13T mutation was also identified in a Danish population (Hougs et al., 2005).
verall, this mutation is associated with a rare HCM phenotype characterized by mid left
entricular obstruction, enlarged papillary muscles and profound septal hypertrophy.

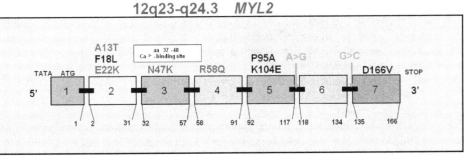

ig. 2. Exon organization of the *MYL2* gene (chromosome 12q23-q24.3) and FHC-linked
utations in human ventricular RLC (Swiss-Prot: P10916). Labeled in red, FHC mutations
escribed in this review; in black, other identified RLC mutations; and in green, intronic
plice site mutations: A (adenine) → G (guanine) transversion in intron 5 and G → C
cytosine) transversion in intron 6.

he F18L mutation arises from a replacement of a bulky nonpolar and hydrophobic
henylalanine by the small uncharged and nonpolar leucine residue. It was found in three
nrelated French families and is associated with a classic phenotype of left ventricular wall
ickening and electrocardiographic (ECG) abnormalities (Richard et al., 2003).

he E22K mutation results from a substitution of a negatively charged glutamate with a
ositively charged lysine leading to potential alterations in the net charge and polarity of the
utation-bearing domain of RLC. The mutation was first identified in three persons (two
rothers and one non-related individual) from two unrelated families screened together
ith 399 unrelated HCM patients (Poetter et al., 1996). Subsequent studies by Kabaeva, et
l. identified seven individuals in a German family carrying the mutation. However, only
ur patients suffered from HCM while the phenotype of the remaining individuals was
efined as "uncertain" (Kabaeva et al., 2002). Based on the latest clinical reports on this
utation, it is known to be associated with moderate septal hypertrophy, late onset of
linical manifestations, and benign to severe disease outcomes.

he N47K mutation results from the replacement of a polar uncharged asparagine residue
y the positively charged lysine. It was first discovered in an individual of Danish descent
Andersen et al., 2001). This mutation is associated with a late onset of the disease and a
apidly progressing phenotype. The proband was diagnosed with HCM at the age of 60, and
uickly progressed to a severe hypertrophic phenotype and diastolic dysfunction. It was
nteresting that septal hypertrophy of this patient increased rapidly (from 31 mm to 45 mm)

in the two years after diagnosis. In 2005, a Danish patient carrying both N47K and a β cardiac myosin heavy chain mutation was identified. The proband bearing both of these mutations displayed a more severe phenotype than patients with either mutation alon (Hougs et al., 2005). However, no incidence of sudden cardiac death (SCD) associated wit this mutation has yet been reported.

The R58Q mutation occurs when the bulky positively charged arginine is replaced by a uncharged but polar glutamine. It was first discovered by Flavigny, et al. in 1998 in thre unrelated French families with HCM (Flavigny et al., 1998). The mutation was associate with a classic form of FHC characterized by left ventricular wall thickness, abnormal EC findings and SCD (Flavigny et al., 1998). In 2002, Kabaeva, et al. detected this R58(mutation in a German proband with a clinical phenotype of moderate septal hypertroph early onset of disease and premature SCD (Kabaeva et al., 2002). In 2003, the R58Q mutatio was once more identified in two independent population studies (from France and Sweden and again was associated with a malignant disease phenotype (Morner et al., 2003; Richar et al., 2003). Out of all identified FHC RLC mutations, the R58Q mutation was found to b the most prevalent, occurring independently in multiple families with different ethni backgrounds. The mutation is associated with a phenotype of severe cardiac hypertroph and multiple incidences of SCD.

The P95A mutation occurs when a bulky hydrophobic proline residue is substituted with smaller alanine residue. It was discovered together with the A13T and E22K mutations in a American family and shares a rare clinical phenotype, similar to that of A13T and E22l positive patients (Poetter et al., 1996).

The K104E mutation results from a replacement of the positively charged lysine with th negatively charged glutamic acid. The mutation was first observed in a Danish family an was mistakenly reported as L103E (Andersen et al., 2001). The parents carrying thi mutation were asymptomatic with a normal ECG pattern. However, their son wa diagnosed with pronounced septal hypertrophy at the age of 17 and progressed to diastoli dysfunction. His sister, 42 years old, was also positive for the mutation, but no typica hypertrophic phenotype was observed in her case. This mutation is associated wit pronounced septal hypertrophy and diastolic filling abnormalities.

The D166V mutation occurs when a negatively charged aspartic acid is substituted with bulky polar valine residue. This mutation was identified in a French proband, with th potential to cause SCD at a young age. It was first mistakenly presented as D166L i Richard, et al., 2003 and later corrected to D166V (Richard et al., 2003; 2004). Similar t R58Q, this mutation is associated with a malignant disease phenotype and SCD.

Intron mutations: Intron 6-1 G>C mutation (IVS 6-1) was discovered along with K104E ii the Danish population and is associated with pronounced septal hypertrophy (Andersen e al., 2001). The other intronic mutation 5-2 A>G, (IVS 5-2) was first discovered in the Frenc population and is associated with a malignant form of FHC (Richard et al., 2003). Th mutation is predicted to lead to a premature codon termination.

The clinical phenotype associated with FHC-linked mutations in the regulatory light chai and current to date literature citations are illustrated in **Table 1**.

This review focuses on the functional phenotypes associated with five (A13T, E22K, N47k R58Q and D166V) RLC mutations extensively studied *in vitro* using RLC-mutan reconstituted muscle systems and *in vivo*, using cardiac muscle preparations from transgeni mice expressing FHC-RLC mutations.

Mutation in RLC	Clinical phenotype	Population	Major findings
A13T	Massive hypertrophy of cardiac papillary muscles, mid-cavity left ventricular obstruction, pronounced septal and ventricular hypertrophy and diastolic filling abnormalities	Danish (Andersen et al., 2001; Hougs et al., 2005); American (Poetter et al., 1996)	Mutation-induced changes in α-helical content and in Ca^{2+} binding properties of RLC (Szczesna et al., 2001). No change in Ca^{2+}sensitivity of myofibrillar ATPase activity (Szczesna et al., 2001). Increased force production in skinned papillary muscle fibers from Tg-A13T mice (unpublished data). Histopathological changes in left ventricles and inter-ventricular septa of Tg-A13T mice (unpublished data)
F18L	Classic form of HCM – increased left ventricular wall thickness, abnormal ECG findings, no mid left ventricular obstruction	French (Flavigny et al., 1998; Richard et al., 2003)	Decrease in Ca^{2+} binding affinity to RLC (Szczesna et al., 2001). Increase in α-helical content of RLC (Szczesna et al., 2001). Decrease in Ca^{2+} sensivity of myofibrillar ATPase activity (Szczesna-Cordary et al., 2004a). Compromised maximal tension, cooperativity and Ca^{2+} sensitivity of force (Roopnarine, 2003).
E22K	Moderate septal hypertrophy, late onset of clinical manifestation or no symptoms of FHC (Kabaeva). Also associated with massive hypertrophy of cardiac papillary muscles and adjacent venstricular tissue causing midcavity obstruction (Poetter)	German (Kabaeva et al., 2002), American (Poetter et al., 1996)	Protein non-phosphorylatable (Szczesna et al., 2001). Mutation induced changes in α-helical content and Ca^{2+} binding properties of RLC (Szczesna et al., 2001). Increase in Ca^{2+} sensitivity of force (Levine et al., 1998; Roopnarine, 2003; Szczesna-Cordary et al., 2004a) and decrease in maximal ATPase and force in skinned fibers from Tg-E22K mice (Szczesna-Cordary et al., 2007). No effect on cross-bridge kinetics (Szczesna-Cordary et al., 2007; (Dumka et al., 2006). Enlarged inter-ventricular septa and papillary muscles (Szczesna-Cordary et al., 2005). No hypertrophy detected in Tg-E22K mice (Sanbe et al., 2000). No changes in ECG (Szczesna-Cordary et al., 2005).
N47K	Pronounced interventricular (septal) and papillary musle hypertrophy; relatively high midventricular flow gradient, diastolic filling abnormalities; late onset disease with a rapidly progressing phenotype	Danish (Andersen et al., 2001; Hougs et al., 2005)	Abolished Ca^{2+} binding to RLC (Szczesna-Cordary et al., 2004a). Increased Ca^{2+} sensivity of myofibrillar ATPase activity (Szczesna-Cordary et al., 2004a). No change in pCa_{50} of force (Szczesna-Cordary et al., 2004a). Prolonged Ca^{2+} transient with no change in force transients in intact papillary muslces (Wang et al., 2006). Decreased isometric force in N47K-myosin based *in vitro* motility assays (Greenberg et al., 2009). Reduction in force and power output under loaded conditions (Greenberg et al., 2010). Decreased cardiac function in isolated perfused working hearts (Abraham et al., 2009).

Mutation in RLC	Clinical phenotype	Population	Major findings
R58Q	Malignant FHC phenotype, early onset of clinical manifestation and high incidence of premature SCD; classic form of HCM - increased left ventricular wall thickness and abnormal ECG findings	German (Kabaeva et al., 2002), French (Flavigny et al., 1998; Richard et al., 2003), Swedish (Morner et al., 2003)	Abolished Ca^{2+} binding to RLC, which was restored upon RLC phosphorylation. (Szczesna et al., 2001). Mutation induced increase in α-helical content of RLC (Szczesna et al., 2001). Increased Ca^{2+} sensitivity of force (Szczesna-Cordary et al., 2004a), and Ca^{2+} and force transient in intact papillary muscles (Wang et al., 2006). Higher ATPase rate and increased activation at submaximal Ca^{2+} (Greenberg et al., 2009). Decreased skewness and kurtosis of fluctuations during contraction (Borejdo et al., 2010). Decreased force (Abraham et al., 2009; Greenberg et al., 2010; Greenberg et al., 2009; Wang et al., 2006). Reduced level of endogenous RLC phosphorylation (Abraham et al., 2009). Decreased cardiac function in isolated perfused working hearts (Abraham et al., 2009). Alterations in diastolic transmitral velocities and increased deceleration time, indicative of diastolic dysfunction (Abraham et al., 2009).
P95A	Rare clinical phenotype, similar to E22K and A13T, of midventricular obstruction	American (Poetter et al., 1996)	Mutation-induced decrease in Ca^{2+} binding to RLC (Szczesna et al., 2001). No significant effect on tension, Ca^{2+} sensitivity, or cooperativity in P95A-reconstituted fibers (Roopnarine, 2003).
K104E	Pronounced septal hypertrophy and diastolic filling abnormalities	Danish (Andersen et al., 2001)	Impaired interaction with IQ-MHC peptide (Szczesna-Cordary et al., 2004b). Slight decrease in binding to RLC-depleted porcine myosin (Huang et al., 2011).
D166V	Malignant FHC phenotype - poor prognosis and SCD at young age	French (Richard et al., 2003; 2004)	Decrease in maximal force and large increase in Ca^{2+} sensitivity in papillary muscle fibers from Tg-D166V mice (Kerrick et al., 2009). Decrease in Ca^{2+} sensitivity of force upon phosphorylation (Muthu et al., 2011). Slower cross bridge kinetics (Borejdo et al., 2010; Mettikolla et al., 2009; Muthu et al., 2010). Reduced level of endogenous RLC phosphorylation (Kerrick et al., 2009). Severe fibrotic lesions in older Tg-D166V mouse hearts (Kerrick et al., 2009).
IVS6-1	Pronounced proximal septal hypertrophy	Danish (Andersen et al., 2001)	G>C transversion in Intron 6 (Andersen et al., 2001).
IVS5-2	Malignant prognosis	French (Richard et al., 2003)	Donor-site splice mutation (A>G) in Intron 5 predicted to lead to a premature termination codon (Richard et al., 2003).

Table 1. Summary of clinical and functional phenotypes of FHC mutations in the regulatory light chain (RLC).

Effect of FHC mutations on the secondary RLC structure and calcium inding properties

his review reports on the studies that were conducted to elucidate the structural and unctional effects of FHC-linked RLC mutations. The RLC protein, labeled in red in **Fig. 3**, raps around the myosin heavy chain (dark blue) and connects the myosin head with the yosin rod region. The three-dimensional (3D) structure of the RLC demonstrates the close roximity of the FHC mutations to either the phosphorylation site of RLC (Ser-15) or the a^{2+} binding site (amino acids 37–48 in the sequence of human ventricual RLC) **(Fig. 3)**. The resence of these two important RLC domains in the RLC structure prompted the studies imed at understanding the effects of the FHC mutations on Ca^{2+} binding to RLC and to etermine how MLCK-dependent phosphorylation of RLC is affected in FHC disease. urthermore, additional studies were conducted to determine the effect of FHC-linked RLC utation and phosphorylation on the secondary RLC structure.

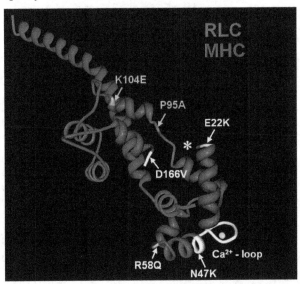

ig. 3. Structure of the regulatory domain of scallop myosin (1WDC) (Houdusse & Cohen, 996): Indicated are the FHC mutations, Ca^{2+}-Mg^{2+} binding site and the phosphorylation ite. The MHC (myosin heavy chain) is labeled in dark blue, and the RLC (regulatory light hain) in red. Asterisks (*) depict the predicted location of A13T and F18L mutations and er-15 phosphorylation site (the region of RLC which is not resolved in all available ertebrate myosin crystal structures).

.1 Circular dichroism study

n order to test the effect of RLC mutations on the secondary structure of RLC, far-UV ircular dichroism (CD) spectra measurements were performed and the α-helical content etermined (Szczesna-Cordary et al., 2004a; Szczesna et al., 2001). Far-UV CD spectra were btained using a 1-mm path quartz cell in a Jasco J-720 spectropolarimeter and were ecorded at 195–250 nm. Mean residue ellipticity ([θ]$_{MRE}$, in degrees *cm^2/dmol) for the pectra were calculated using the following equation:

$$[\theta]_{MRE}=[\theta]/(10^*Cr^*l)$$

where $[\theta]$ is the measured ellipticity in millidegrees, Cr is the mean residue mol concentration, and l is the path length in cm.

The α-helical content for each mutant was calculated using the standard equation for $[\theta]$ 222 nm (Chen & Yang, 1971):

$$[\theta]_{222}=-30,000^*f_H - 2340$$

where f_H is the fraction of α-helical content ($f_H * 100$, expressed in %). Any change above 2 in the α -helical content was considered statistically significant.

As the mutations lie in the proximity of the phosphorylation site (Ser-15) and/or the Ca^2 Mg^{2+} binding site (**Fig. 3**), the α-helical content was measured in the absence (Apo) an presence of Ca^{2+}. In addition, data were collected for phosphorylated RLC (**Table 2**).

Protein	Apo	+Ca²⁺	+P	+P +Ca²⁺
RLC-WT	18	23	18	18
A13T	29	25	19	18
E22K	24	20	No phosphorylation	
N47K	18.7	ND	ND	ND
R58Q	20	22	20	28
P95A	19	23	ND	ND

Table 2. Effect of phosphorylation and Ca^{2+}-binding on the α-helical content of RLC expressed in %. (ND: not determined) (Szczesna-Cordary et al., 2004a; Szczesna et al., 2001)

Based on these results, it was determined that under Apo (no metal) conditions, with th exception of the N47K and P95A mutants, the FHC-linked RLC mutation led to an increase α-helical content compared to RLC-WT (Szczesna-Cordary et al., 2004a; Szczesna et a 2001). It was also observed that upon binding of Ca^{2+} to RLC, the α-helical content wa significantly increased in all proteins including WT (**Table 2**), suggesting that binding c calcium to RLC could be conformation dependent. Interestingly, upon phosphorylatio A13T displayed a significant decrease in the α-helical content compared to nor phosphorylated A13T in the presence or absence of Ca^{2+}. Therefore, phosphorylation of th A13T mutant rescued the secondary structure of the mutant bringing the α-helical content t the level of RLC-WT. The authors concluded that phosphorylation of RLC could reverse th detrimental effect of FHC brought about by the A13T mutation (Szczesna et al., 2001).

2.2 Calcium binding study

As shown above in **Fig. 3**, the N-terminal domain of RLC contains the EF-hand Ca^{2+}-Mg binding site, similar to the EF-hand Ca^{2+}-sites present in troponin C (TnC), parvalbumir calmodulin (CaM) and essential light chain (ELC). To test how these mutations affec calcium binding to the RLC, flow dialysis experiments were conducted and the Ca association/dissociation constant was determined (Szczesna et al., 2001). Radio-labele substrate ($^{45}Ca^{2+}$) was first added into a chamber containing a fixed amount of RLC. Onc the reaction reached steady-state, radio-labeled $^{45}Ca^{2+}$ was chased by unlabeled Ca^{2+}. Th concentrations of bound-Ca^{2+} and free-Ca^{2+} were determined and the K_{Ca} values analyzec Calcium association constant K_{Ca} was extrapolated from the following equation:

$$C_{Ca\text{-}bound}/C_{Ca\text{-}free}/C_p =-K_{Ca}^* \, C_{Ca\text{-}bound}/C_p+ n^*K_{Ca}$$

$C_{Ca-bound}$ and $C_{Ca-free}$ represent the concentration of the bound and free metal, respectively, C_p is
e concentration of the protein, n is the total number of Ca^{2+} binding sites, and K_{Ca} is the Ca^{2+}
inding affinity. $1/K_{Ca}$ represents the apparent calcium dissociation constant K_d (in μM). The
ffect of the mutations on calcium binding to recombinant human cardiac RLC and FHC-
nked mutants is summarized in **Table 3** (Szczesna et al., 2001). **Table 3** also summarizes the
ffect of FHC RLC mutations on calcium binding to myofibrils and skinned muscle fibers
econstituted with WT or FHC-mutant proteins (Szczesna-Cordary et al., 2004a).

RLC protein	Isolated RLC (no Mg²⁺) (μM)	Myofibrils# (2 mM Mg²⁺) (μM)	Fibers# (1 mMMg²⁺) (μM)
RLC-WT	1.50 ± 0.02	0.200 ± 0.009	2.88 ± 0.19
A13T	4.85 ± 0.31	0.191 ± 0.015	3.02 ± 0.06
E22K	25.64 ± 3.48	0.178 ± 0.001	2.63 ± 0.10
N47K	No binding	0.141 ± 0.009	2.51 ± 0.10
R58Q	No binding	0.170 ± 0.004	2.19 ± 0.10
P95A	4.74 ± 1.05	0.200 ± 0.011	2.75 ± 0.25

able 3. Apparent K_d $(1/K_{Ca})$ of isolated RLC-WT and FHC mutants and in mutant-
econstituted myofibrils and skinned porcine muscle fibers (#K_d calculated from the pCa_{50}
alues ±S.E.) (Szczesna-Cordary et al., 2004a).

low dialysis experiments with recombinant RLC-WT and FHC-mutants showed that A13T
nd P95A decreased the K_{Ca} ~3-fold, whereas E22K, N47K and R58Q, changed the Ca^{2+} binding
roperties in a more drastic way. Compared with RLC-WT, the E22K mutation decreased the
$_{Ca}$ value by ~17-fold, whereas both N47K and R58Q mutations eliminated Ca^{2+} binding to RLC
Table 3) (Szczesna et al., 2001). These three Ca^{2+} binding site mutants also showed an increase
1 the Ca^{2+} sensitivity of myofibrillar ATPase activity and force development, with R58Q
emonstrating significantly higher K_{Ca} compared to RLC WT-reconstituted muscle
reparations (Table 3) (Szczesna-Cordary et al., 2004a). Interestingly, flow dialysis studies
howed that the restricted ability of the R58Q mutant to bind calcium was restored upon
hosphorylation (Szczesna et al., 2001). These studies suggested that the phosphorylation and
a^{2+} binding to human cardiac RLC are important for physiological function and that alteration
f any of these properties may contribute to the development of hypertrophic cardiomyopathy.
esults from the *in vitro* studies prompted generation of the animal models of FHC-linked RLC
nutations and subsequent investigations of their functional effects *in vivo*. Studies included
xperiments performed at different levels of complexity; from single molecules to organized
arcomeres in muscle fibers and to the organ and organism levels. Transgenic mice carrying
HC RLC mutations were used in these experiments.

. Animal models of FHC

.1 Generation of transgenic mice

ransgenic (Tg) mouse models expressing wild-type (WT) and FHC-mutated human
entricular cardiac RLC (A13T, E22K, N47K, R58Q and D166V) were generated using the α-
nyosin heavy chain (α-MHC) promoter (clone 26, a generous gift from Dr J. Robbins,
Cincinnati Children's Medical Center, Cincinnati, OH, USA). All of the founders

were bred to non-transgenic (NTg) B6SJL mice. Two types of Tg-WT mice were generated a necessary controls for the transgenic mutant mice; one expressing human ventricula cardiac RLC and another expressing the human ventricular cardiac RLC along with a myc tag sequence. The following transgenic mouse models were produced and used for th experiments described in this review: WT, A13T, E22K, N47K, R58Q and D166V.

3.2 Phenotypic characterization of FHC-RLC animal models
3.2.1 Assessment of cardiac hypertrophy by HW/BW ratio
The heart weight to body weight (HW/BW) ratio was used to examine all generated FHC RLC animal models for heart hypertrophy. **Fig. 4** demonstrates the HW/BW ratio determined for mice carrying A13T, D166V, N47K and R58Q mutations. No evidence c hypertrophy was observed in the majority of mutant mice compared to WT (Kerrick et al 2009; Wang et al., 2006). Differences in HW/BW were only seen between the hearts fror Tg-N47K *versus* Tg-WT mice, but no statistically significant changes were observed.

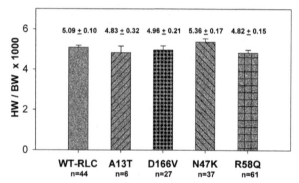

Fig. 4. Heart weight to body weight ratios in transgenic RLC animal models: P-values for al mutant mice (A13T, D166V, N47K and R58Q) *versus* WT-RLC were >0.05.

These results suggested that the histopathological and functional changes observed due t these mutations (discussed later) may be more indicative of the FHC phenotype than overal heart hypertrophy.

3.2.2 Histopathology
The most specific histological feature of hypertrophic cardiomyopathy is an extensive disorganization of the myocyte structure (myocyte disarray). Often observed are abnormall branched (Y-shaped) myocytes with adjacent myocytes arranged perpendicularly o obliquely to each other (Binder et al., 2005). Histological studies were performed t characterize the mutation specific cardiac phenotype at the level of the Tg mouse model an to establish a correlation with the phenotypes observed in patients harboring these FHC RLC mutations. Histopatological evaluation of the hearts from Tg-A13T, Tg-E22K, Tg-W and NTg mice is presented in **Fig. 5**. The upper panel shows longitudinal sections of th whole hearts from Tg-A13T *versus* control mice and the lower panel presents Tg-E22H mouse hearts. As indicated with arrows, a significantly larger LV and inter-ventricula septal mass was observed for both Tg-A13T (unpublished data) and Tg-E22K (Szczesna Cordary et al., 2005) mice compared with Tg-WT or NTg littermates.

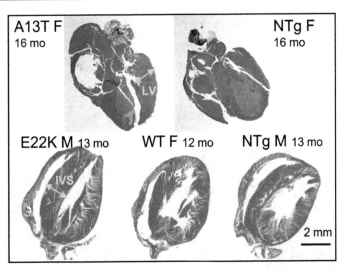

...ig. 5. Longitudinal sections of whole mouse hearts stained with hematoxylin and eosin (H ...c E). Upper panel: Tg-A13T *versus* NTg controls (unpublished data). Bottom panel: Tg-E22K ...nd controls (Szczesna-Cordary et al., 2005). Abbreviations: F, female; M, male; mo, age of ...nice in months; LV, left ventricle; IVS, interventricular septum.

...iross morphological evaluation of the hearts from Tg-A13T and Tg-E22K mice revealed a ...ommon phenotype of enlarged inter-ventricular septa (**Fig. 6**), a phenotype observed in ...atients carrying the A13T and E22K mutations (Poetter et al., 1996). Interestingly, in ...nother study transgenic mice expressing the E22K mutation did not show any features of ...he FHC disease despite almost total replacement of the endogenous WT RLC with mutant ...?LC (Sanbe et al., 2000). No hypertrophy was detected in mature adult animals either when ...hamber weights were determined or at the cellular level (Sanbe et al., 2000).

...)ther RLC FHC mutant mice were examined for histopathological abnormalities, and ...ongitudinal ventricular sections were stained with hematoxylin and eosin to detect any ...issue disorganization and with Masson's trichrome to determine the presence of abnormal ...ollagen deposits and fibrosis. As shown in **Fig. 6**, mice carrying the malignant R58Q ...nutation manifested histopathological changes (myofibrillar disarray and abnormal ...lustering of nuclei) as early as at 4 months of age (**Fig. 6A, B**). The changes seen in older ...~17 months old) mice, presented in Wang et al. were profound in both Tg-R58Q and Tg-...J47K mice (Wang et al., 2006). The changes observed in Tg-N47K mice correlated with the ...henotype found in humans demonstrating a late onset of disease with a rapidly ...rogressing phenotype. Similarly, examination of the older (~17 months of age) Tg-D166V ...nice revealed severe fibrotic lesions present in the left ventricles compared with age ...natched Tg-WT and NTg littermates (**Fig. 6C**). Morphological changes found in the older ...'g-D166V mice suggest that the ventricles of the FHC Tg-D166V mice undergo temporal ...henotypic changes that are not present in the younger mice (~ 7 months of age) (Kerrick et ...l., 2009). These studies suggested that while in Tg-N47K and Tg-D166V animals the ...unctional changes induced by the mutations (evident at 3-6 months of age in mice) may ...recede the development of any detrimental morphological changes; the histopathological ...hanges observed in Tg-R58Q mice paralleled the functional abnormalities.

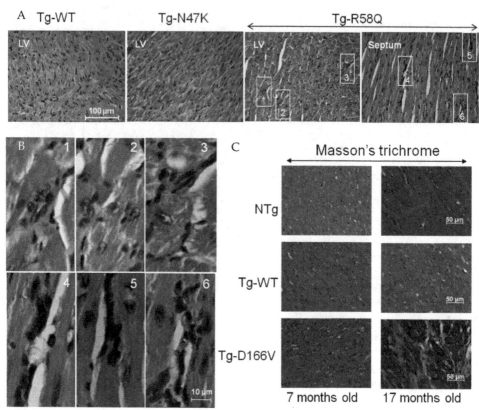

Fig. 6. Histopathology of transgenic mouse hearts. (A) The hearts of representative 4 month-old mice from Tg-WT, Tg-N47K and Tg-R58Q mice were stained with hematoxylin and eosin. Note that nuclei stain blue with hematoxylin, whereas the cells stain pink/red with eosin. Scale bar, 100 μm. (B) Enlarged views of the left ventricle and septal tissues of Tg-R58Q hearts. Scale bar, 10 μm. As indicated, clusters of nuclei could be clearly observed in Tg-R58Q tissues compared to control samples suggesting occurrences of the R58Q-mediated degeneration in Tg-R58Q myocardium. (C) Microscopic views of left ventricles from Tg-D166V and control Tg-WT and NTg mice stained with Masson's trichrome stain (Kerrick et al., 2009). Note the severe fibrotic lesions in the myocardium of older 17 months old Tg-D166V mice. Scale bar, 50 μm.

3.2.3 Echocardiography

Echocardiography, a test in which ultrasound measurements are used to examine the heart, is the least invasive method available to screen for cardiac hypertrophy. The echocardiogram allows for detailed morphological and functional assessment of the heart. Echocardiography examination performed on Tg-E22K mice did not show any major differences between transgenic E22K and control WT and/or NTg hearts (Szczesna-Cordary et al., 2005).

Doppler echocardiography, another technique of ultrasound examination is used to look at how blood flows through the heart chambers, heart valves, and blood vessels. It allows determination of the velocity and direction of blood flow by utilizing the Doppler effect

sed on the cellular findings, Abraham et al. hypothesized that a malignant FHC
enotype associated with the R58Q mutation could be related to diastolic dysfunction of
e R58Q-mutated myocardium (Abraham et al., 2009). Global diastolic haemodynamics
ere evaluated using transmitral Doppler velocities in Tg-R58Q and Tg-N47K mice and
mpared to controls (NTg and Tg-WT). An apical four-chamber view of the heart was
tained. A pulsed Doppler sample was placed at the tip of the mitral leaflets and
ansmitral early (E) and late (A) diastolic velocities and the deceleration time were
easured and used as noninvasive indicators of global diastolic function (Abraham et al.,
09). Interestingly, alterations in diastolic transmitral velocities and prolonged deceleration
ne were only noted in Tg-R58Q myocardium (**Fig. 7**). The authors suggested that the
alignant FHC phenotype associated with R58Q could be related to abnormal relaxation
d diastolic dysfunction of the mutated myocardium. The key conclusion of this study was
at diastolic function is affected earlier in the disease process in the transgenic mouse
odel and may likely be a more sensitive indicator of a malignant FHC phenotype than
pertrophy or systolic dysfunction (Abraham et al., 2009).

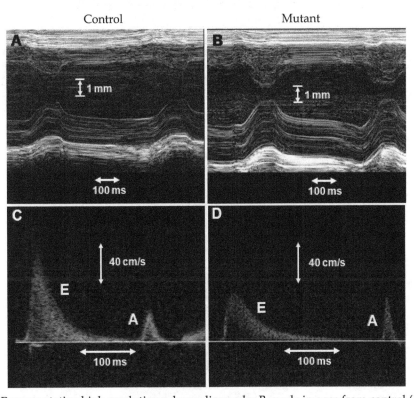

g. 7. Representative high resolution echocardiography B-mode images from control (A)
d Tg-R58Q mice (B) show no significant difference in chamber dimensions or wall
ickness. Representative pulsed Doppler tracings of the mitral valve in controls (C) and Tg-
58Q mice (D) demonstrating reduced E wave velocity and longer deceleration times in the
tter group (Abraham et al., 2009).

3.2.4 Perfused working heart model

The hearts of transgenic mice carrying different RLC mutations were tested for the ability perform work under conditions of physiologically relevant levels of metabolic demands ar for glucose and fatty acid oxidation measured in isolated working hearts (Abraham et al., 200 Szczesna-Cordary et al., 2007). Studies with Tg-E22K mice showed a similar energy metabolis pattern compared to control Tg-WT and NTg mouse hearts, but following 20 minutes of r flow ischemia, the E22K hearts demonstrated a slightly better recovery compared to WT hear (Szczesna-Cordary et al., 2007). In another study with Tg-R58Q and Tg-N47K mice, it w shown that cardiac output, cardiac work and cardiac power were drastically compromise compared with controls, Tg-WT or NTg mice (Abraham et al., 2009). Additional data attaine with Tg-R58Q mice also demonstrated significantly decreased cardiac efficiency in aerobica∎ perfused R58Q hearts compared to controls and poor recovery after an acute ischemic episo confirming greatly compromised cardiac function in Tg-R58Q mice (Abraham et al., 200❡ Results from these studies mirrored the severity of the human phenotypes associated wi R58Q and N47K mutations, with less severe outcomes in N47K patients, while matching t∎ malignant phenotype with multiple cases of SCD in R58Q-positive patients.

3.2.5 Endogenous level of RLC phosphorylation

The highly conserved Ser-15 in RLC can be reversibly phosphorylated *in vivo* by Ca² CaM-activated MLCK. Given the role that RLC phosphorylation can play in affectir thick filament structure and cardiac contractility, examining the mutation induced effe on RLC phosphorylation is important in understanding the effects of any of the FH∎ mutation. Mutations studied in this review can be categorized into two groups based o

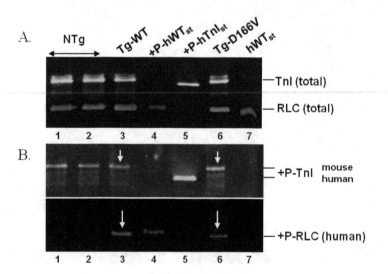

Fig. 8. The effect of the D166V mutation on the phosphorylation status of RLC and Troponi∎ I (TnI) in transgenic mouse ventricular extracts blotted with CT-1 antibody recognizing tota RLC protein and 6F9 antibody recognizing total TnI protein (A) and Mab14 MMS-418R antibody recognizing +P-TnI (top panel) and +P-human RLC antibody recognizing +P-RLC human (Tg) (bottom panel) (B) (Kerrick et al., 2009).

ieir location in the sequence and the 3D organization of RLC (**Fig. 3**): N47K and R58Q-
icated close or within the Ca^{2+} binding site, and A13T, E22K and D166V- located in close
roximity to the phosphorylation site (Ser-15). The status of phosphorylation was
xamined for transgenic mice carrying the R58Q, N47K and D166V mutations (Abraham
: al., 2009; Kerrick et al., 2009; Muthu et al., 2010; Muthu et al., 2011). Mouse extracts
om ventricular tissue were rapidly frozen in liquid nitrogen and analyzed by
nmunoblotting. The phosphorylated Tg-RLC was detected with +P-human RLC
itibodies (generously provided by Dr. Neal Epstein, NIH), specific for the
hosphorylated form of the ventricular RLC; followed by a secondary goat anti-rabbit
itibody conjugated with the fluorescent dye, IR red 800. It was interesting to note that
ie mutations in RLC associated with a malignant phenotype (R58Q and D166V)
isplayed a reduced level of phosphorylation compared to N47K and/or WT.
he decreased level of phosphorylation coincided with those FHC mutations that are
ssociated with a severe phenotype (**Fig. 8**) (Abraham et al., 2009; Kerrick et al., 2009). This
iggested that phosphorylation of the regulatory light chain of myosin could have an
nportant physiological role in the regulation of cardiac muscle contraction.

. Functional studies using cardiac muscle preparations

.1 ATPase assays
.1.1 Actin activated myosin ATPase activity

lyosin's ability to perform mechanical work, powered by the hydrolysis of ATP, requires
iat the enzymatic and mechanical cycles be coupled. Both the hydrolysis of ATP and the
eneration of force and motion are known to be multi-step processes. The cross-bridge cycle
in be broadly divided into states where myosin is strongly or weakly bound to actin. It
:arts with the physiologically short-lived rigor state where myosin is bound strongly to
:tin in the absence of ATP. If ATP or its hydrolysis products are bound (M∘ATP,
1∘ADP∘Pi), myosin shifts to the weakly bound state. Either prior to or following inorganic
hosphate (Pi) release, myosin undergoes its power stroke increasing its affinity for actin.
he actin activated myosin ATPase activity, measured as a function of actin concentration
'as determined for FHC-linked RLC mutants using myosin purified from the mouse hearts
r RLC-depleted porcine myosin reconstituted with WT or FHC RLC mutant protein. The
ssay consisted of titrating myosin with increasing concentrations of skeletal muscle actin.
he data were analyzed with the Michaelis-Menten equation yielding the V_{max} (maximal
TPase rate) and K_m (apparent dissociation constant) parameters.
his assay was performed to understand the effect of the N47K and R58Q mutations on the
ross bridge cycle (Greenberg et al., 2009). The maximal ATPase rates (V_{max}) for NTg (0.43
-1) and Tg-WT (0.43 s^{-1}) were seen to be similar to those of RLC carrying the N47K
iutation (0.43 s^{-1}). However, Tg-R58Q showed a significant increase in V_{max} (0.63 s^{-1}). On
ie other hand, a significant decrease in V_{max} was observed in Tg-A13T mice (0.38 s^{-1})
ompared to Tg-WT (0.51 s^{-1}) or NTg (0.63 s^{-1}) mice (unpublished data). The observed
hanges in the ATPase activity for the mutant RLC compared to controls suggest that the
)tal amount of free ATP in the cell may vary affecting several ATP dependent processes in
ie heart and leading to the development of FHC phenotype. Moreover, as V_{max} represents
ie rate constant of the transition from the weakly to strongly bound myosin cross-bridges,
ie FHC mutations are expected to affect the kinetics of force generating myosin cross-
ridges and muscle contraction.

4.1.2 Myofibrillar ATPase activity

To understand the effect of mutations in RLC at the myofibrillar level, assays wer performed on two types of systems: porcine myofibrils reconstituted with the FHC mutar or cardiac myofibrils prepared from transgenic mice carrying the RLC mutation. For the reconstituted myofibrillar assays, porcine cardiac myofibrils (CMF) were depleted (RLC using Triton and CDTA (Szczesna-Cordary et al., 2004a). The CDTA extraction metho resulted in about 80% depletion of the endogenous RLC. These RLC depleted CMF wer then reconstituted with exogenous recombinant human cardiac RLC-WT and FHC mutant (A13T, F18L, E22K, N47K and R58Q). The authors observed that myofibrils lacking the RL(demonstrated dramatic impairment of the Ca^{2+} regulation of ATPase activity at pCa 8 (lov Ca^{2+}) and 4.5 (high Ca^{2+}) and also demonstrated lower Ca^{2+} sensitivity of ATPase. The latte was determined to be due to partial extraction of troponin C (TnC) that occurs during RL(extraction. Reconstitution of the RLC-depleted CMF with cardiac TnC and RLC (WT or FH(mutant) recovered the Ca^{2+} regulation of ATPase activity, however; the maximal level (ATPase activation was slightly different for various FHC mutants with the highest leve observed for R58Q-reconstituted CMF. As presented in **Table 3**, Ca^{2+} sensitivity (myofibrillar ATPase activity was significantly increased for N47K mutant, slightly increase for E22K and R58Q, slightly decreased for F18L whereas no change was monitored for A13' mutant. It is interesting to note that three of the mutants (N47K, E22K and R58Q) tha increased the Ca^{2+} sensitivity of ATPase were seen to either decrease the affinity for Ca^{2+} (to inactivate the Ca^{2+} binding site of the human cardiac RLC (Szczesna-Cordary et al 2004a; Szczesna et al., 2001).

Myofibrils from mouse ventricular, septal and papillary muscles of NTg, Tg-WT, Tg-E22K Tg-R58Q and Tg-N47K mice were examined for their Ca^{2+} sensitivity of ATPas activity(Abraham et al., 2009; Szczesna-Cordary et al., 2005). Tg-WT and NTg myofibril showed similar pCa_{50} when compared among themselves. This established that the Ca^2 sensitivity was not RLC-isoform (human *versus* mouse)-dependent. A statistically significar increase in the Ca^{2+} sensitivity of myofibrillar ATPase activity was observed between NT or Tg-WT mice and Tg-E22K mice ($\Delta pCa_{50} \cong 0.14$) (Szczesna-Cordary et al., 2004a). Studie on myofibrils from Tg-N47K and Tg-R58Q showed a decrease in the cooperativity of th actin–myosin interaction with a much more dramatic effect exhibited by the R58Q mutatior Though these results reflect what was seen with porcine CMF reconstituted with FH(mutants, the effect seemed to be more pronounced in Tg mice. Recent studies also showe(that the maximal ATPase activity in myofibrils from Tg-D166V mice were significantl lower when compared to WT. However, it is interesting to note that followin phosphorylation, the low levels of ATPase activity observed in Tg-D166V was recovered t the level of Tg-WT (Muthu et al., 2011). The latter study brought to light the beneficial ro that RLC phosphorylation may have on cardiac function. More details on the role of Ca^2 binding and phosphorylation of the regulatory light chain on the cross bridge cycle ar discussed later in this review.

4.2 Studies on cardiac muscle fibers

To test the functional consequence of FHC mutations at higher levels of organizatior cardiac papillary muscle fibers from transgenic mice or RLC-depleted and mutan reconstituted porcine cardiac papillary muscle fibers were used in steady-state force an(ATPase measurements.

Porcine cardiac papillary muscle fibers reconstituted with mutant RLC: Endogenous RLC was depleted from porcine cardiac muscle fiber preparations using CDTA and Triton (Szczesna-Cordary et al., 2004a). Depletion of endogenous RLC resulted in partial extraction of TnC (similar to that seen in porcine CMF). Therefore, TnC was added back along with the mutant RLC during reconstitution. It was observed that depletion of RLC, which was accompanied by a partial extraction of TnC, resulted in a decrease in the maximal level of force development from 100% to ~46%. Reconstitution of RLC-depleted fibers with TnC and RLC-WT restored the maximal level of force to ~84% (Szczesna-Cordary et al., 2004a). FHC mutants (A13T, E22K, N47K and R58Q mutants) were then tested for steady-state force development and the regulation of Ca^{2+} sensitivity of force. The lowest level of recovered force was observed for the E22K mutant (66%) whereas N47K- and R58Q-reconstituted fibers demonstrated 74% and 78%, respectively. Also, The E22K mutation was shown to cause a slight increase while the two Ca^{2+} binding site mutants, N47K and R58Q, showed a significantly large increase in the Ca^{2+} sensitivity of force development (Szczesna-Cordary et al., 2004a). Interestingly, in studies performed on skinned rabbit psoas muscle fibers reconstituted with the E22K mutation, it was observed that the tension at pCa 6.0 and the pCa_{50} value were significantly increased compared to WT-reconstituted psoas fibers (Roopnarine, 2003).

hese results were in accord with the previous studies by Levine et. al on human biopsy amples from patients carrying the E22K mutation. A leftward shift in the tension-pCa curve vas observed signifying a mutation mediated increase in the Ca^{2+} sensitivity of force levelopment (Levine et al., 1998). Levine's group also studied the structure of the thick ilaments carrying the E22K mutation compared to normal human fibers isolated from slow keletal muscle. The authors speculated that because the E22K mutation occurs due to the ubstitution of a positively charged residue for a residue that is acidic, an ordered state of nyosin cross-bridges was expected in both the mutant as well as normal fibers. However, they •bserved a disordered state of the filaments from the mutant biopsy while the wild type ilaments from the normal human sample showed an ordered relaxed state (Levine et al., 1998).

. Transgenic cardiac papillary muscle fibers: To avoid difficulties related to the extraction/replacement of the RLC in porcine muscle preparations, cardiac papillary muscle fibers from transgenic mice expressing RLC mutations were used. The Ca^{2+} sensitivity of force development was first examined in transgenic mice carrying the E22K mutation of RLC and the results compared to WT control mice (Szczesna-Cordary et al., 2005). The mutation was seen to increase the Ca^{2+} sensitivity of force development compared to WT. In addition, a slight gene-dose effect in the force development was observed and the glycerinated skinned muscle fibers from TgE22K L4 expressing 87% transgene demonstrated slightly higher Ca^{2+} sensitivity of force than in Tg-E22K L2 expressing 67% mutant protein (pCa_{50}=5.65 vs. 5.62) (Szczesna-Cordary et al., 2005). The authors concluded that the E22K-mediated structural perturbations in the RLC and altered Ca^{2+}-binding-properties were most likely responsible for the abnormal function of the mutated myocardium and initiation of hypertrophic response and FHC.

iimilar force measurement studies in papillary muscle fibers from Tg-D166V mice revealed hat the presence of the D166V mutation, associated with malignant clinical outcomes, aused a decrease in maximal force as well as a significant leftward shift in myofilament :a²⁺ sensitivity compared to Tg-WT (Muthu et al., 2011). This report was also the first to

demonstrate the physiological effects of RLC phosphorylation in cardiomyopathi
transgenic mouse hearts. As expected, a small leftward shift in the force–pCa dependenc
was observed for Tg-WT papillary muscle fibers (**Fig.9**). In contrast, MLCK-treatment of Tg
D166V fibers resulted in a large decrease in myofilament Ca^{2+} sensitivity (**Fig.9**). Therefore
phosphorylation of D166V- diseased muscle reversed the increased Ca^{2+} sensitivity of forc
and brought it back to the level observed for Tg-WT.

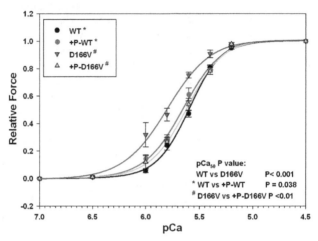

Fig. 9. Effect of RLC phosphorylation on the force–pCa relationship in skinned muscle fibers
from Tg-WT mice and Tg-D166V (Muthu et al., 2011).

In addition to calcium sensitivity, the authors determined the effect of RLC phosphorylation
on maximal steady-state force (Muthu et al., 2011). In contrast to Tg-WT, which displayed a
phosphorylation-induced increase in force, the maximal tension in Tg-D166V papillary
muscle fibers decreased upon phosphorylation. The authors concluded that
phosphorylation of myosin RLC could work as a regulator of the acto–myosin interaction in
both normal and cardiomyopathic hearts. A phosphorylation induced tuning of cardia
function in the diseased heart was seen to be different from the healthy heart and wa
anticipated to vary depending on the type and the level of cardiac insult.

Simultaneous ATPase/force-pCa relationships: Studies were designed to perform simultaneou
force and ATPase measurements in freshly isolated (not glycerinated) skinned papillary
muscle fibers from transgenic mice (Kerrick et al., 2009; Wang et al., 2006). ATPase activity
was measured by the NADH fluorescence method (Guth & Wojciechowski, 1986). In thi
method, the regeneration of ATP from ADP and PEP (phospho-enol-pyruvate) by the
enzyme PK (pyruvate kinase) is coupled to the oxidation of NADH (fluorescent) to NAD
(non-fluorescent) by LDH (Griffiths et al., 1980; Takashi & Putnam, 1979). The decrease in
NADH concentration is detected by a decrease in the fluorescence signal at 450 nm. The
slope of the linear decrease in NADH concentration is used to calculate ATPase activity. In
these measurements, force was recorded simultaneously with ATPase. The concentration o
Ca^{2+} during ATPase/force measurements was measured with Calcium Green-2 fluorescenc
and the data fit to the Hill equation yielding the pCa_{50} and Hill coefficient n_H values (Kerrick
et al., 2009; Wang et al., 2006).

:inned muscle fibers from Tg-E22K mice showed a significant (20%) decrease in maximum
Tpase and force compared to Tg-WT controls (Szczesna-Cordary et al., 2007). However,
ntrary to previously reported studies (Szczesna-Cordary et al., 2005) in glycerinated
.inned muscle fibers, no significant difference in the pCa_{50} of force/ATPase-pCa
ıationships was observed between Tg-E22K and Tg-WT mice. Similar studies on skinned
uscle fibers from Tg-D166V and Tg-R58Q mice showed that compared to Tg-WT, the
utations associated with a malignant disease phenotype (R58Q and D166V) caused large
creases in the Ca^{2+} sensitivity of ATPase and force while those of benign phenotype
J47K) showed no changes in the force/ATPase-pCa dependence (Kerrick et al., 2009; Wang
al., 2006). Simultaneous ATPase/force-pCa measurements using freshly skinned papillary
uscle fibers from Tg-D166V mice demonstrated a large increase in the Ca^{2+} sensitivity of
rce and ATPase compared to control NTg and Tg-WT mice (Kerrick et al., 2009). In
ldition, the maximal ATPase and force per cross-section of muscle fiber were largely
:creased in the mutant Tg-D166V fibers compared to controls. The authors proceeded to
lculate the rate of dissociation of the myosin heads from actin (rate of cross-bridge
ssociation, "g") and showed a mutation-dependent dramatic decrease in g at all levels of
rce activation (Kerrick et al., 2009). Additionally, the energy cost per cross-bridge (fiber
TPase/force) was slightly higher in Tg-D166V fibers compared to controls although the
fference between Tg-D166V and Tg-WT fibers was not statistically significant (Kerrick et
., 2009). The authors speculated that a slower relaxation rate of cycling myosin cross-
idges most likely triggered a series of pathological responses resulting in an abnormal
gulation of cardiac muscle contraction in Tg-D166V mice.

*udies in intact papillary muscle fibers to monitor the rates and amplitudes of $[Ca^{2+}]$ and force
ınsients:* In parallel to skinned fiber studies, the measurements of force and calcium
ınsients were performed in electrically stimulated intact papillary muscle fibers (Kerrick et
., 2009; Wang et al., 2006). These experiments directly addressed potential abnormalities of
.e mutated myocardium of diastolic and systolic function observed in the FHC-mutated
yocardium. Force and Ca^{2+} transients were seen to be significantly shortened in Tg-E22K
tact fibers compared to Tg-WT (Szczesna-Cordary et al., 2007). The authors hypothesized
ıat by changing the properties of the RLC Ca^{2+}-Mg^{2+} binding site, the E22K mutation could
e affecting the function of RLC as a delayed Ca^{2+} buffer. Consequently, a faster Ca^{2+}
·uptake by the sarcoplasmic reticulum proteins and the shorter duration of $[Ca^{2+}]$ and force
ansients could be expected, both indicative of enhanced muscle relaxation. In line with this
xplanation, the R58Q mutation, which was seen to inactivate the RLC calcium binding site
·r Ca^{2+} binding, should induce an opposite effect to E22K in intact papillary muscle fibers.
his was in fact observed and significantly prolonged force and $[Ca^{2+}]$ transients were
ıonitored in Tg-R58Q papillary muscles compared to Tg-WT (Wang et al., 2006). In
ırallel, intact fiber studies on Tg-N47K mutation showed no change in force transients with
nall changes in $[Ca^{2+}]$ transients (Wang et al., 2006).

ı the study on the D166V mutation, the authors investigated whether the slower kinetics of
·rce generating myosin cross-bridges, as determined in Tg-D166V skinned papillary
ıuscle fibers (above), resulted in slower relaxation measured in intact papillary muscles
om Tg-D166V mice (Kerrick et al., 2009). It was observed that the rates of force relaxation
ı Tg-D166V muscles were significantly slower than the rates measured in Tg-WT or NTg
ıpillary muscle fibers. However, the prolonged force transients in Tg-D166V muscle fibers
ere not paralleled by delayed calcium transients and no differences were observed

between [Ca^{2+}] transients of Tg-D166V *versus* Tg-WT or NTg intact muscle fibers (Kerrick al., 2009). Results of this study suggested several potential D166V-mediated factors th. could contribute to FHC when placed *in vivo*. First, a large increase in Ca^{2+} sensitivity cou contribute to decreased ventricular filling at high heart rates when the tail end of the fir Ca^{2+} transient begins to fuse with the second. Secondly, the slow force relaxation rate of tl fibers could also start to fuse with the next contraction when heart rates are high al: contributing to diastolic dysfunction. If severe enough these two factors could affe diastolic filling of the heart sufficiently to result in systolic dysfunction, i.e. decrease i stroke volume. This ultimately would cause the heart to compensate by increasing wa thickness (hypertrophy). Finally, the prediction of decreased twitch force caused by decrease in the time constant for the rate of rise of force would also result in systol dysfunction that could only be compensated for by increases in heart rates.

Overall, studies in skinned and intact muscle fibers from FHC transgenic animals revealed correlation between the mutant-mediated course of the disease in humans and the extent physiological changes observed in the studies with muscle fibers. Prolonged [Ca^{2+}] and for transients in intact Tg-R58Q and Tg-D166V papillary muscles as well as increased Ca sensitivity of ATPase/force observed in skinned fibers correlated with a poor prognosis i R58Q and D166V mutated patients whose phenotype included SCD. Likewise, the slightl prolonged [Ca^{2+}] transient with no alterations in force transient, and no change in Ca sensitivity of ATPase/force observed in Tg-N47K mice, correlated with the phenotype hypertrophic cardiomyopathy described for N47K patients, including lack of SCD.

5. Studies with single molecules

5.1 *In vitro* motility assays

In vitro motility assays were utilized to examine the effects of FHC RLC mutations on tl biochemical and mechanical properties of myosin isolated from the hearts of transgen mice or reconstituted with the recombinant human cardiac WT or FHC mutant. In the stud by Greenberg et al., myosin was purified from Tg-N47K and Tg-R58Q mouse hearts an used in *in vitro* motility assays with Tg-WT myosin as a control (Greenberg et al., 2009 Unregulated motility assays were used to determine whether the mutations caused an changes in the duty cycle and/or actin filament sliding velocity. The principle behind th assay was that the actin filament moves at its maximal velocity when incubated wit enough myosin to ensure that at least one myosin head is interacting with the acti filament at all times. Therefore, the amount of myosin required to achieve maximal velocit would give a qualitative measurement of the duty cycle. The authors observed a significar increase in velocity caused by the R58Q mutation while no major change in actin slidir velocity was observed for Tg-N47K myosin compared to Tg-WT (Greenberg et al., 2009). Additionally, the isometric force of the mutant myosins was studied using a friction loading assay (Greenberg et al., 2009). A low affinity actin binding protein, α-actinin, wa introduced in the assay and the concentration of α-actinin needed to stop the filamer motility was used as a measurement of myosin isometric force. Tg-N47K myosin showed dramatic reduction in isometric force while a less pronounced decrease in force was seen fc Tg-R58Q compared to Tg-WT myosins. The authors also determined the effect of RL mutation on the velocity-pCa dependence using actin complexed with the regulator proteins, troponin and tropomyosin (Greenberg et al., 2009). While Tg-R58Q myosi showed a significant leftward shift in the calcium sensitivity of velocity, Tg-N47K and Tg

T myosins showed no difference in the velocity-pCa curve. This result was consistent with e earlier (Wang et al., 2006) and more recent (Mettikolla et al., 2011) fiber studies using apillary muscles from these mice, where a significant increase in the Ca^{2+} sensitivity of rce was observed for Tg-R58Q mice. Though both Tg-R58Q and Tg-N47K myosins isplayed a reduction in isometric force, the authors concluded that the more extreme henotype for R58Q could stem from an increase in myosin ATPase activity (discussed pove in "Actin activated myosin ATPase assays") (Greenberg et al., 2009). On the other and, study results with myosin isolated from transgenic E22K mice showed no effect of the utation on actin sliding velocity or the velocity-pCa dependence (Szczesna-Cordary et al., 007).

he effect of R58Q and N47K mutations was further tested using porcine myosin depleted f endogenous RLC and reconstituted with the mutant (R58Q or N47K) RLC proteins Greenberg et al., 2010). The authors examined the effects of these mutations on the echanical properties of myosin under both unloaded and loaded conditions. They found at, whereas the mutant myosins were indistinguishable from the controls (WT or native yosin) under unloaded conditions, both R58Q- and N47K-exchanged myosins showed ductions in force and power output compared with WT or native myosin. They also howed that the changes in loaded kinetics resulted from mutation-induced loss of myosin train sensitivity of ADP affinity (Greenberg et al., 2010). The authors concluded that the 58Q and N47K mutations alter the mechanical properties of the myosin neck region, ading to altered load dependent kinetics that may explain the observed mutant-induced HC phenotypes (Greenberg et al., 2010).

2 Single molecule detection (SMD)

he advances in single molecule detection (SMD) by fluorescence techniques were mployed to study some of the earlier discussed FHC-linked RLC mutations. The advantage f SMD includes studying the motion of a small population of myosin cross bridges while orking in their native environment of the sarcomere. Another advantage of this approach the ability to unambiguously determine the behavior (kinetics, orientation, etc.) of the ormal *versus* mutated muscle by observing a few molecules (myosin cross-bridges). Since umans are heterozygous for FHC mutations, the distribution of the healthy and diseased olecules is random and any collection containing more than a few molecules carries a high robability of containing a mixture of healthy and diseased moieties. It is therefore essential use a technique such as SMD which is capable of monitoring properties of single olecules without averaging over ensembles of molecules with different properties.

he E22K substitution was the first FHC-associated mutation in RLC studied by SMD Dumka et al., 2006). Mechanical events were measured by monitoring the anisotropy of ctin labeled with rhodamine phalloidin. The measurements were done on a small opulation of cross bridges in contracting Tg-WT and Tg-E22K cardiac myofibrils. The esults showed that the mutation did not significantly affect the time of cross-bridge issociation and had no major effect on the mechanical performance of the cross bridges. another mutation that was studied using SMD was the D166V mutation associated with a nalignant FHC phenotype (Borejdo et al., 2010; Mettikolla et al., 2009; Muthu et al., 2010). In ne experiment, myofibrils from Tg-D166V mice were labeled with Alexa 488-phalloidin nd the measurements of the fluorescence lifetime (average rate of decay of a fluorescent pecies from its excited state) of the actin attached fluorophores were performed. No differences between lifetimes of Tg-WT and Tg-D166V muscle were observed (Mettikolla (al., 2009). In addition to fluorescence lifetime, a meaningful indicator of the state of muscle that can b studied with SMD is the cross-bridge duty cycle (Mettikolla et al., 2009; Muthu et al., 2010 It was assumed that a cross-bridge is in its strongly attached to actin state for a period c time t_s, while it remains in a dissociated or a weakly attached state for a period of time, t, The ratio $\Psi = t_s/(t_d + t_s)$, was defined as the duty cycle. To measure Ψ, one can follow th changes in the environment of a cross-bridge while it undergoes a cycle of association an dissociation from actin. In the study by Muthu et al. the authors derived the myosin cros: bridge kinetic rates by tracking the orientation of a fluorescently labeled single acti molecule (Muthu et al., 2010). Orientation (measured by polarized fluorescence) oscillate between two states, corresponding to the actin-bound (t_s) and actin-free (t_d) states of th myosin cross-bridge. The rate of cross-bridge attachment during isometric contractio decreased from 3 s^{-1} in myofibrils from Tg-WT to 1.4 s^{-1} in myofibrils from Tg-D166V. Th rate of detachment decreased from 1.3 s^{-1} (Tg-WT) to 1.2 s^{-1} (Tg-D166V). In addition, th average value of the duty cycle in isometrically contracting myofibrils from Tg-WT and Tξ D166V mice was 30% and 50%, respectively (Muthu et al., 2010). The authors hypothesize that the slower kinetics of Tg-D166V myosin cross-bridges could be the result of a mutatior mediated decrease in endogenous phosphorylation of myosin RLC, as was observed in th hearts of Tg-D166V mice (Kerrick et al., 2009). Indeed, the authors showed that the level c RLC phosphorylation was largely decreased in Tg-D166V myofibrils compared to Tg-W' (Muthu et al., 2010). They concluded that the D166V-induced change in the cross-bridg kinetics could further lead to abnormalities in diastolic and/or systolic function that in th long term would result in a compensatory hypertrophy and sudden cardiac death, a observed in patients harboring the D166V mutation in RLC.

The SMD technique was further refined in the study by Borejdo et al. (Borejdo et al., 2010). Th authors analyzed the probability distribution of polarized intensity fluctuations and measure fluctuations by recording the parallel and perpendicular components of fluorescent ligh emitted by an actin-bound fluorophore (Borejdo et al., 2010). The histograms of fluctuations c fluorescent actin molecules in Tg-WT hearts in rigor were represented by perfect Gaussia curves. In contrast, histograms of contracting heart muscle were peaked and asymmetri(suggesting that contraction in the heart driven by the interaction of myosin cross-bridges wit actin occurred in at least two steps (Borejdo et al., 2010). Importantly, there were statisticall significant differences between the histograms of contracting FHC-linked R58Q and D166\ cardiac muscle preparations versus corresponding contracting WT hearts. On the basis of thes results, the authors suggested a simple new method of distinguishing between healthy an FHC R58Q and D166V hearts by analyzing the probability distribution of polarize fluorescence intensity fluctuations of sparsely labeled actin molecules (Borejdo et al., 2010).

Further studies using SMD were performed on cardiac myofibrils from Tg-R58Q mic (Mettikolla et al., 2011). The results showed that the R58Q mutation resulted in a decrease i the rate of cross-bridge binding to actin, dissociation from actin and a decreased rate a which the cross-bridge undergoes the power stroke (Mettikolla et al., 2011). The author hypothesized that slower R58Q cross-bridge kinetics were most likely responsible for th lower force measured in Tg-R58Q skinned muscle fibers. The combined data on the R58(mutation led the authors to conclude that the R58Q hearts may be subject to inefficien energy utilization and compromised heart performance.

Concluding remarks and future directions

'ith the advent of molecular biology and the ability to clone, express and purify myosin LC and the FHC-linked mutations, it has been possible to begin to reconstruct muscle with rious RLC mutants to learn about their function in increasingly more complex systems. he advance of transgenesis has catapulted the researchers to a new era of research where e function of FHC-linked RLC mutations could be studied *in vivo* in transgenic mouse earts. Using various innovative approaches applied at the single molecule, skinned fiber, d intact muscle levels, it has been possible to begin to understand the effect of FHC utations on cardiac function. The presented results indicate that RLC phosphorylation and a²⁺ binding to the RLC EF-hand calcium binding site may play important roles not only in e physiological performance of the heart, but also in muscle contraction of the diseased eart. The MLCK-dependent phosphorylation of RLC was shown to be critical to maintain ormal cardiac function and was suggested to be especially important in the adaptive sponses of the heart to pathophysiological injury. Unraveling the molecular basis of RLC-ediated cardiac dysfunction can ultimately open new possibilities for an effective eatment(s) and efforts should be directed towards developing phosphorylation-mediated scue strategies. Collectively, the results presented in this review provided insight into the echanisms underlying the development of FHC disease caused by the mutations in the rdiac RLC. Future investigations should be focused on the preventive treatments to leviate or reverse the detrimental effects of all identified RLC mutations.

Acknowledgments

his work was supported by grants from the National Institutes of Health (HL071778 and L090786) to Danuta Szczesna-Cordary and the American Heart Association 0POST3420009) to Priya Muthu.

References

braham, T.P.; Jones, M.; Kazmierczak, K.; Liang, H.-Y.; Pinheiro, A.C.; Wagg, C.S.; Lopaschuk, G.D. & Szczesna-Cordary, D. (2009). Diastolic dysfunction in familial hypertrophic cardiomyopathy transgenic model mice. *Cardiovasc Res.* 82:84-92.

lcalai, R.; Seidman, J.G. & Seidman, C.E. (2008). Genetic basis of hypertrophic cardiomyopathy: from bench to the clinics. *J Cardiovasc Electrophysiol.* 19:104-10.

ndersen, P.S.; Havndrup, O.; Bundgaard, H.; Moolman-Smook, J.C.; Larsen, L.A.; Mogensen, J.; Brink, P.A.; Borglum, A.D.; Corfield, V.A.; Kjeldsen, K.; Vuust, J. & Christiansen, M. (2001). Myosin light chain mutations in familial hypertrophic cardiomyopathy: phenotypic presentation and frequency in Danish and South African populations. *J Med Genet.* 38:E43.

inder, W.D.; Fifer, M.A.; King, M.E. & Stone, J.R. (2005). Case records of the Massachusetts General Hospital. Case 26-2005. A 48-year-old man with sudden loss of consciousness while jogging. *N Engl J Med.* 353:824-32.

orejdo, J.; Szczesna-Cordary, D.; Muthu, P. & Calander, N. (2010). Familial hypertrophic cardiomyopathy can be characterized by a specific pattern of orientation fluctuations of actin molecules. *Biochemistry.* 49:5269-77.

Chen, Y.H. & Yang, J.T. (1971). A new approach to the calculation of secondary structures c globular proteins by optical rotatory dispersion and circular dichroism. *Biocher Biophys Res Commun.* 44:1285-91.

Colson, B.A.; Locher, M.R.; Bekyarova, T.; Patel, J.R.; Fitzsimons, D.P.; Irving, T.C. & Moss R.L. (2010). Differential roles of regulatory light chain and myosin binding protein C phosphorylations in the modulation of cardiac force development. *J Physio* 588:981-93.

Ding, P.; Huang, J.; Battiprolu, P.K.; Hill, J.A.; Kamm, K.E. & Stull, J.T. (2010). Cardia myosin light chain kinase is necessary for myosin regulatory light chai phosphorylation and cardiac performance in vivo. *J Biol Chem.* 285:40819-29.

Dumka, D.; Talent, J.; Akopova, I.; Guzman, G.; Szczesna-Cordary, D. & Borejdo, J. (2006 E22K mutation of RLC that causes familial hypertrophic cardiomyopathy i heterozygous mouse myocardium: effect on cross-bridge kinetics. *Am J Physic Heart Circ Physiol.* 291:H2098-2106.

Flavigny, J.; Richard, P.; Isnard, R.; Carrier, L.; Charron, P.; Bonne, G.; Forissier, J.F.; Desnos M.; Dubourg, O.; Komajda, M.; Schwartz, K. & Hainque, B. (1998). Identification o two novel mutations in the ventricular regulatory myosin light chain gene (MYL2 associated with familial and classical forms of hypertrophic cardiomyopathy. *J Mc Med.* 76:208-14.

Geeves, M.A. & Holmes, K.C. (2005). The molecular mechanism of muscle contraction. *Ad Protein Chem.* 71:161-93.

Greenberg, M.J.; Kazmierczak, K.; Szczesna-Cordary, D. & Moore, J.R. (2010 Cardiomyopathy-linked myosin regulatory light chain mutations disrupt myosi strain-dependent biochemistry. *Proc Natl Acad Sci U S A.* 107:17403-8.

Greenberg, M.J.; Watt, J.D.; Jones, M.; Kazmierczak, K.; Szczesna-Cordary, D. & Moore, J.R (2009). Regulatory light chain mutations associated with cardiomyopathy affec myosin mechanics and kinetics. *J Mol Cell Cardiol.* 46:108-115.

Griffiths, P.J.; Guth, K.; Kuhn, H.J. & Ruegg, J.C. (1980). ATPase activity in rapidly activatec skinned muscle fibres. *Pflugers Arch.* 387:167-73.

Guth, K. & Wojciechowski, R. (1986). Perfusion cuvette for the simultaneous measuremen of mechanical, optical and energetic parameters of skinned muscle fibres. *Pfluger Arch.* 407:552-7.

Hartshorne, D.J. & Mrwa, U. (1982). Regulation of smooth muscle actomyosin. *Blood Vessels* 19:1-18.

Houdusse, A. & Cohen, C. (1996). Structure of the regulatory domain of scallop myosin at : A resolution: implications for regulation. *Structure.* 4:21-32.

Hougs, L.; Havndrup, O.; Bundgaard, H.; Kober, L.; Vuust, J.; Larsen, L.A.; Christiansen, M & Andersen, P.S. (2005). One third of Danish hypertrophic cardiomyopath patients have mutations in MYH7 rod region. *Eur J Hum Genet.* . 13:161-165.

Howard, J. & Spudich, J.A. (1996). Is the lever arm of myosin a molecular elastic element *Proc Natl Acad Sci U S A.* 93:4462-4.

Huang, W.; Muthu, P.; Kazmierczak, K. & Szczesna-Cordary, D. (2011). FHC-Linked Myosi Regulatory Light Chain Mutations A13T and K104E Do Not Generate Majo Structural Changes Sufficient to Affect Binding of Myosin to Actin. *Biophysica journal.* 100:110a-111a.

Kabaeva, Z.T.; Perrot, A.; Wolter, B.; Dietz, R.; Cardim, N.; Correia, J.M.; Schulte, H.D Aldashev, A.A.; Mirrakhimov, M.M. & Osterziel, K.J. (2002). Systematic analysis o the regulatory and essential myosin light chain genes: genetic variants and mutations in hypertrophic cardiomyopathy. *Eur J Hum Genet*. 10:741-8.

amm, K.E. & Stull, J.T. (2011). Signaling to Myosin Regulatory Light Chain in Sarcomeres. *Journal of Biological Chemistry*. 286:9941-9947.

errick, W.G.L.; Kazmierczak, K.; Xu, Y.; Wang, Y. & Szczesna-Cordary, D. (2009). Malignant familial hypertrophic cardiomyopathy D166V mutation in the ventricular myosin regulatory light chain causes profound effects in skinned and intact papillary muscle fibers from transgenic mice. *FASEB J*. 23:855-865.

evine, R.J.; Yang, Z.; Epstein, N.D.; Fananapazir, L.; Stull, J.T. & Sweeney, H.L. (1998). Structural and functional responses of mammalian thick filaments to alterations in myosin regulatory light chains. *J Struct Biol*. 122:149-61.

owey, S.; Waller, G.S. & Trybus, K.M. (1993). Skeletal muscle myosin light chains are essential for physiological speeds of shortening. *Nature*. 365:454-6.

ettikolla, P.; Calander, N.; Luchowski, R.; Gryczynski, I.; Gryczynski, Z.; Zhao, J.; Szczesna-Cordary, D. & Borejdo, J. (2011). Cross-bridge kinetics in myofibrils containing familial hypertrophic cardiomyopathy R58Q mutation in the regulatory light chain of myosin. *J Theor Biol*. 284:71-81.

ettikolla, P.; Luchowski, R.; Gryczynski, I.; Gryczynski, Z.; Szczesna-Cordary, D. & Borejdo, J. (2009). Fluorescence Lifetime of Actin in the Familial Hypertrophic Cardiomyopathy Transgenic Heart. *Biochemistry*. 48:1264-1271.

orano, I. (1999). Tuning the human heart molecular motors by myosin light chains. *J Mol Med*. 77:544-55.

orner, S.; Richard, P.; Kazzam, E.; Hellman, U.; Hainque, B.; Schwartz, K. & Waldenstrom, A. (2003). Identification of the genotypes causing hypertrophic cardiomyopathy in northern Sweden. *J Mol Cell Card*. 35:841-849.

uthu, P.; Kazmierczak, K.; Jones, M. & Szczesna-Cordary, D. (2011). The effect of myosin RLC phosphorylation in normal and cardiomyopathic mouse hearts. *J Cell Mol Med*.

uthu, P.; Mettikolla, P.; Calander, N.; Luchowski, R.; Gryczynski, I.; Gryczynski, Z.; Szczesna-Cordary, D. & Borejdo, J. (2010). Single molecule kinetics in the familial hypertrophic cardiomyopathy D166V mutant mouse heart. *J Mol Cell Cardiol*. 48:989-998.

ant, K.; Watt, J.; Greenberg, M.; Jones, M.; Szczesna-Cordary, D. & Moore, J.R. (2009). Removal of the cardiac myosin regulatory light chain increases isometric force production. *FASEB J*. 23:3571-3580.

oetter, K.; Jiang, H.; Hassanzadeh, S.; Master, S.R.; Chang, A.; Dalakas, M.C.; Rayment, I.; Sellers, J.R.; Fananapazir, L. & Epstein, N.D. (1996). Mutations in either the essential or regulatory light chains of myosin are associated with a rare myopathy in human heart and skeletal muscle. *Nat Genet*. 13:63-9.

ayment, I.; Rypniewski, W.R.; Schmidt-Base, K.; Smith, R.; Tomchick, D.R.; Benning, M.M.; Winkelmann, D.A.; Wesenberg, G. & Holden, H.M. (1993). Three-dimensional structure of myosin subfragment-1: a molecular motor. *Science*. 261:50-8.

ichard, P.; Charron, P.; Carrier, L.; Ledeuil, C.; Cheav, T.; Pichereau, C.; Benaiche, A.; Isnard, R.; Dubourg, O.; Burban, M.; Gueffet, J.-P.; Millaire, A.; Desnos, M.; Schwartz, K.; Hainque, B.; Komajda, M. & for the EUROGENE Heart Failure Project (2003). Hypertrophic cardiomyopathy: Distribution of disease genes, spectrum of mutations, and implications for a molecular diagnosis strategy. *Circulation*. 107:2227-2232.

Richard, P.; Charron, P.; Carrier, L.; Ledeuil, C.; Cheav, T.; Pichereau, C.; Benaiche, A
    Isnard, R.; Dubourg, O.; Burban, M.; Gueffet, J.-P.; Millaire, A.; Desnos, M
    Schwartz, K.; Hainque, B.; Komajda, M. & for the EUROGENE Heart Failure Proje
    (2004). Correction to: "Hypertrophic cardiomyopathy: distribution of disease gene
    spectrum of mutations, and implications for a molecular diagnosis strategy
    Circulation. 109:3258.
Robertson, S.P.; Johnson, J.D. & Potter, J.D. (1981). The time-course of Ca^{2+} exchange wit
    calmodulin, troponin, parvalbumin, and myosin in response to transient increase
    in Ca2+. Biophys J. 34:559-69.
Roopnarine, O. (2003). Mechanical Defects of Muscle Fibers with Myosin Light Chai
    Mutants that Cause Cardiomyopathy. Biophys. J. 84:2440-2449.
Sanbe, A.; Nelson, D.; Gulick, J.; Setser, E.; Osinska, H.; Wang, X.; Hewett, T.E.; Klevitsky, R
    Hayes, E.; Warshaw, D.M. & Robbins, J. (2000). In vivo analysis of an essentia
    myosin light chain mutation linked to familial hypertrophic cardiomyopathy. Cii
    Res. 87:296-302.
Small, J.V. & Sobieszek, A. (1977). Ca-regulation of mammalian smooth muscle actomyosi
    via a kinase-phosphatase-dependent phosphorylation and dephosphorylation (
    the 20 000-Mr light chain of myosin. Eur J Biochem. 76:521-30.
Sobieszek, A. (1977). Ca-linked phosphorylation of a light chain of vertebrate smootl
    muscle myosin. Eur J Biochem. 73:477-83.
Szczesna-Cordary, D.; Guzman, G.; Ng, S.S. & Zhao, J. (2004a). Familial hypertroph
    cardiomyopathy-linked alterations in Ca^{2+} binding of human cardiac myosi
    regulatory light chain affect cardiac muscle contraction. J Biol Chem. 279:3535-42.
Szczesna-Cordary, D.; Guzman, G.; Zhao, J.; Hernandez, O.; Wei, J. & Diaz-Perez, Z. (2005
    The E22K mutation of myosin RLC that causes familial hypertroph
    cardiomyopathy increases calcium sensitivity of force and ATPase in transgen
    mice. J Cell Sci. 118:3675-83.
Szczesna-Cordary, D.; Jones, M. & Guzman, G. (2004b). Interaction of Myosin Regulatoi
    Light Chain Mutants Implicated in Familial Hypertrophic Cardiomyopathy wit
    IQ-Myosin Heavy Chain Peptides. Biophys J. 86:393a.
Szczesna-Cordary, D.; Jones, M.; Moore, J.R.; Watt, J.; Kerrick, W.G.L.; Xu, Y.; Wang, Y
    Wagg, C. & Lopaschuk, G.D. (2007). Myosin regulatory light chain E22K mutatio
    results in decreased cardiac intracellular calcium and force transients. FASEB
    21:3974-3985.
Szczesna, D. (2003). Regulatory light chains of striated muscle myosin. Structure, functio
    and malfunction. Curr Drug Targets Cardiovasc Haematol Disord. 3:187-97.
Szczesna, D.; Ghosh, D.; Li, Q.; Gomes, A.V.; Guzman, G.; Arana, C.; Zhi, G.; Stull, J.T. (
    Potter, J.D. (2001). Familial hypertrophic cardiomyopathy mutations in th
    regulatory light chains of myosin affect their structure, Ca^{2+} binding, an
    phosphorylation. J Biol Chem. 276:7086-92.
Takashi, R. & Putnam, S. (1979). A fluorimetric method for continuously assaying ATPas
    application to small specimens of glycerol-extracted muscle fibers. Anal Biochen
    92:375-82.
Wang, Y.; Xu, Y.; Kerrick, W.G.L.; Wang, Y.; Guzman, G.; Diaz-Perez, Z. & Szczesna
    Cordary, D. (2006). Prolonged Ca^{2+} and force transients in myosin RLC transgeni
    mouse fibers expressing malignant and benign FHC mutations. J Mol Biol. 361:286
    299.

10

Role of Genetic Factors in Dilated Cardiomyopathy

Cieslewicz Artur and Jablecka Anna
Karol Marcinkowski Medical University in Poznan, Department of Clinical Pharmacology
Poland

. Introduction

)ilated cardiomyopathy (DCM) is a heart muscle disease characterized by cardiac chamber nlargement and impaired systolic (and almost always diastolic) function. It is usually ssociated with heart failure, arrhythmias and/or conduction system disease and hromboembolic disease but may also be asymptomatic. DCM is diagnosed in the presence ɔf left ventricular enlargement and systolic dysfunction (left ventricular ejection fraction less han 50% or fractional shortening of less than 25-30%). It is considered one of the most ommon causes of heart failure, resulting in considerable morbidity and mortality. Patients vith DCM suffer from heart failure, arrhythmia and are at risk of premature death. The ɔrevalence of dilated cardiomyopathy is one case out of 2500 patients with an incidence of 7/100 000/year and it is 3 times more frequent in blacks and males than whites and females Bender et al., 2011, Hershberger et al., 2007, Taylor et al., 2006).

)CM may appear sporadic in a single member of family and is called then idiopathic DCM IDC). Dilated cardiomyopathy may be also inherited and is termed familial DCM (FDC), ɔntributing for 20-48 % of DCM. According to Mestroni et al. (1999), the diagnosis of FDC s made in the presence of two or more affected individuals in a single family or in the ɔresence of a first-degree relative of a dilated cardiomyopathy patient with well locumented unexplained sudden death at < 35 years of age. The principle causes of FDC are ;enetic mutations affecting cardiac myocytes (Taylor et al., 2006). Knowledge about genes nvolved in development of dilated cardiomyopathy can be used to create genetic tests for ɪssessing the risk of DCM.

ʌs DCM is a multigenic disorder, there are many genes contributing to development of this lisease. More than 30 genes, coding a variety of proteins such as nuclear envelope proteins, ardiac sarcomere units, ion channels, transcription factors, or dystrophin-associated ytoskeletal complex, were identified as causes of dilated cardiomyopathy (Hershberger et ɪl., 2009a). Some of these genes (discussed in this chapter) are presented in Table 1. For ɪdditional information see Hershberger et al. (2010) and UpToDate® website.

?.Major genetic causes of DCM

?.1 Lamins A/C (LMNA)

ʎuclear lamins (see Figure 1) are intermediate filament-type proteins that are major ɔuilding blocks of the nuclear lamina – a meshwork underlying the inner nuclear membrane. They can also be localized in the nuclear interior. Nuclei assembled *in vitro* in the absence of lamins are fragile, indicating the role of lamins in stabilizing the cell nucleus Lamins also take part in DNA replication, chromatin organization, spatial arrangement c nuclear pore complexes, nuclear growth and anchorage of nuclear envelope protein (Stuurman et al., 1998). Patients carrying mutations in LMNA gene are known to be at ris of conduction disorders and arrhythmic events in addition to ventricular dilatation an heart failure (Haugaa et al., 2009).

Gene	Encoded protein	Function
Major genetic factors		
LMNA	lamins A/C	building blocks of nuclear lamina
TNNT2	cardiac troponin T (cTnT)	regulation of muscle contraction
β-MYH7	β-myosin heavy chain	conversion of chemical energy into mechanical force
Other genetic factors		
SCN5A	alpha subunit of type V voltage-gated sodium channel	control of the flow of sodium ions into cardiac muscle cells
TCAP	titin-cap (telethonin)	regulation of sarcomere assembly
HBEGF	heparin-binding epidermal growth factor	regulation of cell growth and differentiation
SRA1	steroid receptor RNA activator 1	stimulation of proliferation and apoptosis
IK	cytokine	down-regulation of expression of HLA class II antigens
TPM1	α-tropomyosin	regulation of actin-myosin interaction
PSEN 1/2	presenilin 1 / 2	multi-pass transmembrane proteins
Dnm1l	dynamin-1-like	establishing mitochondrial morphology
LDB3	LIM domain binding 3	interaction with α-actinin-2 and protein kinase C

Table 1. Genes associated with dilated cardiomyopathy

Many studies suggest that defects in LMNA gene, encoding lamins A/C, are one of the mos significant genetic causes of dilated cardiomyopathy. According to Colombo et al. (2008), th LMNA gene is involved in up to 30-50% of patients with cardiac conduction disorders an DCM. Arbustini et al. (2002) were one of the first to reveal the role of LMNA mutations i developing dilated cardiomyopathy. The researchers investigated the prevalence of LMN gene defects in familial and idiopathic DCM associated with atrioventricular block o increased serum creatine-phosphokinase (sCPK). 73 cases of DCM (15 with atrioventricula block) were analysed, revealing five LMNA mutations (K97E, E111X, R190W, E317K and base pair insertion at 1713 cDNA) in five cases of familial autosomal dominant DCM wit atrioventricular block (33%). The role of LMNA mutations was further confirmed by Hermida Prieto et al. (2004) in the study on 67 consecutive patients with DCM (18 with FDC, 17 wit possible FDC and 32 with idiopathic DCM). The researchers observed two disease-causin mutations in LMNA gene, a novel R349L substitution and R190W (the same as in Arbustini e al. study). Both mutations were associated with severe forms of familial DCM. Anothe scovery concerning lamins was brought by Kärkkäinen et al. (2006). The study was carried ut on 66 DCM patients, who received heart transplant. DNA sequencing revealed 6 utations in LMNA gene (A132P, S143P, R190W, T1085 deletion, G1493 deletion, and R541S) hich explained DCM in 9% patients. Moreover, one of these mutations (S143P) explained 7 % f all cases in an unselected DCM population.

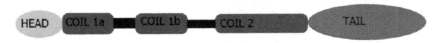

ig. 1. Structure of human lamin.

order to investigate mechanism responsible for electrophysiologic and myocardial henotypes caused by dominant human LMNA mutations, an experiment was carried out n heterozygous *Lmna* +/- mice (Wolf et al., 2008). Cardiac function and electrophysiology ere examined in heterozygous mice which underwent a targeted deletion of LMNA gene sulting in reduced level of lamin A/C protein in hearts. The researchers found out that espite normal structure and function in young *Lmna* +/- mice, older mice had altered trioventricular nodal architecture, functional electrophysiological deficits and arrhythmias. oreover, aged *Lmna* +/- mice, similar to humans with LMNA mutations, developed DCM, metimes without overt conductions system disease. 50-week old *Lmna* +/- mice had nlarged ventricular chambers in systole (p=0.01) and diastole (p=0.002) corresponding to gnificantly decreased fractional shortening (p=0.02). Cardiac sections of these mice also howed more fibrosis than wildtype mice. Cell and sarcomere shortening were decreased in *mna* +/- myocytes compared to wildtype (p<0.001) with ventricular dilatation and epressed cardiac contractility consistent with DCM in aged *Lmna* +/- mice. These findings onfirmed lamin A/C haploinsufficency as a possible mechanism leading to DCM.

arks et al. (2008) were one of the first to carry out a research concerning lamins A/C utation on a large group of patients. DNA from 324 patients with DCM (187 with FDC) as sequenced for nucleotide alterations in LMNA gene. 18 protein-altering variants (14 ovel) were identified in 5.9% cases (7.5% of FDC and 3.6% of IDC). 11 alterations were issense mutations (which changed conserved amino acid), three were nonsense, another ree were insertion/deletion and one was a splice site alteration. Conduction system isease and DCM were common among the carriers of these LMNA variants. These findings ere further investigated by Cowan et al. (2010), who expressed in COS7 cells GFP-relamin A constructs including 13 LMNA variants identified by Parks et al. (see Table 2). onfocal immunofluorescence microscopy was then used to characterize GFP-lamin A calization and nuclear morphology. Abnormal phenotypes were observed for 10 out of 13 nalyzed variants, providing evidence which supported pathogenicity of these variants. ecently, Botto et al. (2010) described additional novel LMNA mutation in FDC. Sequencing f the patient's LMNA coding exons revealed heterozygous missense mutation cytosine to nymine at nucleotide 565 in exon 3 which caused a substitution of arginine to hydrophobic ryptophan (R189W mutation) in a conserved residue located in the coil 1b of the alpha-elical rod domain. This mutation was located near the most prevalent lamin A/C mutation 190W, suggesting a "hot-spot" region at exon 3 and was not identified in a group of 50 ealthy volunteers. Moreover, the mutation was identified in 3 relatives of patient, who will hen benefit from regular clinical cardiac follow-up and early treatment.

LMNA variant	Mutation type	Pathogenicity of mutation (+/-)
R89L	substitution: Arg to Leu	+
R101P	substitution: Arg to Pro	+
R166P	substitution: Arg to Pro	+
R190Q	substitution: Arg to Gln	+
E203K	substitution: Glu to Lys	+
I210S	substitution: Ile to Ser	+
L215P	substitution: Leu to Pro	+
A318T	substitution: Ala to Thr	-
R388H	substitution: Arg to His	+
R399C	substitution: Arg to Cys	-
S437Hfsx1	substitution: Ser to His, frameshift, STOP codon (nonsense)	+
R471H	substitution: Arg to His	-
R654X	STOP codon (nonsense)	+

Table 2. LMNA variants inspected in patients with DCM (Cowan et al., 2010).

2.2 Cardiac troponin T (TNNT2)

Troponin T is the tropomyosin-binding protein in the troponin regulatory complex located on the thin filament of the contractile apparatus (see Figure 2). There are three isotype forms of troponin T: fast skeletal muscle, slow skeletal muscle and cardiac troponin T. These muscle-specific isoforms are expressed by different genes. Further diversity of troponin T comes from alternative splicing of RNA molecule (Katus et al., 1992).

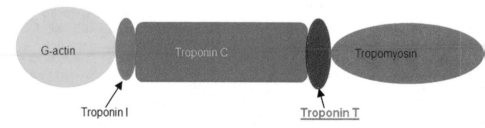

Fig. 2. Location of troponin T in the troponin regulatory complex.

Cardiac troponin T is encoded by TNNT2 gene, which alterations significantly contribute to dilated cardiomyopathy. Kamisago et al. (2000) were one of the first to show the role of TNNT2, identifying a deletion of AGA triplet resulting in deletion of lysine in residue 210 (K210 deletion) of troponin T protein chain in samples from two unrelated families suffering DCM. K210 mutation is one of the most frequent variants observed in patients suffering DCM. Otten et al. (2010) carried out a study, identifying 6 DCM patients carrying K210 deletion from 4 Dutch families. These patients showed severe form of DCM with early disease manifestation (mean age of DCM manifestation was 33 years) Moreover, heart transplantation was required in three patients at ages 12, 18 and 1 years.

he evidence from large cohort of patients was further provided by Mogensen et al. (2004). he researchers performed the study on 235 patients suffering DCM (102 with FDC). lutation analysis of TNNT2 resulted in identification of three novel mutations (R131W, 205L and D270N) and one reported previously(K210 deletion) in 13 patients from 4 ımilies. Three out of 13 patients received cardiac transplants, three died of heart failure, nother three died suddenly and four remained stable on conventional heart failure therapy. ll mutations segregated with the disease in each family and were absent in the control roup and in the group of patients with hypertrophic cardiomyopathy (HCM). Identified ıutations were considered disease-causing, because they co-segregated with disease in each ımily, were absent in control and HCM groups and were localized in conserved and ınctionally important regions of gene. Moreover, functional studies of mutated protein ›vealed altered troponin protein-protein interactions.

dditional data concerning the role of TNNT2 mutations in DCM was delivered by lershberger et al. (2009b). The researchers carried out bidirectional sequencing of TNNT2 sing DNA samples from 313 unrelated probands with DCM (183 with FDC and 130 with)C). Six protein-altering mutations were identified in 9 probands (2.9% of all patients). Ione of these variants were present in control group (253 patients). Five variants were ıissense mutations altering highly conserved amino acids (four novel mutations: R134G, 151C, R159Q, R205W and one previously reported in HCM:E244D)and one was K210 eletion. All of these mutations were considered possibly or likely disease-causing based on ıe clinical, pedigree and molecular genetic data (see Table 3). Additional functional studies f these mutations, carried out in cardiac myocytes reconstituted with mutant troponin T roteins revealed decreased Ca^{2+} sensitivity of force development (a hallmark of DCM), ıpporting disease-causing potential of these genetic variants.

TNNT2 variant	Mutation type	Disease-causing
R134G	substitution: Arg to Gly	yes (segregated with disease in other affected family members)
R151C	substitution: Arg to Cys	yes (homozygous mutation associated with aggresive disease)
R159Q	substitution: Arg to Gln	yes (replacement of conserved amino acid)
R205W	substitution: Arg to Trp	yes (similar to disease-causing R205L mutation reported by Mogensen et al., 2004)
E244D	substitution: Glu to Asp	yes (reported as disease-causing in patient with HCM)
K210del	deletion of lysine	yes (reported as disease-causing in several cases)

able 3. Disease-causing TNNT2 variants observed in patients with DCM (Hershberger et ı., 2009b)

1utations in TNNT2 may be also associated with more than one type of cardiomyopathy. or example, Menon et al. (2008) study conducted on a family with autosomal dominant eart disease variably expressed as restrictive cardiomyopathy (RCM), HCM and DCM ›vealed cosegregation of TNNT2 mutation with disease phenotype. Sequencing of TNNT2 lentified a heterozygous missense mutation resulting in I79N substitution inherited by all 9 affected family members but none of the six unaffected relatives. Mutation carriers wer diagnosed with RCM (2 patients), HCM (3 patients), DCM (2 patients), mixe cardiomyopathy (1 patient) and mild concentric left ventricular hypertrophy (1 patient). An experiment on mice, carried out by Ahmad et al. (2008) revealed the role of cardia troponin T quantity and function in development of heart and in dilated cardiomyopathy The researchers created heterozygous TNNT2+/- mice (i.e. lacking one TNNT2 allele) an then crossbred them to obtain homozygous null TNNT2-/- embryos. Moreover, transgeni mice overexpressing wildtype (TGWT) or mutant (TGK210Δ: K210 deletion) TNNT2 were als generated and used to create individuals lacking one allele of TNNT2 and carrying wildtyp (TNNT2+/-/ TGWT) or mutant (TNNT2+/-/ TGK210Δ) transgenes. The scientists found out tha TNNT2+/- mice compared to wildtype had significantly reduced transcript but not protein Moreover, TNNT2+/- mice had normal hearts. On the other hand TNNT2+/-/ TGK210Δ mic had severe DCM while TGK210Δ only mild DCM, suggesting the role of greater ratio c mutant to wildtype TNNT2 transcript in TNNT2+/-/ TGK210Δ mice compared to TGK210 individuals. TNNT2+/-/ TGK210Δ also showed muscle Ca2+ desenization but no difference i maximum force generation. The TNNT2-/- embryos had normally looped hearts but thi ventricular walls, large pericardial effusions, noncontractile hearts and severe disorganized sarcomers.

2.3 β-myosin heavy chain (MYH7)

Myosin is a protein that converts chemical energy into mechanical force through hydrolysi of ATP. Within the cell, it is organized as a pair of heavy chains and two pairs of ligh chains. The myosin heavy chain is a highly asymmetric molecule with a predominantl globular head and a rod-like tail, which is formed of two α-helices and accounts for th formation of the thick filament backbone (see Figure 3). The globular head contains a ligh chain-binding domain and a catalytic domain with actin and ATP-binding sites (Kabaev 2002).

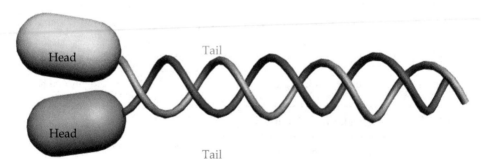

Fig. 3. A pair of myosin heavy chains.

Currently, more than 70 different mutations have been identified in MYH7 gene in associatio with DCM (Tanjore et al., 2010). Moreover, mutations in MYH7 have been reported in 4.2% cases of dilated cardiomyopathy (Hershberger et al., 2008). Clinical evaluations carried out i 21 kindreds with FDC delivered first data suggesting the role of MYH7 mutations in dilate cardiomyopathy (Kamisago et al., 2000). A genome-wide linkage study revealed genetic locu for mutations associated with DCM located at chromosome 14q11.2-13, encoding the gene fo ardiac β-myosin heavy chain. Disease-causing dominant mutations of MYH7 (S532P and '764L) were identified in 4 kindreds, resulting in early-onset ventricular dilatation (average ge: 24 years) and diminished contractile function. 'wo novel mutations were identified in the study conducted by Kärkkäinen et al. (2004), arried out on 52 DCM Finnish patients. Screening of MYH7 coding regions resulted in .dentification of R1053Q and R1500W mutations in two patients. The R1500W mutation was ssociated with typical DCM phenotype. On the other hand, patient with R1053Q variant ad dilated left ventricle and impaired systolic function, but other family members carrying his mutation had septal hypertrophy, suggesting that this variant was primarily an HCM nutation which could also lead to DCM.

Additional MYH7 mutations were identified by Villard et al. (2005). The researchers creened all coding regions of MYH7 and TNNT2 gene in 96 independent patients (54 with 'DC and 42 with IDC), identifying seven new mutations in MYH7 gene (see Table 4). Moreover, contrasting clinical features were observed between MYH7 and TNNT2 mutation arriers: mean age at diagnosis was late, penetrance was incomplete in adults and mean age t major cardiac event was higher in MYH7 mutation carriers compared to TNNT2.

MYH7 variant	Mutation type	Affected part of myosine heavy chain
I201T	substitution: Ile to Thr	head
T412N	substitution: Thr to Asn	head
A550V	substitution: Ala to Val	head
T1019N	substitution: Thr to Asn	tail
R1193S	substitution: Arg to Ser	tail
E1426K	substitution: Glu to Lys	tail
R1634S	substitution: Arg to Ser	tail

Table 4. Disease-causing MYH7 variants observed in patients with DCM (Villard et al., 2005)

Hershberger et al. (2008) in a study carried out on a cohort of 313 patients identified 12 mutations in MYH7 gene (9 novel): R237W, V964L, A970V, R1045C, D1096Y, R1359C, R1500W, E1619K, V1692M, G1808A, H1901Q and R1863Q. These variants were observed in .3 out of 313 probands (4.2%), revealing that MYH7 was the most commonly mutated gene n studied group. All observed variants were considered possibly or likely disease-causing. Additional two mutations were described by Boda et al. (2009) in the group of 100 DCM patients. Screening of MYH7 gene revealed a substitution G377R in one DCM patient, liagnosed at the age of 11 years and R787H substitution in another patient, diagnosed at the ge of 7 years. Møller et al. (2009) identified three MYH7 mutations (K637E, resulting in charge change in actin cleft, L1038P introducing helix-breaking proline in the rod and R1832C resulting in loss of plus charge in light meromyosin and introduction of reactive ysteine) in one-quarter of studied DCM patients.

Tanjore et al. (2010) in the study carried out on 292 individuals (100 healthy controls, 95 HCM and 92 DCM) revealed common genetic variation (5 SNPs) in exons 7, 12, 19 and 20 of MYH7 gene for DCM and HCM patients. However, three out of 5 variants were heterozygous in HCM, whereas the same SNPs were found to be homozygous in DCM patients, revealing the dose effect of the protein with the gross anatomical variations in the ventricles leading to heart failure in DCM cases.

Rare mutations explain only a small percentage of DCM cases. Rampersaud et al. (2009) assumed that more common variants may also play a role in increasing susceptibility to DCM, similarly to observations in other common complex diseases. To verify that hypothesis, case-control analyses were performed on all DNA polymorphic variation identified in a resequencing study of six genes associated with DCM carried out on 477 individuals (289 probands with DCM and 188 controls). Multivariate analyses revealed that a block of 9 MYH7 variants was strongly associated with DCM.

3. Other genes involved in development of DCM

Variation in three genes discussed above is considered to explain abut 10% of DCM cases. There are however other genetic factors that can also play role in development of dilated cardiomyopathy.

SCN5A gene encodes alpha subunit of type V voltage-gated sodium channel (see Figure 4) which is abundant in cardiac muscle and controls the flow of sodium ions into cardiac muscle cells, playing major role in signalling start of each heartbeat, coordinating the contractions of the upper and lower chambers of heart and maintaining normal heart rhythm.

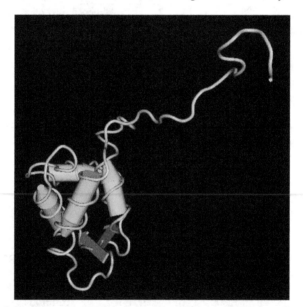

Fig. 4. Structure of the C-terminal Ef-hand domain of human cardiac sodium channel. Available from http://www.ncbi.nlm.nih.gov/Structure/mmdb/mmdbsrv.cgi?uid=68594 (Chagot et al., 2009).

Mutations in SCN5A has been described as causative in long QT syndrome and dilated cardiomyopathy. McNair et al. (2004) carried out a research on a large family affected by an autosomal cardiac conduction disorder associated with sinus node dysfunction, arrhythmia and ventricular dilatation and dysfunction. Linkage analyses mapped the disease phenotype to a region on chromosome 3p22-p25, containing cardiac sodium channel gene SCN5A. SCN5A gene was screened in 21 subjects, revealing a heterozygous G to A substitution at osition 3823, changing aspartic acid to asparagine (D1275N) in highly conserved residue. he mutation was present in all affected family members (19 patients), while being absent in 00 control chromosomes, and predicted a change of charge within the S3 segment of rotein domain III. All of mutations changed conserved amino acids. Two novel variants egregated with FDC in families and were considered likely disease-causing. On the other and, two variants associated also with Brugada syndrome (R526H) and long QT-syndrome A572D) did not segregate with DCM.

SCN5A variant	Mutation type	Pathogenicity of mutation (+/-)	Also associated with
S216L	substitution: Ser to Leu	+	LQT syndrome
R222Q	substitution: Arg to Gln	+	-
R526H	substitution: Arg to His	-	Brugada syndrome
A572D	substitution: Ala to Asp	-	LQT syndrome
P648L	substitution: Pro to Leu	+	LQT syndrome
I1835T	substitution: Ile to Thr	+	-
P2005A	substitution: Pro to Ala	+	LQT syndrome

able 5. SCN5A variants observed in patients with DCM (Hershberger et al., 2008)

A study performed on 338 DCM patients from Familial Cardiomyopathy Registry evealed 5 missense SCN5A mutations, including novel E446K, F1520L, V1279I and lready described D1275 and R222Q. Mutations were detected in 1.7% of DCM families. Most of them were localized to the highly conserved homologous S3 and S4 ransmembrane segments , suggesting a shared mechanism of disruption of the voltage-ensing mechanism of this channel leading to DCM. Patients carrying SCN5A mutations howed strong arrhythmic pattern that had clinical and diagnostic implications (McNair t al., 2011).

itin-cap (or telethonin), encoded by **TCAP** gene, is a protein regulating sarcomere ssembly. It has kinase activity and serves as attachment for myofibrils and other muscle-elated proteins (Valle et al., 1997). Mutations in TCAP gene were described in association vith cardiomyopathies. Hayashi et al. (2004) analyzed TCAP genotype in 346 patients vith HCM and 136 with DCM (34 FDC, 102 IDC), revealing two mutations in patients vith HCM and one (E132Q substitution) in patient with DCM. Moreover, the researchers lemonstrated that HCM-associated mutations augmented the ability of titin-cap to nteract with titin and calsarcin-1, whereas DCM-associated mutations impaired the nteraction of titin-cap with muscle LIM protein, titin and calsarcin-1. The role of TCAP in levelopment of DCM was also confirmed by Hershberger et al. (2008), who found three rotein-altering variants of TCAP in 3 out of 313 DCM patients (with two variants egregating with disease).

.DB3 (LIM domain binding 3), also known as ZASP or CYPHER is another gene associated vith DCM. It encodes a protein containing PDZ domain which interacts with α-actinin-2 hrough its N-terminal PDZ domain and with protein kinase C through C-terminal LIM lomains (a cysteine-rich motif containing two zinc-binding modules). It also interacts with nyozenin family members.

irst data revealing the role of LDB3 in DCM was delivered by Vatta et al. (2003). The esearch was carried out on 100 DCM probands and resulted in identification of 5 mutations (substitutions: S196L, I352M, D117N, K136M and T213I) in 6 patients (two families and four sporadic cases). None of these mutations were identified in the control group (200 individuals). 5 out of 6 mutations resulted in substitutions in conserved regions and all lie within the linker between PDZ and LIM domains. *In vitro* studies showed cytoskeletor disarray in cells transfected with mutated LDB3. One additional mutation in LDB3 was discovered by Arimura et al. (2004) in the study carried out on 96 unrelated Japanes patients with DCM. D626N substitution located within the LIM domain was identified in a familial case but not in the unrelated controls. A family study showed that all affecter siblings had the same mutation, associated with late onset cardiomyopathy. A yeast two hybrid assay demonstrated that described mutation increased the affinity of LIM domain for protein kinase C, suggesting a novel biochemical mechanism of the pathogenesis of DCM Hershberger et al. (2008) identified two mutations in the LIM domain of LDB3 (A371T and A698T). Second mutation was identified in two unrelated probands and was predicted to change highly conserved amino acid; therefore it was considered disease-associated.

TPM1 is a gene encoding tropomyosin α-1 protein and another candidate gene for DCM Tropomyosines are highly conserved actin-binding proteins involved in the contractile system of striated and smooth muscles and cytoskeleton of non-muscle cells. TPM1 form predominant tropomyosine of striated muscle and functions in association with troponin complex to regulate calcium-dependent interaction of actin and myosin during muscle contraction. Mutations in this gene are associated with HCM and also DCM. Lakdawala et al. (2010) performed direct sequencing of 6 sarcomere genes on 334 probands with DCM revealing D230N missense mutation in TPM1 gene, which segregated with DCM in two large unrelated families. Additional *in vitro* studies demonstrated major inhibitory effects or sarcomere function with reduced Ca^{2+} sensitivity, maximum activation and Ca^{2+} affinity compared to wildtype TPM1.

A role of **presenilin** genes in dilated cardiomyopathy was described by Li et al. (2006) Presenilins are multi-pass transmembrane proteins which function as a part of γ-secretase intramembrane protease complex. There are two presenilin genes in human genome: **PSEN** and **PSEN2**, both showing conservation between species. Mutations in these genes are the most common cause of Alzheimer's disease. They are also expressed in the heart and play critical role in cardiac development. The researchers analyzed sequence variation of PSEN and PSEN2 in 315 patients with DCM, revealing novel PSEN1 mutation D333G in one family and a single PSEN2 mutation S130L in two other families. Both mutations segregated with DCM and heart failure. PSEN1 mutation was associated with complete penetrance and progressive disease that resulted in the necessity of cardiac transplantation or in death whereas carriers of PSEN2 mutation showed partial penetrance, milder disease and more favourable prognosis. Moreover, calcium signalling was altered in cultured fibroblasts from mutation carriers.

Genes that are associated with complex diseases can also be organized as linkage disequilibrium clusters that are often inherited together. Friedriechs et al. (2009) described such 600-kb region of linkage disequilibrium on 5q31.2-3 chromosome, harboring multiple genes to be associated with DCM in three independent Caucasian populations. Functiona assessments in zebrafish demonstrated that at least three genes from this region (**HBEGF** - heparin-binding epidermal growth factor, **IK** cytokine and **SRA1** - steroid receptor RNA activator 1) resulted independently in a phenotype of myocardial contractile dysfunction under the condition of reduced expression.

ost of the genes associated with DCM phenotype are present in nuclear genome. There are wever examples of mitochondrial genes that can also contribute to development of lated cardiomyopathy. Ashrafian et al. (2010) described C452F mutation in highly nserved region of the M domain of **Dnm1l** (dynamin1-like gene) in mice, resulting in duced levels of mitochondria enzyme complexes in hearts, which then suffered from ATP epletion (energy deficiency that might contribute to DCM).

Conclusions

is always difficult to find genetic cause of multigenic disorders, such as dilated rdiomyopathy, especially if it is considered that mutations in genome are only one of ctors contributing to disease. Nevertheless, knowledge about genetic basis underlying ich diseases proves to be very useful both in diagnostics and treatment, providing the ossibility of early diagnosis and thus increasing the chance of successful therapy.

References

hmad F, Banerjee SK, Lage ML, Huang XN, Smith SH, Saba S, Rager J, Conner DA, Janczewski AM, Tobita K, Tinney JP, Moskowitz IP, Perez-Atayde AR, Keller BB, Mathier MA, Shroff SG, Seidman CE & Seidman JG (2008). The role of cardiac troponin t quantity and function in cardiac development and dilated cardiomyopathy. *PLoS ONE*, Vol.3, No.7, pp. e2642

rbustini E, Pilotto A, Repetto A, Grasso M, Negri A, Diegoli M, Campana C, Scelsi L, Baldini E, Gavazzi A & Tavazzi L (2002). Autosomal dominant dilated cardiomyopathy with atrioventricular block: a lamin A/C defect-related disease. *J Am Coll Cardiol*, Vol.39, No.6, pp. 981-90

rimura T, Hayashi T, Terada H, Lee SY, Zhou Q, Takahashi M, Ueda K, Nouchi T, Hohda S, Shibutani M, Hirose M, Chen J, Park JE, Yasunami M, Hayashi H & Kimura A (2004). A Cypher/ZASP mutation associated with dilated cardiomyopathy alters the binding affinity to protein kinase C. *J Biol Chem*, Vol.279, No.8, pp. 6746-52.

shrafian H, Docherty L, Leo V, Towlson C, Neilan M, Steeples V, Lygate CA, Hough T, Townsend S, Williams D, Wells S, Norris D, Glyn-Jones S, Land J, Barbaric I, Lalanne Z, Denny P, Szumska D, Bhattacharya S, Griffin JL, Hargreaves I, Fernandez-Fuentes N, Cheeseman M, Watkins H & Dear TN (2010). A mutation in the mitochondrial fission gene dnm1l leads to cardiomyopathy. *PLoS Genet*, Vol.6, No.6, pp. e1001000

ender JR, Russel KS, Rosenfeld L & Chaudry S (Eds.). (2011) *Oxford American handbook of Cardiology*. Oxford University Press, Inc., ISBN 978-0-19-538969-2, New York

oda U, Vadapalli S, Calambur N & Nallari P (2009). Novel mutations in beta-myosin heavy chain, actin and troponin-I genes associated with dilated cardiomyopathy in Indian population. *J Genet*, Vol.88, No.3, pp. 373-7

otto N, Vittorini S, Colombo MG, Biagini A, Paradossi U, Aquaro G & Andreassi MG (2010). A novel LMNA mutation (R189W) in familial dilated cardiomyopathy: evidence for a 'hot spot' region at exon 3: a case report. *Cardiovasc Ultrasound*, Vol.8, No.9, available from
http://www.cardiovascularultrasound.com/content/8/1/9

Chagot B, Potet F, Balser JR & Chazin WJ (2009). Solution NMR structure of the C-termin. EF-hand domain of human cardiac sodium channel Nav1.5. *J Biol Chem*, Vol.28 No.10, pp. 6436-45

Colombo MG, Botto N, Vittorini S, Paradossi U & Andreassi MG (2008). Clinical utility (genetic tests for inherited hypertrophic and dilated cardiomyopathies. *Cardiova. Ultrasound*, Vol.6, No.62, available from http://www.cardiovascularultrasound.com/content/6/1/62

Cowan J, Li D, Gonzalez-Quintana J, Morales A & Hershberger RE (2010). Morphologic analysis of 13 LMNA variants identified in a cohort of 324 unrelated patients wi idiopathic or familial dilated cardiomyopathy. *Circ Cardiovasc Genet*, Vol.3, No. pp. 6-14

Friedrichs F, Zugck C, Rauch GJ, Ivandic B, Weichenhan D, Müller-Bardorff M, Meder B, Mokhtari NE, Regitz-Zagrosek V, Hetzer R, Schäfer A, Schreiber S, Chen Neuhaus I, Ji R, Siemers NO, Frey N, Rottbauer W, Katus HA & Stoll M (2009 HBEGF, SRA1, and IK: Three cosegregating genes as determinants (cardiomyopathy. *Genome Res*, Vol.19, No.3, pp. 395-403

Genes associated with nonsyndromic dilated cardiomyopathy. UpToDate.com Availab from http://www.uptodate.com/contents/image?imageKey=CARD%2F29266 topicKey=CARD%2F4911&source=see_link

Haugaa KH, Leren TP & Amlie JP (2009). Genetic testing in specific cardiomyopathie *F1000 Med Rep*, Vol1, No.52, available from http://f1000.com/reports/m/1/52

Hayashi T, Arimura T, Itoh-Satoh M, Ueda K, Hohda S, Inagaki N, Takahashi M, Hori F Yasunami M, Nishi H, Koga Y, Nakamura H, Matsuzaki M, Choi BY, Bae SW, Yo CW, Han KH, Park JE, Knöll R, Hoshijima M, Chien KR & Kimura A (2004). Tca gene mutations in hypertrophic cardiomyopathy and dilated cardiomyopathy. *Am Coll Cardiol*, Vol.44, No.11, pp. 2192-201

Hermida-Prieto M, Monserrat L, Castro-Beiras A, Laredo R, Soler R, Peteiro J, Rodríguez Bouzas B, Alvarez N, Muñiz J & Crespo-Leiro M (2004). Familial dilate cardiomyopathy and isolated left ventricular noncompaction associated with lami A/C gene mutations. *Am J Cardiol*, Vol.94, No.1, pp. 50-4

Hershberger RE, Kushner JD & Parks SB (2007). Dilated cardiomyopathy overview, In: *Ger Reviews* (1993-2011), Pagon RA, Bird TD, Dolan CR & Stephens K (Ed.). Availab from http://www.ncbi.nlm.nih.gov/books/NBK1309/?&log$=disease6_name

Hershberger RE, Parks SB, Kushner JD, Li D, Ludwigsen S, Jakobs P, Nauman D, Burgess [Partain J & Litt M (2008). Coding sequence mutations identified in MYH7, TNNT. SCN5A, CSRP3, LBD3, and TCAP from 313 patients with familial or idiopath dilated cardiomyopathy. *Clin Transl Sci*, Vol.1, No.1, pp. 21-26

Hershberger RE, Cowan J, Morales A & Siegfried JD (2009a). Progress with geneti cardiomyopathies: Screening, counseling, and testing in dilated, hypertrophic an arrhythmogenic right ventricular dysplasia/cardiomyopathy. *Circ Heart Fail*, Vol.: No.3, pp. 253-261

Hershberger RE, Pinto JR, Parks SB, Kushner JD, Li D, Ludwigsen S, Cowan J, Morales / Parvatiyar MS & Potter JD (2009b). Clinical and functional characterization (TNNT2 mutations identified in patients with dilated cardiomyopathy. *Ci Cardiovasc Genet*, Vol.2, No.4, pp. 306-313

Iershberger RE, Morales MS & Siegfried MS (2010). Clinical and genetic issues in dilated cardiomyopathy: A review for genetics professionals. *Genet Med*, Vol.12, pp: 655-67

amisago M, Sharma SD, DePalma SR, Solomon S, Sharma P, Mcdonough B, Smoot L, Mullen MP, Woolf PK, Wigle ED, Seidman JG & Seidman CE (2000). Mutations in sarcomere protein genes as a cause of dilated cardiomyopathy. *N Engl J Med*, Vol.343, No.23, pp. 1688-96

ärkkäinen S, Heliö T, Jääskeläinen P, Miettinen R, Tuomainen P, Ylitalo K, Kaartinen M, Reissell E, Toivonen L, Nieminen MS, Kuusisto J, Laakso M & Peuhkurinen K (2004). Two novel mutations in the beta-myosin heavy chain gene associated with dilated cardiomyopathy. *Eur J Heart Fail*, Vol.6, No.7, pp. 861-8

ärkkäinen S, Reissell E, Heliö T, Kaartinen M, Tuomainen P, Toivonen L, Kuusisto J, Kupari M, Nieminen MS, Laakso M & Peuhkurinen K (2006). Novel mutations in the lamin A/C gene in heart transplant recipients with end stage dilated cardiomyopathy. *Heart*, Vol.92, No.4, pp. 524-6

atus HA, Looser S, Hallermayer K, Remppis A, Scheffold T, Borgya A, Essig U & Geuss U (1992). Development and in vitro characterization of a new immunoassay of cardiac troponin T. *Clin Chem*, Vol.38, No.3, pp. 386-93.

habaeva Z. Genetic analysis in hypertrophic cardiomyopathy: missense mutations in the ventricular myosin regulatory light chain gene. Humboldt University, Berlin, 2002

akdawala N, Dellefave L, Redwood CS, Sparks E, Cirino AL, Depalma S, Colan SD, Funke B, Zimmerman RS, Robinson P, Watkins H, Seidman CE, Seidman JG, McNally EM & Ho CY (2010). Familial dilated cardiomyopathy caused by an alpha-tropomyosin mutation: the distinctive natural history of sarcomeric dcm. *J Am Coll Cardiol*, Vol.55, No.4, pp. 320–329

i D, Parks SB, Kushner JD, Nauman D, Burgess D, Ludwigsen S, Partain J, Nixon RR, Allen CN, Irwin RP, Jakobs PM, Litt M & Hershberger RE (2006). Mutations of presenilin genes in dilated cardiomyopathy and heart failure. *Am J Hum Genet*, Vol.79, No.6, pp. 1030–1039

AcNair WP, Ku L, Taylor MR, Fain PR, Dao D, Wolfel E & Mestroni L (2004). SCN5A mutation associated with dilated cardiomyopathy, conduction disorder, and arrhythmia. *Circulation*, Vol.110, No.15, pp. 2163-7

AcNair WP, Sinagra G, Taylor MR, Di Lenarda A, Ferguson DA, Salcedo EE, Slavov D, Zhu X, Caldwell JH & Mestroni L (2011). SCN5A mutations associate with arrhythmic dilated cardiomyopathy and commonly localize to the voltage-sensing mechanism. *J Am Coll Cardiol*, Vol.57, No.21, pp. 2160-8

Aenon SC, Michels VV, Pellikka PA, Ballew JD, Karst ML, Herron KJ, Nelson SM, Rodeheffer RJ & Olson TM (2008). Cardiac troponin T mutation in familial cardiomyopathy with variable remodeling and restrictive physiology. *Clin Genet*, Vol.74, No.5, pp. 445-54

Aestroni L, Maisch B, McKenna WJ, Schwartz K, Charron P, Rocco C, Tesson F, Richter A, Wilke A & Komajda M (1999). Guidelines for the study of familial dilated cardiomyopathies. Collaborative Research Group of the European Human and Capital Mobility Project on Familial Dilated Cardiomyopathy. *Eur Heart J*, Vol.20, No.2, pp. 93-102

Aogensen J, Murphy RT, Shaw T, Bahl A, Redwood C, Watkins H, Burke M, Elliott PM & McKenna WJ (2004). Severe disease expression of cardiac troponin C and T mutations in patients with idiopathic dilated cardiomyopathy. *J Am Coll Cardio* Vol.44, No.10, pp. 2033-40

Møller DV, Andersen PS, Hedley P, Ersbøll MK, Bundgaard H, Moolman-Smook Christiansen M & Køber L (2009). The role of sarcomere gene mutations in patient with idiopathic dilated cardiomyopathy. *Eur J Hum Genet*, Vol.17, No.10, pp. 1241-9

Otten E, Lekanne dit Deprez RH, Weiss MM, van Slegtenhorst M, Joosten M, van der Smagt JJ, de Jonge N, Kerstjens-Frederikse WS, Roofthooft MTR, Balk AHMM, van der Berg MP, Ruiter JS & van Tintelen JP (2010). Recurrent and founder mutations i the Netherlands: mutation p.K217del in troponin T2, causing dilate cardiomyopathy. *Neth Heart J*, Vol.18, No.10, pp. 478-485

Parks SB, Kushner JD, Nauman D, Burgess D, Ludwigsen S, Peterson A, Li D, Jakobs P, Li M, Porter CB, Rahko PS & Hershberger RE (2008). Lamin A/C mutation analysis i a cohort of 324 unrelated patients with idiopathic or familial dilate cardiomyopathy. *Am Heart J*, Vol.156, No.1, pp. 161-169

Parks SB, Kushner JD, Nauman D, Burgess D, Ludwigsen S, Peterson A, Li D, Jakobs P, Li M, Porter CB, Rahko PS & Hershberger RE (2008). Lamin A/C mutation analysis i a cohort of 324 unrelated patients with idiopathic or familial dilate cardiomyopathy. *Am Heart J*, Vol.156, No.1, pp. 161-9

Rampersaud E, Kinnamon DD, Hamilton K, Khuri S, Hershberger RE, & Martin ER (2010) Common susceptibility variants examined for association with dilate cardiomyopathy. *Ann Hum Genet*, Vol.74, No.2, pp. 110-116

Stuurman N, Heins S & Aebi U (1998). Nuclear lamins: their structure, assembly, an interactions. *J Struct Biol*, Vol.122, pp. 42-66

Tanjore R, RangaRaju A, Vadapalli S, Remersu S, Narsimhan C & Nallari P (2010). Geneti variations of β-MYH7 in hypertrophic cardiomyopathy and dilate cardiomyopathy. *Indian J Hum Genet*, Vol.16, pp. 67-71

Taylor MRG, Carniel E & Mestroni L (2006). Cardiomyopathy, familial dilated. *Orph J Rar Dis*, Vol.1, No.27, available from http://www.ojrd.com/content/1/1/27

Valle G, Faulkner G, De Antoni A, Pacchioni B, Pallavicini A, Pandolfo D, Tiso N, Toppo S Trevisan S & Lanfranchi G (1997). Telethonin, a novel sarcomeric protein of hear and skeletal muscle. *FEBS Lett*, Vol.415, No.2, pp. 163-8

Vatta M, Mohapatra B, Jimenez S, Sanchez X, Faulkner G, Perles Z, Sinagra G, Lin JH, V TM, Zhou Q, Bowles KR, Di Lenarda A, Schimmenti L, Fox M, Chrisco MA Murphy RT, McKenna W, Elliott P, Bowles NE, Chen J, Valle G & Towbin J (2003). Mutations in Cypher/ZASP in patients with dilated cardiomyopathy an left ventricular non-compaction. *J Am Coll Cardiol*, Vol.42, No.11, pp. 2014-27

Villard E, Duboscq-Bidot L, Charron P, Benaiche A, Conraads V, Sylvius N & Komajda N (2005). Mutation screening in dilated cardiomyopathy: prominent role of the bet myosin heavy chain gene. *Eur Heart J*, Vol.26, No.8, pp. 794-803

Wolf CM, Wang L, Alcalai R, Pizard A, Burgon PG, Ahmad F, Sherwood M, Branco DM Wakimoto H, Fishman GI, See V, Stewart CL, Conner DA, Berul CI, Seidman CE & Seidman JG (2008). Lamin A/C haploinsufficiency causes dilated cardiomyopath and apoptosis-triggered cardiac conduction system disease. *J Mol Cell Cardio* Vol.44, No.2, pp. 293-303

Permissions

The contributors of this book come from diverse backgrounds, making this book a truly international effort. This book will bring forth new frontiers with its revolutionizing research information and detailed analysis of the nascent developments around the world.

We would like to thank Josef Veselka, MD, PhD, for lending his expertise to make the book truly unique. He has played a crucial role in the development of this book. Without his invaluable contribution this book wouldn't have been possible. He has made vital efforts to compile up to date information on the varied aspects of this subject to make this book a valuable addition to the collection of many professionals and students.

This book was conceptualized with the vision of imparting up-to-date information and advanced data in this field. To ensure the same, a matchless editorial board was set up. Every individual on the board went through rigorous rounds of assessment to prove their worth. After which they invested a large part of their time researching and compiling the most relevant data for our readers. Conferences and sessions were held from time to time between the editorial board and the contributing authors to present the data in the most comprehensible form. The editorial team has worked tirelessly to provide valuable and valid information to help people across the globe.

Every chapter published in this book has been scrutinized by our experts. Their significance has been extensively debated. The topics covered herein carry significant findings which will fuel the growth of the discipline. They may even be implemented as practical applications or may be referred to as a beginning point for another development. Chapters in this book were first published by InTech; hereby published with permission under the Creative Commons Attribution License or equivalent.

The editorial board has been involved in producing this book since its inception. They have spent rigorous hours researching and exploring the diverse topics which have resulted in the successful publishing of this book. They have passed on their knowledge of decades through this book. To expedite this challenging task, the publisher supported the team at every step. A small team of assistant editors was also appointed to further simplify the editing procedure and attain best results for the readers.

Our editorial team has been hand-picked from every corner of the world. Their multi-ethnicity adds dynamic inputs to the discussions which result in innovative outcomes. These outcomes are then further discussed with the researchers and contributors who give their valuable feedback and opinion regarding the same. The feedback is then collaborated with the researches and they are edited in a comprehensive manner to aid the understanding of the subject.

Apart from the editorial board, the designing team has also invested a significant amoun of their time in understanding the subject and creating the most relevant covers. The scrutinized every image to scout for the most suitable representation of the subject an create an appropriate cover for the book.

The publishing team has been involved in this book since its early stages. They wer actively engaged in every process, be it collecting the data, connecting with the contributor or procuring relevant information. The team has been an ardent support to the editoria designing and production team. Their endless efforts to recruit the best for this project, ha resulted in the accomplishment of this book. They are a veteran in the field of academic and their pool of knowledge is as vast as their experience in printing. Their expertise an guidance has proved useful at every step. Their uncompromising quality standards hav made this book an exceptional effort. Their encouragement from time to time has bee an inspiration for everyone.

The publisher and the editorial board hope that this book will prove to be a valuabl piece of knowledge for researchers, students, practitioners and scholars across the globe

List of Contributors

Angelos Tsipis
1st Department of Pathology, Medical School, University of Athens, Greece

Akihiro Hirashiki and Toyoaki Murohara
Nagoya Graduate School of Medicine, Japan

Zhong-Hui Duan
Department of Computer Sciences, University of Akron, Akron, OH, USA

Manveen K. Gupta, Sadashiva S. Karnik and Sathyamangla V. Naga Prasad
Department of Molecular Cardiology, Lerner Research Institute, Cleveland Clinic, Cleveland, OH, USA

Maegen A. Ackermann, Li-Yen R. Hu and Aikaterini Kontrogianni-Konstantopoulos
Department of Biochemistry and Molecular Biology, University of Maryland, School of Medicine, Baltimore, MD, USA

Byambajav Buyandelger and Ralph Knöll
British Heart Foundation – Centre for Research Excellence, National Heart & Lung Institute, Imperial College, London, UK

Laura Dewar, Bo Liang, Yueh Li, Shubhayan Sanatani and Glen F. Tibbits
Simon Fraser University, Canada

Cornelia Jaquet and Andreas Mügge
Molecular Cardiology & Clinic of Cardiology, St. Josef-Hospital & Bergmannsheil, University Hospitals of the Ruhr-University of Bochum, Germany

Lilienbaum Alain
Univ. Paris Diderot-Paris 7, Unit of Functional and Adaptive Biology (BFA) affiliated with CNRS (EAC4413), Laboratory of Stress and Pathologies of the Cytoskeleton, Paris, France

Vernengo Luis
Clinical Unit, Department of Genetics, Faculty of Medicine, University of the Republic, Montevideo, Uruguay

Priya Muthu, Wenrui Huang, Katarzyna Kazmierczak and Danuta Szczesna-Cordary
University of Miami Miller School of Medicine, Miami, FL, USA

Cieslewicz Artur and Jablecka Anna
Karol Marcinkowski Medical University in Poznan, Department of Clinical Pharmacology, Poland

Printed in the USA
CPSIA information can be obtained
at www.ICGtesting.com
JSHW011431221024
72173JS00004B/761

9 781632 420701